The Natural Immun

Humoral Fa

The Natural Immune System

Humoral Factors

Edited by
E D I T H   S I M
Department of Pharmacology, University of Oxford

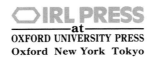
OXFORD UNIVERSITY PRESS
Oxford New York Tokyo

Oxford University Press, Walton Street, Oxford OX2 6DP
Oxford   New York   Toronto
Delhi   Bombay   Calcutta   Madras   Karachi
Kuala Lumpur   Singapore   Hong Kong   Tokyo
Nairobi   Dar es Salaam   Cape Town
Melbourne   Auckland   Madrid
and associated companies in
Berlin   Ibadan

Oxford is a trade mark of Oxford University Press

Published in the United States
by Oxford University Press Inc., New York

A catalogue record for this book is available from the British Library

Library of Congress Cataloging in Publication Data
Humoral factors / edited by Edith Sim.
(The natural immune system)
Includes bibliographical references and index.
1. Blood proteins.   2. Inflammation—Mediators.   3. Complement (Immunology).
4. Cytokines.   5. Tumor necrosis factors.   6. Acute phase proteins.
I. Sim, E. (Edith)   II. Series.
[DNLM: 1. Complement—physiology.   2. Immune System—physiology.
3. Immunity, Natural.   4. Infection—immunology.   QW 541 H925]
QR185.4.H85   1993   616.07'9—dc20   92—49146
ISBN 0–19–963336–3 (pbk.)
ISBN 0–19–963335–5 (hbk.)

Typeset by Apex Products, Singapore
Printed in Great Britain by
Information Press Ltd., Eynsham, Oxford

This volume is dedicated to the memory of
Alan F. Williams
an outstanding scientist and generous friend

Preface

In this series of books natural immunity has been defined as the immunological response of the host without prior sensitization to microbes, neoplasms,
and pathological states. The response of the host to these diverse challenges
involves many defence mechanisms acting in concert and includes both cells
and soluble mediators. The soluble mediators can have short-range effects
in cell–cell interactions and some circulating components have longer range
effects. Although the distinction is not entirely clear-cut, these mediators which
are released into the circulation are termed the humoral factors and it is these
humoral mediators which are considered in this volume. As well as having a
role in defence, many of these components are also important in homeostasis.
Humoral factors can destroy foreign material or damaged tissue and also act
as middlemen between phagocytes and their targets. This go-between activity
is referred to as opsonization. There is thus a dynamic interplay of humoral
mediators and cells in natural immunity and initial activation of circulating
components can result in recruitment of phagocytic cells and other cellular
components such as lymphocytes, mast cells, and platelets.

As well as providing a first line of defence in natural immunity, it is now
beginning to be understood that many of the humoral factors have a longer-
acting more subtle role in regulating the specific immune response.

It is the aim of this volume to present a molecular overview of humoral
factors involved in response to infection, disease, or injury and to discuss their
role in homeostasis. Recognition and controlled activation are key elements
in all defence mechanisms and these aspects of humoral factors in natural
immunity will be emphasized. Selected topics have been chosen to highlight
the systems involved.

The book covers four major classes of humoral factors in natural immunity.
(1) The acute phase refers to an increased synthesis of factors which control a
vast range of functions from fever to destruction of neoplasms which occurs
in response to infection, neoplasia, and trauma. (2) The plasma complement
system is activated in response to infection, tissue damage, and probably neoplasia.
(3) Activation of the clotting cascade systems limits the spread of infection and
localizes inflammation. It is a key humoral mechanism activated in tissue damage
and activation products of blood coagulation are important in controlling access
of other effector cells. (4) The final section deals with lipid mediators which are
produced in response to the humoral factors described in the earlier sections.

Introductory chapters to the acute phase response and to the complement
system are presented in Chapters 1 and 5. Extensive cross-references between

the individual chapters is a reflection of the interdependence of the systems which are covered.

During the period the book was being prepared at least five of the authors changed address but nevertheless produced manuscripts (mostly) without prodding. I am grateful to the staff of OUP who used just the right level of encouragement. I thank Mike Kerr for help in the early stages of planning, Kevin Butcher and Joanna Plowman for dedicated secretarial assistance, and B.F.G. for bearing with my many weekend absences.

Oxford   E. S.
July 1992

Contents

5   The complement system

K. WHALEY AND C. LEMERCIER

6 C1q and related molecules in defence

K. B. M. REID AND S. THIEL

7   C3 and C4 as opsonins in natural immunity

M. K. HOSTETTER

8   Complement-derived anaphylatoxins in natural immunity

R. BURGER AND G. ZILOW

11 Platelet adhesion molecules in natural immunity

K. T. PREISSNER AND P. G. DE GROOT

12 Eicosanoids in defence

J. STANKOVA AND M. ROLA-PLESZCZYNSKI

13   Lipid mediators in defence mechanisms

Z. HONDA AND T. SHIMIZU

Contributors

H. U. Beuscher Institut für Klinische Mikrobiologie der Universität Erlangen-Nurnberg, Wasserturmstrasse 3, D-8520 Erlangen, Germany.

S. Bhakdi Institute of Medical Microbiology, Johannes-Gutenberg-University, D-6500 Mainz, Germany.

R. Burger Robert Koch Institut des Bundesgesundheitsamtes, Nordufer 20, D-1000 Berlin 65, Germany.

P. G. de Groot Department of Haematology, University Hospital, Heidelberglaan 100, Box 85 500, NL-3508 GA Utrecht, The Netherlands.

W. Fiers Laboratory of Molecular Biology, State University of Ghent, Ledeganckstraat 35, B-9000 Ghent, Belgium.

P. C. Heinrich Institut für Biochimie der RWTH Aachen, Klinikum Pauwelstrasse, D-5100 Aachen, Germany.

Z. Honda Department of Internal Medicine and Physical Therapy, Faculty of Medicine, University of Tokyo, 7–3–1 Hongo, Bunkyo-ku, Tokyo 113, Japan.

M. K. Hostetter Departments of Pediatrics and Microbiology, University of Minnesota Medical School, Minneapolis, Minnesota, USA.

C. Lemercier Department of Immunology, University of Leicester, Leicester Royal Infirmary, Leicester LE2 7LX, UK.

J. H. McVey Haemostasis Research Group, CRC, Watford Road, Harrow, Middlesex HA1 3UJ, UK.

D. P. O'Brien Haemostasis Research Group, CRC, Watford Road, Harrow, Middlesex HA1 3UJ, UK.

K. T. Preissner Department of Haemostasis Research, Kerckhoff Klinik, Max-Planck-Gesellschaft, Sprudelhof 11, D-6350 Bad Nauheim, Germany.

K. B. M. Reid MRC Immunochemistry Unit, Department of Biochemistry, University of Oxford, South Parks Road, Oxford OX1 3QU, UK.

M. Rola-Pleszczynski Immunology Division, Department of Paediatrics, Faculty of Medicine, University of Sherbrooke, Sherbrooke, QC J1H 5N4, Canada.

M. Röllinghoff Institut für Klinische Mikrobiologie der Universität Erlangen-Nurnberg, Wasserturmstrasse 3, D-8520 Erlangen, Germany.

S. Rose-John Institut für Biochimie der RWTH Aachen, Klinikum Pauwelstrasse, D-5100 Aachen, Germany.

T. Shimizu Second Department of Biochemistry, Faculty of Medicine, University of Tokyo, 7–3–1 Hongo, Bunkyo-ku, Tokyo 113, Japan.

J. Stankova Immunology Division, Department of Paediatrics, Faculty of Medicine, University of Sherbrooke, Sherbrooke, QC J1H 5N4, Canada.

D. M. Steel Department of Genetics, Trinity College, University of Dublin, Dublin 2, Ireland.

S. Thiel Department of Immunology, Institute of Medical Microbiology, University of Aarhus, DK-8000 Aarhus C, Denmark.

K. Whaley Department of Immunology, University of Leicester, Leicester Royal Infirmary, Leicester LE2 7LX, UK.

A. S. Whitehead Department of Genetics, Trinity College, University of Dublin, Dublin 2, Ireland.

G. Zilow Institut für Immunologie, Universität Heidelberg, Im NeuenheimerFeld 305, 6900 Heidelberg, Germany.

Abbreviations

α1AT	alpha-1-antitrypsin
AA	A component of amyloid
ACTH	adrenocorticotrophic hormone
ADP	adenosine diphosphate
AP	P component of amyloid
APC	activated protein C
APR	acute phase reactant
ARDS	adult respiratory distress syndrome
A-SAA	acute phase serum amyloid A
AT	anaphylatoxins
ATIII	anti-thrombin III
ATP	adenosine triphosphate
AP	anti-plasmin
BCG	bacillus Calmette–Guérin
BP	TNF-binding proteins
C1q	
C1r	
C1s	
C2	
C3	
C4	complement components
C5	
C6	
C7	
C8	
C9	
C1qR	C1q receptor
C3a desArg	C3a lacking the N-terminal arginine residue
C4bp	C4b binding protein
cAMP	cyclic 3′5′ adenosine monophosphate
CHO	Chinese hamster ovary
CNS	central nervous system
CO	cyclo-oxygenase
CP-4	collagenous protein 4 (same as SPD)
cPLA$_2$	cytoplasmic phospholipase A$_2$

CR1   complement receptor type 1 (CD 35/C3b receptor)
CR2   complement receptor type 2 (CD 21/C3d receptor)
CR3   complement receptor type 3 (CD 11b,CD18/iC3b receptor)
CRD   carbohydrate recognition domain
CRF   corticotrophin releasing factor
CRP   C-reactive protein
C-SAA   constitutive serum amyloid A

Da   daltons
DAF   decay accelerating factor (CD55)
DAG   diacylglycerol
DFP   di-isopropylfluorophosphonate

EGF   epidermal growth factor
ELAM   endothelial leucocyte adhesion molecule

FV
FVII
FVIII   } blood coagulation factors
FIX
FX
FLAP   5-lipoxygenase activating protein
fMLP N-formyl-methionylleucylphenylalanine

GalNAc N-acetylgalactosamine
GAP   GTP hydrolase activating protein
Gla   gamma-carboxyglutamic acid
G-CSF   granulocyte colony-stimulating factor
GM-CSF   granulocyte macrophage colony-stimulating factor
GPC   glycerophosphocholine
GPI   glycerophosphatidylinositol
Gi   guanosine nucleotide binding inhibitory protein
Gp   guanosine nucleotide binding protein involved in control of
            phospholipase C
GlcNAc N-acetylglucosamine
Gs   guanosine nucleotide binding stimulatory protein
GTP   guanosine triphosphate

HDL   high density lipoprotein
HIV   human immunodeficiency virus
HPETE   hydroperoxyeicosatetraenoic acid
HRF   homologous restriction factor

IAP   pertussis toxin

ICAM	intercellular adhesion molecule
IFN	interferon
Ig	immunoglobulin
IκB	inhibitor of nuclear factor kappa B
IL	interleukin
IL-1R	receptor for interleukin-1
IL-1ra	interleukin-1 receptor antagonist
IP$_3$	inositol-1,4,5-triphosphate
LBP	lipopolysaccharide binding protein
LCAT	lecithin–cholesterol acyltransferase
LDL	low density lipoprotein
LFA-1	lymphocyte function associated molecule type 1 (CD11a, CD18)
LGL	large granular lymphocytes
LO	lipoxygenase
LPS	lipopolysaccharide (endotoxin)
LT	leukotriene
MAC	membrane attack complex
MACIP	membrane attack complex inhibitory protein
Man	mannose
MBP	mannan-binding protein
MCP	membrane cofactor protein (CD 40)
MDP	muramyldipeptide
MethA	mediator derived from methylcholanthrene-induced tumour
MHC	major histocompatibility complex
MIRL	membrane inhibitor of reactive lysis
MOF	multi-system organ failure
MPIF	monocyte pro-coagulant inducing activity
MTT	3-(4,5-dimethythiazol-2-yl)-2,5-diphenyltetrazolium bromide
NC	natural cytotoxic lymphocytes
NDGA	nordihydroguaiaretic acid (lipoxygenase inhibitor)
NFκB	nuclear factor kappa B
NK	natural killer lymphocytes
PAF	platelet activating factor
PAI-1	plasminogen activator inhibitor type 1
PG	prostaglandin
PIP$_2$	phosphatidyl inositol-4,5-biphosphate
PKC	protein kinase C
PLA$_2$	phospholipase A$_2$
PLC	phospholipase C
PMA	phorbol 12-myristate 13-acetate

PNH	paroxysmal nocturnal haemoglobinuria
RaRF	Ra reactive factor
RCA	regulation of complement activation
SAA	serum amyloid A
SAP	serum amyloid P
SDS-PAGE	sodium dodecylsulfate-polyacrylamide gel electrophoresis
SOD	superoxide dismutase
SP-A	lung surfactant protein A
SP-D	lung surfactant protein D
SP40-40	clusterin
TCR	T cell receptor
TF	tissue factor
TGFβ	transforming growth factor beta
T_H	helper T lymphocytes
TNFα	tumour necrosis factor alpha
TNFβ	tumour necrosis factor beta or lymphotoxin
TNF-R55	tumour necrosis factor receptor subunit of 55 kDa
TNF-R75	tumour necrosis factor receptor subunit of 75 kDa
TPA	12-O-tetradecanoyl-phorbol-13-acetate
TXA	thromboxane
VSV	vesicular stomatitis virus

1 The acute phase response

D. M. STEEL AND A. S. WHITEHEAD

1 Introduction

Homeostasis is the combination of physiological variables that permits the individual of a species to function optimally under the conditions normally encountered. Consequently, the long-term maintenance of homeostasis enhances the capacity of both the individual and the species to survive and the regulatory mechanisms that determine the contributing biochemical and metabolic parameters are subject to strong selective pressures. An 'acute phase' stimulus such as infection or trauma, however, represents a potentially debilitating and therefore life-threatening short-term challenge to the individual during which there is an overriding need to eliminate the cause underlying the stimulus and to re-establish homeostasis. To achieve this the 'acute phase response', in which the biochemical and metabolic variables are reset, has evolved to counteract 'natural' challenges such as infection and tissue trauma by direct and indirect action, and to promote rapid recovery. The acute phase response can be considered the body's first line of systemic defence and begins to act well in advance of any antibody-mediated immune responses.

The mammalian response to an acute phase stimulus necessarily involves a wide ranging complex of physiological changes. It is of short duration (a few days) and is characterized by fever, alterations in hormone and electrolyte levels, increased vascular permeability, changes in metabolic and catabolic rates, and elevated circulating concentrations of acute phase reactants (APRs). The acute phase response is initiated by, and co-ordinated by, a large number of diverse inflammatory mediators (including cytokines, anaphylatoxins, glucocorticosteroids). Some are released initially at the site of inflammation and have potent local and systemic effects; the ensuing cascade induces proliferation, altered phenotype and behaviour, and modified biosynthetic capacities, of target cells and tissues (Figure 1.1).

In addition to the 'natural' inflammatory stimuli mentioned above, the acute phase response is also elicited by clinically important conditions such as myocardial infarction and neoplasms, and by surgery. Many of the clinically important stimuli would be fatal or heavily selected against without modern medical intervention. Such stimuli have therefore played little or no role in directing the evolution of the acute phase response, and the physiological, biochemical, and metabolic variables, optimized by evolution for the 'natural' challenge, may not always be optimal for the patient. Similarly, chronic inflammation renders the individual unfit and unlikely to survive long in the

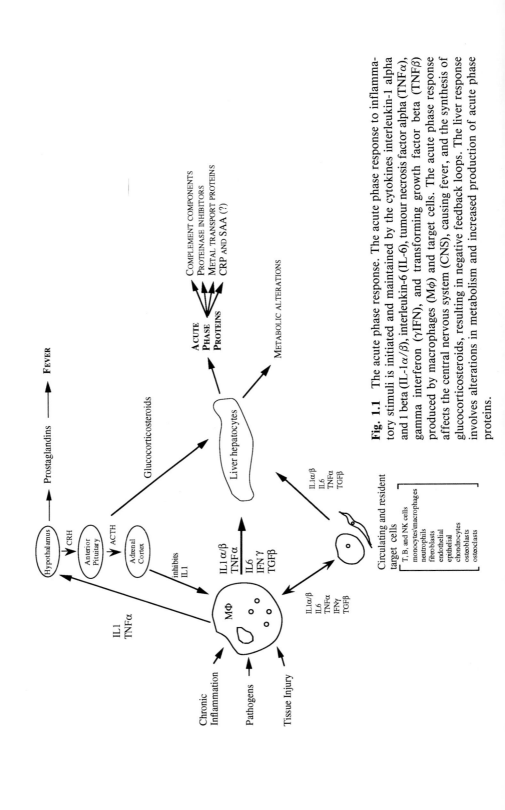

Fig. 1.1 The acute phase response. The acute phase response to inflammatory stimuli is initiated and maintained by the cytokines interleukin-1 alpha and 1 beta (IL–1α/β), interleukin-6 (IL-6), tumour necrosis factor alpha (TNFα), gamma interferon (γIFN), and transforming growth factor beta (TNFβ) produced by macrophages (Mφ) and target cells. The acute phase response affects the central nervous system (CNS), causing fever, and the synthesis of glucocorticosteroids, resulting in negative feedback loops. The liver response involves alterations in metabolism and increased production of acute phase proteins.

absence of medical and social support, and therefore the parameters of the acute phase response sustained in chronic inflammatory diseases are also unlikely to have arisen as the result of evolutionary selection; rather they represent an aberrant continuation of some aspects of the acute phase response beyond a few days. This explains in part the negative consequences of some chronic inflammatory diseases. For example, the availability of increased concentrations of complement components in acute infection is of obvious benefit in providing the means to deal directly with the causative infectious agent via alternative pathway activation and subsequent opsonization, whereas the activation of elevated levels of complement components in chronic inflammatory conditions such as rheumatoid arthritis contribute to the underlying inflammation and the tissue damage manifested by the disease.

In the following sections we outline the processes associated with the establishment and maintenance of the acute phase response, and the contributions of the changes apparent during the acute phase response in terms of host survival.

2   The role of cytokines in the acute phase response

The acute phase response is triggered by cytokines produced by activated mononuclear phagocytes, lymphocytes, and other differentiated cell types in response to an inflammatory stimulus. Cytokines act locally and systemically to recruit and activate target cells including some that produce additional cytokines. This results in a cascade of events controlled and co-ordinated principally by the various cytokines elicited. The ensuing activation and proliferation of target cells and tissues, with the consequent alteration in cellular phenotype, enhances host survival by neutralizing the inflammatory agent, and by promoting repair processes and a return to homeostasis. This section focuses on our current understanding of the local and systemic effects of inflammatory cytokines. These include interleukin-1 (IL-1), interleukin-6 (IL-6), tumour necrosis factor-α (TNFα), interferon-γ (IFNγ), and transforming growth factor-β (TGFβ). The many activities of these cytokines are discussed briefly below, and IL-1, IL-6, and TNF-α are reviewed in more detail in Chapters 2–4.

2.1   Interleukin-1 (IL-1)

Interleukin-1 is generally regarded as the pro-inflammatory cytokine that is of central importance in the initiation and maintenance of the acute phase response (reviewed in 1 and see Chapter 2). Originally named 'endogenous pyrogen' for its ability to induce fever (2), IL-1 has, over the past 20 years, had other acronyms based on its multiple biological activities. These include lymphocyte activating factor (3), thymocyte proliferation factor, and helper peak-1 for its ability to induce thymocyte activation and proliferation; B cell activating factor for its ability to stimulate direct activation of plasma cells (4); leucocyte endogenous mediator for its ability to induce acute phase protein synthesis (reviewed in 5); and mononuclear cell factor (6), monocyte derived recruiting activity (7), catabolin (8), osteoclast-activating factor (9), and haemopoietin-1 (10) which reflect its role in a wide range of additional physiological processes. All of the above functions were eventually attributed to a 17.5 kDa protein which was given the inclusive name of interleukin-1 (11). There are two isoforms of human IL-1: IL-1α of pI 5.0 and IL-1β of pI 7.0. Both isoforms have been cloned and sequenced (12, 13) establishing that both molecules are synthesized as pro-peptides of approximately 31 kDa that are processed to the mature 17.5 kDa products. The generation of the mature IL-1β molecule from its pro-peptide requires a proteolytic cleavage event that is mediated by a specific, apparently unique enzyme, the interleukin-1β converting enzyme, which has recently been defined at the molecular level (14). The existence of such an enzyme implies a precise control mechanism governing the production of the active form of this cytokine, and indicates the likelihood that the production of this, and other active inflammatory mediators, is subject to specific and finely tuned control pathways.

Although IL-1 is considered primarily a product of activated mononuclear phagocytes, given the proper stimulatory signal it is synthesized by a number of other differentiated cell types, including lymphocytes (helper T cells, B cells, NK cells, neutrophils, and large granular lymphocytes); vascular cells (smooth muscle and endothelial cells); epithelial cells of the cornea and thymus; skin cells (keratinocytes, Langerhans cells); brain cells (astrocytes, microglial cells, glioma cells); dendritic cells; mesangial cells of the kidney; fibroblasts; and chondrocytes (reviewed in 15, 16). Mononuclear phagocytes can be stimulated to produce IL-1 in response to a number of activating stimuli such as contact with T cells (during antigen presentation), viruses, bacteria, antigen–antibody complexes, and some chemicals (reviewed in 16).

IL-1 also acts directly on the central nervous system (CNS) by stimulating the hypothalamus and by synergizing with prostaglandins, thereby modulating the firing rate of thermoregulatory neurons in the brain and causing fever (1, 17). This brings about the production of corticotrophin releasing factor (CRF) and adrenocorticotrophic hormone (ACTH) which results in glucocorticosteroid synthesis (18). The induction of elevated levels of glucocorticosteroids by IL-1 in turn creates a negative feedback regulatory loop, since IL-1 synthesis in activated macrophages is inhibited by glucocorticosteroids (19). The initiation of the above cascade and its pro-inflammatory sequelae therefore sets the programme which, if uninterrupted, leads to a return to homeostasis.

A return to homeostasis is probably also promoted by the induction, possibly by IL-1 itself, of the interleukin-1 receptor antagonist protein (IL-1rn/ IL-1ra/IRAP) (20). IL-1ra inhibits IL-1 agonist activity by binding to the IL-1 receptors on target cells thereby directly blocking the engagement of IL-1 and the consequent transduction of signals via the receptors (20). IL-1ra is synthesized at increased levels in the livers of mice undergoing experimentally induced inflammation at a time when the hepatic synthesis of acute phase reactants is at its maximum (21). The induction of the antagonist therefore coincides with the peak of the systemic acute phase response when the pro-inflammatory role of IL-1 (and other cytokines) has been fulfilled.

During the acute phase response, IL-1 triggers cell-mediated, humoral, and natural immune responses by acting on T cells, B cells, or NK cells directly, or by stimulating these target cells indirectly by inducing the synthesis of other cytokines that can provide them with additional positive or negative regulatory signals (reviewed in 15). IL-1 is also important for B cell maturation and antibody production (22). Circulating IL-1 co-ordinates cellular mobilization by accelerating the release of mature neutrophils from the bone marrow into the bloodstream, and by acting as a chemoattractant, drawing neutrophils, T cells, and monocytes to sites of inflammation (23). At the site of inflammation, IL-1 induces proliferation of fibroblasts and epithelial cells and enhances the adherence of lymphocytes to sites of tissue damage by inducing the synthesis of the intercellular adhesion molecule-1 (ICAM-1) on endothelial cells and epithelial cells (24). IL-1 promotes wound healing by stimulating the synthesis of the clotting factors plasminogen activator and its inhibitor (25), pro-coagulant (26), platelet activating factor (27), collagens (28), and collagenase (29).

In summary IL-1 behaves as a multi-functional hormone by signalling a variety of cells to make more IL-1 and/or other cytokines; by stimulating the CNS; by inducing hepatic APR synthesis; and by co-ordinating local cell signalling at the site of inflammation.

2.2   Interleukin-6 (IL-6)

Interleukin-6 (IL-6) is a 26 kDa protein (reviewed in 30) that has also previously been named according to its several functions: interferon-β2 for its anti-viral activity (31); B cell stimulatory factor-2 or B cell differentiation factor for its ability to induce the differentiation of B cells into antibody producing plasma cells (32, 33); hybridoma or hybridoma/plasmacytoma growth factor (34); cytotoxic differentiation factor for its ability (in synergy with IL-2 and IFNγ) to induce differentiation of thymocytes to cytotoxic T lymphocytes (35), and hepatocyte-stimulating factor for its ability to stimulate hepatic acute phase protein synthesis (36). IL-6 is made by activated mononuclear phagocytes, T cells, B cells, fibroblasts, epithelial cells, some plasmacytomas, and probably many other cell types, if the proper stimulus is given (reviewed in 30; see Chapter 3). As is the case for IL-1, IL-6 stimulates other immune and non-immune cell types to differentiate and to secrete additional cytokines. IL-6 is thought to participate in the regulation of haemopoiesis in the bone marrow by stimulating granulocyte and macrophage colony formation from progenitor cells (37). The growth and differentiation activities of IL-6 have been the subject of numerous reviews (30, 38, 39).

2.3   TNFα/cachectin

TNFα/cachectin is a 17 kDa protein of pI 4.7 produced primarily by activated mononuclear phagocytes in response to bacterial lipopolysaccharide and some viruses, and was originally identified by, and named for, its tumouricidal properties and its association with the severe wasting (cachexia) that occurs during some neoplastic and infectious diseases (reviewed in 40 and Chapter 4). TNFα induces fever, although it is not as pyrogenic as IL-1, and shares many of the *in vitro* and *in vivo* target cells and actions of IL-1; however, its synthesis is probably restricted to activated monocytes (41), NK cells (42), and mast cells (43). Like IL-1, TNF has many diverse biological functions (reviewed in 40), which include: promoting B cell proliferation thereby augmenting antibody production; inhibition of thrombomodulin and induction of pro-coagulant factor synthesis in endothelial cells, thereby promoting clot formation; induction of IL-1, IL-6, GM-CSF, and prostaglandin synthesis by macrophages, endothelial cells, and fibroblasts; induction of collagenase synthesis in osteoclasts and fibroblasts; enhancing leucocyte binding to endothelium by inducing ICAM-1 synthesis; and increasing adhesiveness, phagocytosis, and degranulation of neutrophils. The TNFα gene is closely linked (44) to the gene encoding lymphotoxin (TNFβ), a related cytokine which is the product of stimulated lymphocytes (45). The location of these genes between the Class I and Class II regions of the human major histocompatibility complex (MHC) and adjacent to other immunologically important loci of the Class III region, i.e. C2, C4, and factor B, is of considerable interest. The maintenance of close genetic linkage among the highly polymorphic genes of the MHC such that they are generally inherited 'en bloc' has prompted speculation about the relative contributions of particular combinations of alleles of immune function molecules to host defence under different types of challenges. Little work has been done to date on the differential function of polymorphic variants of cytokines, a potentially important area of research with relevance to both the acute phase response and the study of the maintenance of the pro-inflammatory processes acting in chronic inflammation.

2.4   IFNγ and TGFβ

IFNγ is synthesized by T cells and NK cells in response to mitogens, antigens, and IL-2 (46), and is generally anti-proliferative for many cell types. Other names historically given to IFNγ include: 'immune interferon' for its anti-viral properties (47) and 'macrophage activating factor' for its enhanced tumouricidal, anti-microbial, and antigen presenting activities (48). IFNγ inhibits B cell differentiation and proliferation, enhances immunoglobulin production, and has been shown to inhibit IL-4-mediated immunoglobulin class switching (49).

TGFβ is produced in many tumour cell lines (50) and normal tissues including human platelets (51) and placenta (52). It too is multi-functional: it directly inhibits the growth of many neoplastic and normal cells including vascular smooth muscle and endothelial cells, epithelial cells, keratinocytes, myoblasts, T cells and B cells, and additionally inhibits the activity of a number of growth factors (reviewed in 53). TGFβ also acts as a chemo-attractant for fibroblasts (54) and monocytes (55) and stimulates the synthesis of collagen and collagenase (56), plasminogen activator (57), and fibronectin (58), thereby promoting tissue repair.

Together the above activities of IFNγ and TGFβ may help to limit the extent and progression of inflammation.

3   Cytokine signal transduction

Cytokines modulate gene expression in target tissues by first binding to specific receptors on the target cell surface. The ligand–receptor complex then provides a signal that is transduced from the inner face of the plasma membrane to the nucleus. The mechanism by which this signal is transduced may be specific to the target cell. In this section we shall consider our current understanding of the interactions of the IL-1 molecules with their receptors and examine the models proposed for signal transduction (reviewed in 59, 60).

There are two distinct membrane receptors for IL-1 (61): an 80 kDa (type 1) receptor present on T cells, fibroblasts, and connective tissue cells, and a 67 kDa (type 2) receptor, found only on B cells. Both receptors have an extracellular domain, a short transmembrane domain, and a cytoplasmic domain. Both bind IL-1α and IL-1β; however, only the 80 kDa receptor is capable of interaction with the IL-1 receptor antagonist protein (IL-1rn) (20).

Cytokines modulate cellular activities by activating protein kinases via at least two major pathways. One pathway involves the conversion of ATP to cAMP, a second messenger that is generated by membrane adenylate cyclase. The other mechanism involves the hydrolysis of the membrane lipid phosphatidylinositol-4,5-triphosphate by phospholipase C, which yields diacylglycerol (DAG) and inositol-1,4,5-triphosphate (IP$_3$) (62). Phospho-inositide hydrolysis results in DAG binding to protein kinase C. Activated cAMP and DAG are capable of modifying the activity of protein kinases A and C respectively. With regard to IL-1 signal transduction, some investigators report the involvement of cAMP or DAG as second messengers while others dispute the involvement of either (reviewed in 59, 60, 63). This controversy is extended to whether or not activation of IL-1 responsive genes occurs via different signalling pathways in different cell types (reviewed in 63). Recent evidence suggests that the signal transduction pathway leading to the activation of IL-1 responsive genes in fibroblasts and connective tissue cells involves phosphorylation events mediated by a novel serine kinase (reviewed in 63).

Many receptor–ligand complexes are coupled to guanosine nucleotide binding proteins (G proteins, e.g. Gs, Gi, Go, Gt) which bind GTP and transduce signals from the occupied receptors to effector enzymes such as adenylate cyclase, phospholipase C or phospholipase A_2 (see Chapter 13). G proteins have been implicated in mediating the generation of DAG by the modulation of phospholipase C activity. Activation of G proteins is accompanied by enhanced GTP binding and GTPase activity, and their roles in IL-1 signal transduction can be analysed experimentally using radiolabelled GTP analogues or measuring GTP hydrolysis in IL-1 treated cells or membrane preparations. For most receptor–ligand complexes, pre-treatment of cells with pertussis toxin (IAP) causes G proteins to uncouple. This is due, in the case of 'classical' G proteins, to ribosylation of ADP by the A subunit of the toxin. IL-1α and IL-1β cause increased GTPase activity and activation of G proteins in membranes prepared from thymoma cells due to an increased affinity for GTP (64). Pre-treatment of thymomas and B cells with intact pertussis toxin partially inhibits the IL-1 induced G protein activity. However, the B subunit of the toxin, which does not contain ADP ribosylating activity, inhibits G protein activation as efficiently as the intact pertussis toxin (65). Inhibition of G protein activation by IL-1 is therefore not attributable to ADP ribosylation. It appears, therefore, that pertussis toxin inhibition of IL-1 signal transduction does not involve inactivation of a classical G protein, but may be due to the inactivation of some other 'G-like' protein (Chapter 13). Such non-classical pertussis-sensitive G protein activation has been demonstrated for IL-2, TNF, and GM-CSF signalling mechanisms (reviewed in 63).

Although the early signals required for IL-1 signal transduction remain under debate, the increased transcription of APR RNAs consequent to IL-1–receptor interactions requires the activation of factors that bind to the 5' regulatory regions of the IL-1 responsive genes. The activation of the cytoplasmic transcription factor nuclear factor kappa B (NFκB) (66) is via the IL-1-induced phosphorylation and dissociation of its associated inhibitor protein IκB (67) thereby allowing it to enter the nucleus and bind to DNA. NFκB is centrally involved in the IL-1 directed gene activation of a number of APR genes. Thus IL-1 signalling involves the mobilization of pre-existing transcription factors. In addition, the induction of gene expression in IL-1 responsive genes can be achieved with phorbol myristate acetate (PMA) which activates the transcription factors *c-fos/c-jun* that bind to AP1 sites in the promoters (68). As both PMA and IL-1 can stimulate the synthesis of these DNA binding proteins the capacity of IL-1 to increase the absolute levels of transcription factors represents an additional means of control of gene expression (reviewed in 63).

4   Acute phase proteins

One of the most dramatic consequences of the acute phase response is the radically altered biosynthetic profile of the liver (reviewed in 30). Under normal conditions the liver synthesizes a characteristic range of plasma proteins at steady state concentrations. Many of these proteins have important functions that are required during the acute phase response and consequently are induced following an inflammatory stimulus. Conversely others, in particular albumin, are down-regulated to allow an increase in the capacity of the liver to synthesize the induced 'acute phase reactants' (APRs). APRs have a wide range of activities that contribute to host defence (reviewed in 30, 69): they stimulate and participate in immune responses; sequester essential cofactors and cell types, and direct them to sites of tissue damage; directly neutralize inflammatory agents, and help to minimize the extent of tissue damage locally; and participate in tissue repair and regeneration.

4.1   Activities of APRs

Proteins that participate in the complement, coagulation, and contact (kinin-forming) cascades that increase in plasma concentration during the acute phase enhance the host's ability to destroy invading micro-organisms and provide essential blood clotting components. The induced complement components include C2, C3, C4, C5, C9, C4 binding protein (C4bp), and factor B. In addition to their cytolytic activity, complement proteins have a wide range of activities in natural immunity (see Chapters 5–10 and reference 70). Activation of the complement cascade ultimately results in the local accumulation of neutrophils, macrophages, and plasma proteins that participate in the killing of infectious agents, the clearance of foreign and host cellular debris, and the repair of damaged tissue. Plasma levels of fibrinogen, the precursor to the clot-forming protein fibrin (see Chapter 11), are increased during the acute phase response (71) to provide an ample supply of one of the critical proteins involved in limiting local tissue damage and the entry of pathogens, and in promoting wound healing. Fibrinogen levels have, in addition, been useful clinically in determining the 'erythrocyte sedimentation rate', an important indicator of inflammation as the absolute concentration of fibrinogen correlates with the rate at which erythrocytes sediment (72).

A number of proteinase inhibitors are APRs, including α1-antitrypsin, α1-antichymotrypsin, α2-antiplasmin, C1 inhibitor, and inter-α-trypsin inhibitor (73). These inhibitors help to neutralize the lysosomal hydrolases released following the infiltration and activation of macrophages and neutrophils (73). Thus inappropriate collateral damage to healthy host tissues is kept to a minimum.

The plasma levels of metal transport proteins such as haptoglobin, haemopexin, and caeruloplasmin are increased during the acute phase response (reviewed in 74). Haptoglobin and haemopexin bind haemoglobin and the haem moiety, respectively, and prevent iron loss during infection and injury. In addition they minimize the levels of haem iron available for uptake by bacteria thereby depriving the infectious agent of an essential nutrient and further increasing the host's resistance to infection. Caeruloplasmin is involved in copper and iron transport and acts as a scavenger for the removal of oxygen-free radicals released by macrophages and neutrophils which can cause further tissue damage.

The plasma proteins albumin, pre-albumin, transferrin, apolipoprotein AI, and apolipoprotein AII are decreased during the acute phase response and are therefore termed 'negative APRs'.

A subset of APRs are massively induced. Serum amyloid A protein (SAA) and one of the pentraxins, either C-reactive protein (CRP) or serum amyloid P component (SAP) depending on species, are increased by up to a thousand-fold during inflammation. These 'major' APRs are considered in more detail later.

4.2   Magnitude of APR synthesis

The changes in the plasma concentrations of individual APRs are variable, and probably reflect differences in the amount of each protein that is required to participate effectively in the acute phase response. The magnitude of increase (or decrease) in APR plasma concentration varies (Table 1.1) from only 50 per cent (caeruloplasmin, C3), to a moderate 2–4-fold (proteinase inhibitors, haptoglobin, fibrinogen), to over 1000-fold (CRP, SAA) (reviewed in 30, 69, 73). The kinetics of human APR induction are characterized by increased plasma levels of CRP, SAA, and α1-antichymotrypsin within the first 12 hours after the acute stimulus, followed by α1-antitrypsin, α1-acid glycoprotein, haptoglobin, and factor B levels increasing approximately 24 hours later. CRP and SAA proteins have very short half-lives (5–7 hours), whereas most APRs have half-lives of 3–5 days (reviewed in 75). After the acute phase response, plasma concentrations of APRs return to their normal values; some APRs, however, remain elevated indefinitely in the case of chronic inflammation. Patterns of the acute phase response in various infectious diseases and inflammatory conditions have been extensively reviewed by others (75, 76).

APR induction profiles differ greatly between species, although APRs in different species share a high degree of structural and functional homology. For example, CRP but not SAP is a major APR in humans; conversely, in mice (undergoing experimentally induced inflammation) SAP is a major APR whereas CRP is only a minor APR (reviewed in 77). Humans, mice, and rabbits exhibit a dramatic induction of SAA during the acute phase response but rats do not. Moreover, the proteinase inhibitor α_2-macroglobulin does not increase in plasma concentration in humans during the acute phase response but in mice and rats it is a significantly induced APR (78).

Table 1.1 Human acute phase reactants and relative change in plasma concentration during the acute phase response

Acute phase reactant	Fold change
Complement and clotting components	
C2	+
C3	+
C4	++
C4 binding protein (C4bp)	++
C9	++
Factor B (FB)	+++
Fibrinogen (FGN)	+++
Proteinase inhibitors	
α2-Antiplasmin (α2AP)	++
α1-Antitrypsin (α1AT)	+++
α1-Antichymotrypsin (α1ACT)	+++
C1 Inhibitor (C1inh)	+++
Inter-α-trypsin inhibitor (IαTinh)	+
Metal transport proteins	
Caeruloplasmin (CER)	++
Haptoglobin (HP)	+++
Haemopexin (HXN)	++
Major APRs	
α1-Acid glycoprotein (α1AGP)	+++
C-Reactive protein (CRP)	++++
Serum amyloid A (SAA)	++++
Negative APRs	
Albumin (Alb)	−
Apolipoprotein AI (ApoAI)	−
Apolipoprotein AII (ApoAII)	−
Transferrin (TFN)	−

+, <1.5-fold increase; ++, 1.5–2-fold increase;
+++, 2–5-fold increase; ++++, >1000-fold increase;
−, 1.5–2-fold decrease.

4.3   Heterogeneity of APR gene regulation

Our present knowledge of the kinetics and magnitude of APR biosynthesis in response to *in vivo* inflammatory stimuli is based largely on studies using rodent models. In the early studies, rabbits and mice were injected with bacterial lipopolysaccharide (LPS) or an inflammatory chemical stimulus such as turpentine, azocaesein, or thioglycollate, and plasma and tissue levels of APR protein and mRNA were determined. Purified and recombinant cytokines became available thereafter and allowed the effects of individual cytokines on the acute phase response in general, and APR synthesis in particular, to be analysed *in vivo*. However, these studies are complicated by the additional inflammatory processes elicited by cytokines which produce a spectrum of responses (as detailed earlier) that are secondary or consequent to the direct effect of the agent under test. Primary hepatocyte cultures have been used by a number of investigators; however, it is also often difficult to differentiate between primary and secondary effects in these studies as liver cell cultures can contain a number of other cell types such as fibroblasts and Kupffer cells which may become stimulated by test cytokines to produce additional factors that can synergize with or inhibit the mediator being analysed. Cultured hepatoma cell lines such as PLC/PRF/5, HepG2, Hep3B, and HuH-7 provide useful models for the study of individual APR genes by inflammatory mediators under culture conditions. However the APRs expressed by these cell lines can respond very differently to cytokine treatments in terms of their capacity to be induced and their magnitude of induction, and in some instances different investigators have reported conflicting results using the same cell line. Human hepatoma/hepatocyte cultures nevertheless do constitute useful models for the study of common mechanisms by which defined cytokines, alone or in combinations, modulate human APR gene expression.

The differential response of individual APRs to recombinant inflammatory mediators is summarized in Table 1.2 (reviewed in 30, 79). IL-1, IL-6, and TNF are each capable of inducing the biosynthesis of a number of human APRs, (e.g. α1-antichymotrypsin, α1-acid glycoprotein, caeruloplasmin, C3, factor B, SAA) and causing a decrease in the biosynthesis of others, (e.g. alpha fetoprotein). IL-1, but not IL-6 or TNF, also decreases the synthesis of C1 inhibitor and SAP in human hepatoma cells. With respect to the synthesis of other APRs the responses of hepatoma cells to each of these cytokines is heterogeneous: for some APRs, biosynthesis is induced only by IL-6 and not by IL-1, (e.g. C4bp, SAP, haemopexin, haptoglobin, fibrinogen). Co-treatment of cells with IL-1 plus IL-6 has an additive or synergistic effect on some APR genes (α-acid glycoprotein, CRP, C3, factor B, haptoglobin, SAA). Alternatively one cytokine can exert an inhibitory effect which over-rides the action of an inducing cytokine; for example IL-1 and TNF can inhibit the up-regulation by IL-6 of C1 inhibitor and SAP synthesis, and of CRP, haptoglobin, fibrinogen, and SAA synthesis, respectively.

The glucocorticosteroid dexamethasone greatly enhances the response of some APRs to cytokines in cell culture systems (80), though it is generally unable to induce APR synthesis on its own. This emphasizes an important feature of the acute phase response: as discussed earlier, IL-1 stimulates the CNS to produce glucocorticosteroids that enhance the capacity of IL-1 to induce APR synthesis in the liver while at the same time down-regulating further IL-1 synthesis by activated monocytes. Dexamethasone, a synthetic glucocorticosteroid, is therefore often routinely included at approximately

Table 1.2 Regulation of human acute phase reactants by cytokines

	IL-1	IL-6	TNFα	TGFβ	IFNγ
α1ACT	+	+	+	+	−
α1AGP	+	+	+		
α1AT	+	+		+	
αFP	−	−	−	−	
Alb	−	−	−	−	
ApoAI				−	
ApoAII				−	
C1inh	−	+			
C2	+				+
C3	+	+	+		
C4					+
C4bp		+	+		
CER	+	+	+		
CRP		+			
FB	+	+	+		+
FGN		+	−	−	
FN		−	−		+
HP	+	+	+		−
HXN		+			
1αTinh	+				
SAA	+	+			+
SAP	−	+			
TFN	−		−		

+, up-regulation; −, down-regulation. No symbol is either no change or not tested. See Table 1.1 for abbreviations.

physiological concentrations in the experimental cytokine treatment protocols to augment their inductive effects.

IFNγ has more limited effects than IL-1, IL-6, and TNF on APR synthesis. Most studies of IFNγ APR induction have used mouse L cells transfected with the APR gene of interest. In these studies the biosynthesis of SAA (81), C2 and factor B (82), and C4 (83) can be induced. IFNγ also induces the synthesis of human factor B and C2 genes in primary monocytes (82). It has been suggested that IFNγ alters hepatocyte responsiveness indirectly by modulating the number of cellular cytokine receptors (84). TGFβ has also recently been shown to regulate the synthesis of a number of APRs (85).

5   The major APRs

Serum amyloid A protein (SAA), C-reactive protein (CRP), and serum amyloid P component (SAP) can be induced to up to a thousand-fold of their normal plasma concentrations (reviewed in 69) during the acute phase, and therefore constitute a distinct subgroup of APRs. They are often referred to as 'major' acute phase proteins. Studies of SAA, CRP, and SAP illustrate many of the challenges posed by research into the organization, structure, function, and control of expression of APRs. The extreme alterations in the biosynthesis of these major APRs indicate that they are of considerable biological interest. Although their precise physiological roles remain undefined and are the subject of considerable debate the magnitude and rapidity of their induction following an acute phase stimulus, together with their short half-lives (around six hours, whereas those of other APRs are measured in days), suggest that there is a particular requirement for these proteins very early in the establishment of host defence. They are therefore likely to be of considerable clinical importance and are likely to have a critical protective role.

5.1   CRP and SAP

CRP and SAP are pentraxins, proteins with a characteristic pentameric configuration of five subunits arranged as a disc (reviewed in 77). Generally only one pentraxin is a major APR in a given species, the other being expressed essentially constitutively. In man (86) and rabbit (87) CRP is the inducible pentraxin whereas in the mouse it is SAP (88). The apparent paradox of the species-specific alternate expression of pentraxins is unresolved though it is likely that the requirement for an acute phase pentraxin during inflammation is met by some common physiological activity invested in the particular molecule induced. Such a common function has not yet been defined.

CRP was originally named for its ability to bind the C-polysaccharide of pneumococcus (89). Subsequently it has been shown to function *in vitro* as an opsonin for bacteria, parasites, and immune complexes; in addition it can initiate the complement cascade and enhance macrophage tumouricidal activity (reviewed in 69). The exquisite responsiveness of CRP to an acute phase stimulus and its wide concentration range, together with ease of measurement have led to CRP plasma levels being used to monitor accurately the severity of inflammation and the efficacy of disease management.

SAP was originally named because it is found in serum and is the circulating form of the amyloid P (AP) component (90). AP is one of the two major constituents of the amyloid deposits which are the occasional consequence of a range of chronic recurrent inflammatory diseases (91) (see below). It is a normal component of basement membranes (92) and has the capacity to bind to fibronectin (93). Unlike CRP, it has no obvious immune-related function.

CRP and SAP display about 50 per cent amino acid identity (94) confirming the relatedness implied by their gross structural similarities. The genes encoding CRP and SAP have remained in close physical and genetic linkage in man and mouse (95). They map to syntenic regions in both species: band q2.1 of chromosome 1 and the distal portion of chromosome 1 in man (96) and mouse (97) respectively. Flanking loci in both species include many genes with immune and inflammation related roles: all of the Fc receptors to date have been mapped to the same regions (reviewed in 98) as have a group of interferon inducible products in mouse (99). It is likely therefore that the entire region around the pentraxin genes will be of considerable scientific and clinical importance and fine mapping studies are being undertaken in the authors' and other laboratories. CRP and SAP from a number of mammalian species have been cloned and sequenced. Computer based evolutionary analyses have revealed that their genes probably duplicated from a common ancestral pentraxin gene early in mammalian evolution (approximately 200 million years ago, prior to the time of the divergence of eutherian mammals and marsupials). The proteins are evolving at twice the rate of most other products of gene duplication in mammals (100). Future studies to identify the putative pentraxin activity that is essential in conferring a protective function during the acute phase response should therefore be directed towards the regions of the molecules that have retained much higher levels of similarity than those displayed by CRP and SAP as a whole. One candidate activity is suggested by the capacity of both pentraxins to bind to chromatin (101, 102). The ability to bind to and effect the clearance of nuclear material released from necrotic tissue during inflammation would provide an efficient means of precluding the initiation of auto-immune processes directed towards nuclear antigens and would explain, at least in part, the required presence of high circulating levels of pentraxins during inflammation.

The acute phase expression of CRP and SAP has been extensively studied *in vivo* and *in vitro*. In a recent study (103), mice given a single experimental acute phase stimulus, for example via intraperitoneal injection of thioglycollate or subcutaneous injection of azocaesein, show massive increases in hepatic SAP mRNA levels within 2–4 hours and peak concentrations by 8–12 hours. These are superseded by dramatically elevated circulating SAP protein levels peaking around 24–36 hours. Background levels of both hepatic mRNA and plasma protein are re-established by 72 hours in accord with the transient nature of the acute phase response. The magnitude and kinetics of SAP mRNA and protein induction is stimulus-specific, indicating that the cytokine cascade and the counterbalancing controls that modify, reduce, and terminate the consequent pro-inflammatory signalling are themselves subject to exquisite control and do not merely follow a pre-set programme.

In vitro studies using human hepatoma cultures treated with inflammatory mediators such as monocyte conditioned medium and recombinant IL-1β and recombinant IL-6 have revealed some of the intrinsic genetic elements and biosynthetic controls which are important in determining the level of pentraxin expression (104, 105). In such studies CRP mRNA and protein synthesis is induced by IL-6. Although no significant change is elicited by IL-1β alone, in combination with IL-6 there is a massively enhanced response compared with that to IL-6 alone (105, 106). The location of the IL-6 response elements have been fine mapped in the CRP promoter (105). SAP mRNA can be induced in human PLC/PRF/5 cells by treatment with recombinant IL-6; treatment with recombinant IL-1β down-regulates SAP mRNA synthesis, an effect which predominates when both cytokines are present (106). This suggests that, although human SAP is not considered to be a significant acute phase protein, there may be conditions, especially at local sites, under which the relative cytokine proportions present would promote increased non-hepatic SAP synthesis. The above *in vitro* results show that the cytokine-specific responses of related liver products differ during the acute phase response. That the differential responses of the same liver protein between species are generally dependent upon intrinsic genetic control elements is illustrated by the capacity of mice, in which CRP is a very minor APR (107), to induce greatly a human CRP transgene using the endogenous mouse cytokine, signal transduction, and cellular biosynthetic pathways (108).

5.2   SAA

SAA is a major acute phase protein in most mammalian species, and is the most dramatically induced (reviewed in 69). The kinetics of its induction by different inflammatory stimuli in mouse *in vivo* studies parallel those discussed above for SAP (103). SAA is a small apolipoprotein (104 amino acids in human) which, during the acute phase response, associates with high density lipoprotein (HDL) (109), in particular HDL3. SAA can become the predominant apolipoprotein associated with HDL3, exceeding apolipoprotein AI (110). SAA is the product of multiple related genes in several species. These genes have a common organization, four exons and three introns, which is reminiscent of several other apolipoprotein genes. In humans two acute phase SAA (A-SAA) genes have been described: *SAA1* and *SAA2* are almost identical with respect to the primary structures of their specified products, their gene organizations and sequences, and their mode of expression (111, 112). They are undoubtedly the result of an ancestral gene duplication followed by regular gene conversion events. In addition there is a third gene (*SAA3*) (113) for which no mRNA or protein product has been described. Although it was originally reported to have the structural integrity of an authentic transcribed gene (113), the presence of an in-frame stop codon was subsequently identified indicating that it is in fact a pseudogene (114). Recently, we have identified the product of a fourth SAA gene: C-SAA ('constitutive' SAA) is present on normal HDL3 and is minimally induced, if at all, during acute inflammation (115). Its expression is therefore radically different from that of the A-SAAs. Sequence analysis of a C-SAA cDNA clone predicts a mature molecule of 112 amino acids with only 55 per cent identity to the SAA1 and SAA2 proteins. The extra 8 amino acids present in C-SAA reside in an octapeptide that is positioned relative to the A-SAA sequence between residues 69 and 70.

Although, based on sequence identity and content, and on induction capacity, C-SAA is a more distantly related member of the SAA superfamily than the A-SAA genes *SAA1* and *SAA2*, it is nevertheless closely linked to these genes. We have mapped the C-SAA gene (112) to the *SAA4* locus (111) located 9 kb downstream from the *SAA2* locus. In addition the *SAA1* locus is located on the same 350 kb *Not*I restriction fragment as the *SAA2/SAA4* linked pair. The *SAA3* pseudogene is not on this fragment although it has been mapped to the short arm of chromosome 11 (G. C. Sellar and A. S. W., unpublished) as has a putative fifth SAA gene (G. C. Sellar and A. S. W., unpublished). It is likely, therefore, that an extensive cluster of SAA superfamily genes, displaying different degrees of relatedness and different induction characteristics exists. The existence of such a cluster is supported by the close linkage on a syntenic region of mouse chromosome 7 (116) of the two major acute phase SAA genes (*SAA1* and *SAA2*), a minor acute phase gene (*SAA3*) and an SAA pseudogene (ψSAA) (117, 118), the first three being approximately analogous to their similarly numbered human counterparts. No C-SAA has been identified to date in mouse. However, an octapeptide in a position similar to that present in human C-SAA is present in the massively induced A-SAAs of a range of species including dog, cat, horse, and mink. When compared to the octapeptide-containing A-SAAs of other mammals, the human C-SAA presents a paradox since it is the only one which is constitutively expressed.

The differential expression of SAA superfamily members constitutes one of the best systems for the study of comparative control mechanisms in APR genes and their products. Woo *et al.* (119) have demonstrated that IL-1 can induce the expression of human A-SAA following transfection into mouse fibroblasts of a human *SAA2* gene. Edbrooke *et al.* (120) subsequently demonstrated that the IL-1 responsive region of the *SAA2* promoter region contained a NFκB binding site and established that this transcription factor was intimately involved in controlling expression of the gene. We have analysed SAA expression in the human hepatoma cell line PLC/PRF/5 (106, 121) and have shown that IL-6 can also induce SAA mRNA and protein expression, though not by the same magnitude as IL-1β. When IL-1β and IL-6 are used together they show a dramatic synergistic induction that is of the same magnitude and kinetics as that produced by monocyte conditioned medium, a relatively physiological stimulus (121). This established that for A-SAA, IL-1β and IL-6 (in combination) are the cytokines that are both necessary and sufficient for maximum induction. Our studies with PLC/PRF/5 cells have confirmed that the principal means of exercising control of SAA expression following an inflammatory stimulus is via increased transcription and the accumulation of mRNA (121). At the time when induced SAA mRNA levels are at their peak, however, the capacity of the cells to synthesize SAA protein is less than would be expected from a strictly proportional use of the absolute levels of accumulated SAA mRNA when compared with earlier times post-stimulus. This suggests a modulating role for post-transcriptional control. This modulation does not appear to be due to progressive variation in the A-SAA export capacities of the cells at different times post-stimulus, as is the case for CRP (122), or differential engagement of A-SAA mRNA by the cellular translation apparatus, i.e. ribonucleoproteins, monosomes, and polysomes, as is the case for ferritin heavy and light chain mRNAs (123). Although the cellular levels of A-SAA mRNA decrease rapidly after reaching their peak, the A-SAA mRNA itself is intrinsically stable. Our current efforts to define the biosynthesis of A-SAA are focused on the mRNA poly (A) tail which shows a progressive, controlled shortening from the length present at the time of the appearance of induced mRNA concentrations: this may affect specific mRNA degradation processes and/or the efficiency of its translation. In contrast to A-SAA, C-SAA is minimally induced by IL-1β and IL-6. Although its genetic organization is grossly the same as that of the A-SAA genes the sequence and motifs contained in its promoter region and introns are radically different (112). A comparative analysis of A-SAA and C-SAA promoter activity will be useful in further defining the intrinsic genetic elements required for the induction of major APRs.

5.3   The clinical consequences of major APR induction

SAA and SAP are archetypal examples of plasma proteins that are beneficial in the transient acute phase response but that have detrimental effects in chronic inflammation. The causative or associated involvement of these major acute phase proteins in a number of clinical conditions has been implicated directly or circumstantially as outlined briefly below.

5.3.1   Secondary amyloidosis

Secondary, or reactive, amyloidosis is the occasional consequence of a number of chronic and recurrent inflammatory diseases (91), for example leprosy, tuberculosis, systemic lupus erythematosus, and rheumatoid arthritis. It is characterized by the ultimately fatal progressive deposition of insoluble fibrils in a variety of tissues including spleen, liver, and kidney. Secondary amyloid deposits are composed principally of amyloid A (AA) (124), which is derived, probably by proteolysis, from the precursor SAA (125), in association with amyloid P component (AP) (90) which is the localized form of SAP. The pathogenesis of secondary amyloidosis is poorly understood, however AA is deposited as β-pleated sheets and AP, which has been shown to be capable of acting as an elastase inhibitor (126), may protect the deposits against degradation by proteolytic enzymes. Alternatively, SAP may act as a nucleating agent in fibril deposition via its binding to fibronectin. Whatever the precise mechanism, it is clear that high circulating and local levels of SAA and SAP such as those that are maintained in mice undergoing chronic experimental inflammation (127) are likely to contribute to amyloidogenesis. Although not a major APR in humans, as mentioned above SAP may be induced locally or systemically by different combinations of cytokines. Recent studies have shown that there is a dynamic interchange of SAP between the circulation and the deposits in patients with secondary amyloidosis (128) and there are anecdotal reports of regression and even disappearance of deposits in some patients. It is therefore important to devise strategies to down-regulate specifically SAA and/or SAP during chronic inflammation not only to halt or slow down the progression of amyloid deposition, but to reduce the concentration of these major APRs to below an 'amyloidogenic threshold' and permit the action of physiological corrective and clearance mechanisms, if they exist, to predominate.

5.3.2 Cardiovascular disease

The association of SAA with HDL3 suggests another area in which chronic high SAA concentrations may promote clinical disease. Elevated HDL levels correlate inversely with susceptibility to atherosclerosis (129). HDL is central to the process of reverse cholesterol transport, and there is a significant decrease in plasma HDL cholesterol during inflammation (110). It is likely that during inflammation the association of A-SAA with HDL modifies the particle and equips it for a protective host defence role for which there is an overriding short term requirement. High SAA levels on HDL3 are achieved at the expense of apolipoprotein AI, the associated concentration of which is much reduced. HDL is the major substrate for lecithin-cholesterol acyltransferase (LCAT), one of the critical enzymes involved in cholesterol esterification. As apolipoprotein AI is required as an activator for the LCAT reaction (130) A-SAA may interfere with this reaction by displacing apoAI (directly or indirectly) from the HDL particle which could radically alter HDL metabolism during inflammation. Thus SAA may diminish the functional capacity of HDL for reverse cholesterol transport. We would further speculate that C-SAA on normal HDL contributes to its normal physiological role in reverse cholesterol transport. The chronic persistence of A-SAA on HDL in chronic inflammatory diseases could compromise the function of HDL over significant periods of time. Together with the concomitant sustained decrease in total HDL this would constitute a major risk factor for the development of atherosclerosis and could provide a molecular explanation for the increased mortality from cardiovascular disease observed in patients with active systemic rheumatoid arthritis (131).

5.3.3 Connective tissue disease

Recently the rabbit SAA3 molecule has been shown to be a product of synovial fibroblasts that can be induced with either phorbol esters or IL-1. The rabbit SAA3 appears to function as an autocrine collagenase inducer (132). As collagenase is the central component involved in the enzymatic breakdown of collagens I, II, and III in the connective tissue of rheumatoid arthritis and osteoarthritis patients, some SAAs may play a critical role in the pathogenesis of these diseases. If other SAA superfamily members are also local or systemic signal molecules, the rapidity and magnitude of their induction suggests that they would be important in driving the acute phase response and in mediating the continuation of potentially detrimental processes in chronic inflammation.

In summary, a thorough examination of the structure, expression, and molecular genetics of all of the members of the SAA superfamily is likely, therefore, to be of considerable clinical, as well as biological, importance.

6 Summary

The acute phase response represents a radical departure from the normal metabolic processes that maintain homeostasis. The ability of an organism to respond quickly and effectively to a physical challenge has evolved as a short term survival strategy. The many physiological changes that take place immediately following such a challenge are initiated, maintained, and co-ordinated principally by a complex network of cytokines. These cytokines act in concert to modulate their own synthesis and to alter the metabolic and biosynthetic profiles of some of the major systems of the body: immune, haemopoietic, CNS, and the liver. The combined effects of the acute phase is to neutralize the pro-inflammatory actions of the stimulus; to physically kill and/or remove the stimulating agent and the tissue debris generated by the stimulus; to promote tissue repair; and to facilitate a rapid return to homeostasis. Researchers are only now beginning to understand the complexities of the acute phase response and flexibility of the reaction elicited by a range of stimulating agents and to realize that it is of great clinical as well as scientific interest. Considerable effort will continue to be made to define the parameters that shape the acute phase response more completely in order to be able to optimize the treatment of infectious disease and trauma. In addition, we need to discover more about the mechanisms whereby some acute phase processes continue to act, with devastating medical and social consequences, in chronic inflammatory conditions.

Acknowledgement

We thank Clarissa Uhlar for assistance with the preparation of the manuscript.

References

1   Dinarello, C. A. (1984). Interleukin-1. *Rev. Infect. Dis.*, **6**, 51–95.
2   Atkins, E. (1960). Pathogenesis of fever. *Physiol. Rev.*, **40**, 580–646.

3 Gery, I. and Waksman, B. H. (1972). Potentiation of the T lymphocyte response to mitogens. II. The cellular source of potentiating mediator(s). *J. Exp. Med.*, **136**, 143–55.

4 Wood, D. D. and Cameron, P. M. (1976). Stimulation of the release of a B cell-activating factor from human monocytes. *Cell. Immunol.*, **21**, 133–45.

5 Kampschmidt, R. F. (1981). Leucocytic endogenous mediator/endogenous pyrogen. In *The physiologic and metabolic responses of the host* (ed. M. C. Powanda and P. G. Canonico), pp. 55–74. Elsevier/North-Holland.

6 Krane, S. M., Dayer, J.-M., Simon, L. S., and Byrne, M. S. (1985). Mononuclear cell-conditioned medium containing mononuclear cell factor (MCF), homologous with interleukin-1, stimulates collagen and fibronectin synthesis by adherent rheumatoid synovial cells: effects of prostaglandin E_2 and indomethacin. *Collagen Rel. Res.*, **5**, 99–117.

7 Broxmeyer, H. E. (1986). Biomolecule–cell interactions and the regulation of myelopoiesis. *Int. J. Cell Cloning*, **4**, 378–405.

8 Saklatvala, J., Sarsfield, S. J., and Townsend, Y. (1985). Pig interleukin-1. Purification of two immunologically different leucocyte proteins that cause cartilage resorption, lymphocyte activation, and fever. *J. Exp. Med.*, **162**, 1208–22.

9 Dewhirst, F. E., Stashenko, P. P., Mole, J. E., and Tsurumachi, T. (1985). Purification and partial sequence of human osteoclast-activating factor: identity with interleukin-1 beta. *J. Immunol.*, **135**, 2562–8.

10 Stanley, E. R., Bartocci, A., Patinkin, D., Rosendall, M., and Bradley, T. R. (1986). Regulation of very primitive, multipotent, haemopoietic cells by haemopoietin-1. *Cell*, **45**, 667–74.

11 Aarden, L. A., Brunner, T. K., Cerottini, J.-C., Dayer, J.-M., de Weck, A. L., Dinarello, C. A., Dissabato, G., Farrar, J. J., Gery, I., Gillis, S., Handschumacher, R. E., Henney, C. S., Hoffmann, M. K., Koopman, W. J., Krane, S. M., Lachman, L. B., Lefkowits, I., Mishell, R. I., Mizel, S. B., Oppenheim, J. J., Paetkau, V., Plate, J., Rollinghoff, M., Rosenstreich, D., Rosenthal, A. S., Rosenwasser, L. J., Schimpl, A., Shim, H. S., Simon, P. L., Smith, K. A., Wagner, H., Watson, J. D., Wecker, E., and Wood, D. D. (1979). Revised nomenclature for antigen non-specific T cell proliferation and helper factors [letter]. *J. Immunol.*, **123**, 2928–9.

12 Auron, P. E., Webb, A. C., Rosenwasser, L. J., Mucci, S. F., Rich, A., Wolff, S. M., and Dinarello, C. A. (1984). Nucleotide sequence of human monocyte interleukin-1 precursor cDNA. *Proc. Natl. Acad. Sci. U.S.A.*, **81**, 7907–11.

13 March, C. J., Mosley, B., Larsen, A., Cerretti, D. P., Braedt, G., Price, V., Gillis, S., Henney, C. S., Kronheim, S. R., Grabstein, K., Conlon, P. J., Hopp, T. P., and Cosman, D. (1985). Cloning, sequence, and expression of two distinct human interleukin-1 complementary DNAs. *Nature*, **315**, 641–7.

14 Cerretti, D. P., Kozlosky, C. J., Mosley, B., Nelson, N., Van Ness, K., Greenstreet, T. A., March, C. J., Kronheim, S. R., Druck, T., Cannizzaro, L. A., Huebner, K., and Black, R. A. (1992). Molecular cloning of the interleukin-1β converting enzyme. *Science*, **256**, 97–100.

15 Durum, S. K., Oppenheim, J. J., and Neta, R. (1990). Immunophysiologic role of interleukin-1. In *Immunophysiology: the role of cells and cytokines in immunity and inflammation* (ed. J. J. Oppenheim and E. M. Shevach), pp. 210–25. Oxford University Press.

16 DiGiovine, F. S. and Duff, G. W. (1990). Interleukin-1: the first interleukin. *Immunol. Today*, **11**, 13–20.

17 Bernheim, H. A., Gilbert, T. M., and Stitt, J. T. (1980). Prostaglandin E levels in third ventricular cerebrospinal fluid of rabbits during fever and change in body temperature. *J. Physiol.*, **301**, 69–78.

18 Besedovsky, H., Del Rey, A., Sorkin, E., and Dinarello, C. A. (1986). Immunoregulatory feedback between interleukin-1 and glucocorticoid hormones. *Science*, **233**, 652–4.

19 Kern, J. A., Lamb, R. J., Reed, J. C., Daniele, R. P., and Nowell, P. C. (1988). Dexamethasone inhibition of IL-1β production by human monocytes post-transcriptional mechanisms. *J. Clin. Invest.*, **8**, 237–44.

20 Hannum, C. H., Wilcox, C. J., Arend, W. P., Joslin, F. G., Dripps, D. J., Heindahl, P. L., Armes, L. G., Sommer, A., Eisenberg, S. P., and Thompson, R. C. (1990). Interleukin-1 receptor antagonist activity of a human interleukin-1 inhibitor. *Nature*, **343**, 336–41.

21 Zahedi, K., Seldin, M. F., Rits, M., Ezekowitz, R. A. B., and Whitehead, A. S. (1991). The mouse interleukin-1 receptor antagonist protein (IL-1rn): molecular characterization, gene mapping, and mRNA synthesis *in vitro* and *in vivo*. *J. Immunol.*, **146**, 4228–33.

22 Falkoff, R. J. M., Butler, J. L., Dinarello, C. A., and Fauci, A. S. (1984). Direct effects of a monoclonal B cell differentiation factor and of purified interleukin-1 on B cell differentiation. *J. Immunol.*, **133**, 692–6.

23 Cybulsky, M. I., Colditz, I. G., and Movat, H. Z. (1986). The role of interleukin-1 in neutrophil leucocyte emigration induced by endotoxin. *Am. J. Pathol.*, **124**, 367–72.

24 Dustin, M. L., Rothlein, R., Bhan, A. K., Dinarello, C. A., and Springer, T. A. (1986). Induction by interleukin-1 and interferon gamma, tissue distribution, biochemistry, and function of a natural adherence molecule (ICAM-1). *J. Immunol.*, **137**, 245–54.

25 Nachman, R. L., Hajjar, K. A., Silverstein, R. L., and Dinarello, C. A. (1986). Interleukin-1 induces endothelial cell synthesis of plasminogen activator inhibitor. *J. Exp. Med.*, **163**, 1595–600.

26 Bevilacqua, M. P., Pober, J. S., Majeau, G. R., Cotran, R. S., and Gimbrone Jr, M. A. (1984). Interleukin-1 induces biosynthesis and cell surface expression of procoagulant activity on human vascular endothelial cells. *J. Exp. Med.*, **160**, 618–23.

27 Dejana, E., Brevario, F., Erroi, A., Bussolino, F., Mussoni, L., Gramse, M., Pintucci, G., Casali, B., Dinarello, C. A., Van Damme, J., and Mantovani, A. (1987). Modulation of endothelial cell function by different molecular species of interleukin-1. *Blood*, **69**, 695–9.

28 Wahl, S. M., Wahl, L. M., and McCarthy, J. B. (1978). Lymphocyte-mediated activation of fibroblast proliferation and collagen production. *J. Immunol.*, **121**, 942–6.

29 Postlethwaite, A. E., Lachman, L. B., Mainardi, C. L., and Kang, A. H. (1983). Interleukin-1 stimulation of collagenase production by cultured fibroblasts. *J. Exp. Med.*, **157**, 801–6.

30 Fey, G. H. and Gauldie, J. (1989). The acute phase response of the liver in inflammation. In *Progress in liver diseases* Vol. 9 (ed. H. Popper and F. Schaffner), pp. 89–116. WB Saunders, Philadelphia.

31 Sehgal, P. B. and Sagar, A. D. (1980). Heterogeneity of poly(I).poly(C)-induced human fibroblast interferon mRNA species. *Nature*, **288**, 95–7.

32 Hirano, T., Yasukawa, K., Harada, H., Taga, T., Watanabe, Y., Matsuda, T., Kashiwamura, S-I., Nakajima, K., Koyama, K., Iwamatsu, A., Tsunasawa, S.,

Sakiyama, F., Matsui, H., Takahara, Y., Taniguchi, T., and Kishimoto, T. (1986). Complementary DNA for a novel human interleukin (BSF-2) that induces B lymphocytes to produce immunoglobulin. *Nature,* **324,** 73–6.

33 Kishimoto, T. (1985). Factors affecting B cell growth and differentiation. *Annu. Rev. Immunol.,* **3,** 133–57.

34 Aarden, L. A., de Groot, E. R., Schaap, O. L., and Lansdorp, P. M. (1987). Production of hybridoma growth factor by human monocytes. *Eur. J. Immunol.,* **17,** 1411–16.

35 Takai, Y., Wong, G. G., Clark, S. C., Burakoff, S. J., and Herrmann, S. H. (1988). B cell stimulatory factor 2 is involved in the differentiation of cytotoxic T lymphocytes. *J. Immunol.,* **140,** 508–12.

36 Gauldie, J., Richards, C., Harnish, D., Lansdorp, P., and Baumann, H. (1987). Interferon β2/B cell stimulating factor type 2 shares identity with monocyte-derived hepatocyte-stimulating factor and regulates the major acute phase protein response in liver cells. *Proc. Natl. Acad. Sci. U.S.A.,* **84,** 7251–5.

37 Chiu, C.-P., Moulds, C., Coffman, R. L., Rennick, D., and Lee, F. (1988). Multiple biological activities are expressed by a mouse interleukin-6 cDNA clone isolated from bone marrow stromal cells. *Proc. Natl. Acad. Sci. U.S.A.,* **85,** 7099–103.

38 Wong, G. G. and Clark, S. C. (1988). Multiple actions of interleukin-6 within a cytokine network. *Immunol. Today,* **9,** 137–9.

39 Billiau, A. (1988). Interferon-β2 as a promoter of growth and differentiation of B cells. *Immunol. Today,* **8,** 84–7.

40 Beutler, B. and Cerami, A. (1990). Cachectin (tumor necrosis factor): an endogenous mediator of shock and inflammatory response. In *Immunophysiology: the role of cells and cytokines in immunity and inflammation* (ed. J. J. Oppenheim and E. M. Shevach), pp. 226–37. Oxford University Press.

41 Aggarwal, B., Kohr, W. J., Haas, P. E., Moffat, B., Spencer, S. A., Henzel, W. J., Bringman, T. S., Nedwin, G. E., Goeddel, D. V., and Harkins, R. N. (1985). Human tumour necrosis factor. Production, purification, and characterization. *J. Biol. Chem.,* **260,** 2345–54.

42 Degliantoni, G., Murphy, M., Kobayoshi, M., Francis, M. K., Perussia, B., and Trinchieri, G. (1985). Natural killer (NK) cell-derived haematopoietic colony-inhibiting activity and NK cytotoxic factor. Relationship with tumour necrosis factor and synergism with immune interferon. *J. Exp. Med.,* **162,** 1512–30.

43 Palladino Jr, M. A. and Finkle, B. S. (1986). Immunopharmacology of tumour necrosis factors α and β. *Trends Pharmacol. Sci.,* **7,** 388-9.

44 Nedwin, G. E., Naylor, S. L., Sakaguchi, A. Y., Smith, D., Jarret-Nedwin, J., Pennica, D., Goeddel, D. V., and Gray, P. W. (1985). Human lymphotoxin and tumour necrosis factor genes: structure, homology, and chromosomal localization. *Nucleic Acids Res.,* **13,** 6361–73.

45 Aggarwal, B. B., Moffat, B., and Harkins, R. N. (1984). Human lymphotoxin: production by a lymphoblastoid cell line, purification, and initial characterization. *J. Biol. Chem.,* **259,** 686–91.

46 Farrar, W. L., Johnson, H. M., and Farrar, J. J. (1981). Regulation of the production of immune interferon and cytotoxic T lymphocytes by interleukin-2. *J. Immunol.,* **126,** 1120–5.

47 Wheelock, E. F. (1965). Interferon-like virus-inhibitor induced in human leucocytes by phytohaemagglutinin. *Science,* **149,** 310–11.

48   Nathan, C. F., Murray, H. W., Wiebe, M. E., and Rubin, B. Y. (1983). Identification of interferon-gamma as the lymphokine that activates human macrophage oxidative metabolism and anti-microbial activity. *J. Exp. Med.*, **158**, 670–89.

49   Coffman, R. L. and Carty, J. (1986). A T cell activity that enhances polyclonal IgE production and its inhibition by interferon-γ. *J. Immunol.*, **136**, 949–54.

50   Dart, L. L., Smith, D. M., Meyers, C. A., Sporn, M. B., and Frolik, C. A. (1985). Transforming growth factors from a human tumour cell: characterization of transforming growth factor-β and identification of high molecular weight transforming growth factor-α. *Biochemistry*, **24**, 5925–31.

51   Assoian, R. K., Komoriya, A., Meyers, C. A., Miller, D. M., and Sporn, M. B. (1983). Transforming growth factor-β in human platelets. Identification of a major storage site, purification, and characterization. *J. Biol. Chem.*, **258**, 7155–60.

52   Frolik, C. A., Dart, L. L., Meyers, C. A., Smith, D. M., and Sporn, M. B. (1983). Purification and initial characterization of a type β transforming growth factor from human placenta. *Proc. Natl. Acad. Sci. U.S.A.,* **80**, 3676–80.

53   Ellingsworth, L. R. (1990). Effect of growth factors on immunity and inflammation. In *Immunophysiology: the role of cells and cytokines in immunity and inflammation* (ed. J. J. Oppenheim and E. M. Shevach), pp. 320–35. Oxford University Press.

54   Postlethwaite, A. E., Keski-Oja, J., Moses, H. L., and Kang, A. H. (1987). Stimulation of the chemotactic migration of human fibroblasts by transforming growth factor beta. *J. Exp. Med.*, **165**, 251–6.

55   Wahl, S. M., Hunt, D. A., Wakefield, L. M., McCartney-Francis, N., Wahl, L. M., Roberts, A. B., and Sporn, M. B. (1987). Transforming growth factor type 2 induces monocyte chemotaxis and growth factor production. *Proc. Natl. Acad. Sci. U.S.A.*, **84**, 5788–92.

56   Chua, C. C., Geiman, D. E., Keller, G. H., and Ladda, R. L. (1985). Induction of collagenase secretion in human fibroblast cultures by growth promoting factors. *J. Biol. Chem.*, **260**, 5213–16.

57   Laiho, M., Saksela, O., and Keski-Oja, J. (1986). Transforming growth factor beta alters plasminogen activator activity in human skin fibroblasts. *Exp. Cell. Res.*, **164**, 399–407.

58   Ignotz, R. A. and Massague, J. (1986). Transforming growth factor-β stimulates the expression of fibronectin and collagen and their incorporation into the extracellular matrix. *J. Biol. Chem.*, **261**, 4337–45.

59   O' Neill, L. A. J., Bird, T. A., and Saklatvala, J. (1990). Interleukin-1 signal transduction. *Immunol. Today*, **11**, 392–4.

60   Mizel, S. B. (1990). How does interleukin-1 activate cells? Cyclic AMP and interleukin-1 signal transduction. *Immunol. Today*, **11**, 390–1.

61   Chizzonite, R., Truitt, T., Kilian, P. L., Stern, A. S., Nunes, P., Parker, K. P., Kaffka, K. L., Chua, A. O., Lugg, D. K., and Gubber, U. (1989). Two high affinity interleukin-1 receptors represent separate gene products. *Proc. Natl. Acad. Sci. U.S.A.*, **86**, 8029–33.

62   Farrar, W. L., Ferris, D. K., and Harel-Bellan, A. (1991). Lymphokine-induced molecular signal transduction. In *Immunophysiology: the role of cells and cytokines in immunity and inflammation* (ed. J. J. Oppenheim and E. M. Shevach), pp. 67–87. Oxford University Press.

63 Saklatvala, J. and O'Neill, L. (1991). Interleukin-1 signal transduction. In *Cytokine interactions and their control* (ed. A. Baxter and R. Ross), pp. 15–26. John Wiley and Sons Ltd.

64 O'Neill, L. A. J., Bird, T. A., Gearing, A. J. H., and Saklatvala, J. (1991). Interleukin-1 signal transduction: increased GTP binding and hydrolysis in membranes of a murine thymona lina (EL4). *J. Biol. Chem.*, **265**, 3146–52.

65 O'Neill, L. A. J., Ikebe, T., Sarsfield, S. J., and Saklatvala, J. (1992). The binding subunit of pertussis toxin inhibits IL-1 induction of IL-2 and prostaglandin production. *J. Immunol.*, **148**, 1474–79.

66 Sen, R. and Baltimore, D. (1986). Multiple nuclear factors interact with the immunoglobulin enhancer sequences. *Cell*, **46**, 705–16.

67 Baeurle, P. A. and Baltimore, D. (1988). IκB: A specific inhibitor of the NFκB transcription factor. *Science*, **242**, 540–6.

68 Curran, T. and Franza, B. R. (1988). Fos and jun: the AP-1 connection. *Cell*, **55**, 395–7.

69 Kushner, I., Volanakis, J. E., and Gewurz, H. (ed.) (1982). C-reactive protein and the plasma protein response to tissue injury. *Ann. N. Y. Acad. Sci.*, **389**, 235–74.

70 Law, S. K. A. and Reid, K. B. M. (1988). Complement. IRL Press Ltd., Oxford.

71 Mossesson, M. W. and Doolittle, R. F. (ed.) (1983). Molecular biology of fibrinogen and fibrin. *Ann. N. Y. Acad. Sci.*, **408**, 1–672.

72 Talstad, J. and Haugen, H. F. (1979). The relationship between the erythrocyte sedimentation rate (ESR) and plasma proteins in clinical materials and models. *Scand. J. Clin. Lab. Invest.*, **39**, 519–24.

73 Gordon, A. H. and Koj, A. (ed.) (1985). In *The acute phase response to injury and infection, research monographs in cell and tissue physiology*, Vol. 10. Elsevier.

74 Sipe, J. D. (1990). The acute phase response. In *Immunophysiology: the role of cells and cytokines in immunity and inflammation* (ed. J. J Oppenheim and E. M. Shevach), pp. 259–73. Oxford University Press.

75 Laurent, P. E. (1989). Clinical measurement of acute phase proteins to detect and monitor infectious diseases. In *Acute phase proteins in the acute phase response* (ed. M. B. Pepys), pp. 150–60. Springer-Verlag.

76 Van Riiswijk, M. H. and Van Leeuwen, M. A. (1989). C-reactive protein: clinical aspects. In *Acute phase proteins in the acute phase response* (ed. M. B. Pepys), pp. 161–8. Springer-Verlag.

77 Pepys, M. B. and Baltz, M. L. (1983). Acute phase proteins with special reference to C-reactive protein and related proteins (pentraxin) and serum amyloid A protein. *Adv. Immunol.*, **34**, 141–212.

78 Lonberg-Holm, K., Reed, D. L., Roberts, R. C., Herbert, R. R., Hillmann, M. C., and Kutney, R. M. (1987). Three high molecular weight proteinase inhibitors of rat plasma. Isolation, characterization, and acute phase changes. *J. Biol. Chem.*, **262**, 438–45.

79 Gauldie, J. (1989). Interleukin-1 in the acute phase response. In *Acute phase proteins in the acute phase response* (ed. M. B. Pepys), pp. 1–22. Springer-Verlag.

80 Baumann, H., Richards, C., and Gauldie, J. (1987). Interaction among hepatocyte-stimulating factors, interleukin-1, and glucocorticoids for regulation of acute phase plasma proteins in human hepatoma (HepG2) cells. *J. Immunol.*, **139**, 4122–8.

81 Edbrooke, M. R. and Woo, P. (1989). Regulation of human SAA gene expression by cytokines. In *Acute phase proteins in the acute phase response* (ed. M. B. Pepys), pp. 21–7. Springer-Verlag.

82 Strunk, R. C., Cole, F. S., Perlmutter, D. H., and Colten, H. R. (1985). Gamma interferon increases expression of Class III complement genes C2 and factor B in human monocytes and in murine fibroblasts transfected with human C2 and factor B genes. *J. Biol. Chem.*, **260**, 15280–5.

83 Miura, N., Prentice, H., Schneider, P. M., and Perlmutter, D. H. (1987). Synthesis and regulation of the two human complement C4 genes in stable transfected mouse fibroblasts. *J. Biol. Chem.*, **262**, 7298–305.

84 Aggarwal, B. B., Essalu, T. E., and Hass, P. E. (1985). Characterization of receptors for human tumour necrosis factor and their regulation by γ-interferon. *Nature*, **318**, 665–7.

85 Mackiewicz, A., Ganapathi, M. K., Schultz, D., Brabanec, A., Weinstein, J., Kelley, M. F., and Kushner, I. (1990). Transforming growth factor beta 1 regulates production of acute phase proteins. *Proc. Natl. Acad. Sci. U.S.A.*, **87**, 1491–5.

86 Kushner, I., Broder, M. L., and Karp, D. (1978). Control of the acute phase response. Serum C-reactive protein kinetics after acute myocardial infarction. *J. Clin. Invest.*, **61**, 235–42.

87 Kushner, I. and Feldman, G. (1978). Control of the acute phase response. Demonstration of C-reactive protein synthesis and secretion by hepatocytes during acute inflammation in the rabbit. *J. Exp. Med.*, **148**, 466–77.

88 Pepys, M. B., Baltz, M. L., Gomer, K., Davies, A. J. S., and Doenhoff, M. (1979). Serum amyloid P component is an acute phase reactant in the mouse. *Nature*, **278**, 259–61.

89 Tillet, W. S. and Francis Jr, T. (1930). Serological reactions in pneumonia with non-protein somatic fraction of pneumococcus. *J. Exp. Med.*, **52**, 561–71.

90 Cathcart, E. S., Comerford, F. R., and Cohen, A. S. (1965). Immunologic studies on a protein extracted from human secondary amyloid. *N. Engl. J. Med.*, **273**, 143–6.

91 Cohen, A. S. and Calkins, E. (1959). Electron microscopic observation of a fibrous component in amyloid of diverse origins. *Nature*, **183**, 1202–3.

92 Dyck, R. F., Lockwood, M., Kershaw, M., McHugh, N., Duance, V., Baltz, M. L., and Pepys, M. B. (1980). Amyloid P component is a constituent of normal glomerular basement membrane. *J. Exp. Med.*, **152**, 1162–74.

93 DeBeer, F. C., Baltz, M. L., Holford, S., Feinstein, A., and Pepys, M. B. (1981). Fibronectin and C4 binding protein are selectively bound by aggregated amyloid P component. *J. Exp. Med.*, **154**, 1134–49.

94 Woo, P., Korenberg, J. R., and Whitehead, A. S. (1985). Characterization of genomic and complementary DNA sequence of human C-reactive protein, and comparison with the complementary DNA sequence of serum amyloid P component. *J. Biol. Chem.*, **260**, 13384–8.

95 Yunis, I. and Whitehead, A. S. (1990). The mouse C-reactive protein gene maps to distal chromosome 1 and, like its human counterpart, is closely linked to the serum amyloid P component gene. *Immunogenetics*, **32**, 361–3.

96 Floyd-Smith, G., Whitehead, A. S., Colten, H. R., and Francke, U. (1986). The human C-reactive protein gene (CRP) and serum amyloid P component gene (APCS) are located on the proximal long arm of chromosome 1. *Immunogenetics*, **24**, 171–6.

97 Whitehead, A. S., Rits, M., and Michaelson, J. (1988). Molecular genetics of mouse serum amyloid P component (SAP): cloning and gene mapping. *Immunogenetics*, **28**, 388–90.

98 Lalley, P. A., Davisson, M. T., Graves, J. A. M., O'Brien, S. J., Womack, J. E., Roderick, T. H., Creau-Goldberg, A. L., Hillyard, D. P., and Rogers, J. A. (1989). Report on the committee on comparative mapping. *Cytogenet. Cell Genet.*, **51**, 503–32.

99 Kingsmore, S. F., Snoddy, J., Choubey, D., Lengyel, P., and Seldin, M. F. (1989). Physical mapping of a family of interferon-activated genes, serum amyloid P component and α-spectrin on mouse chromosome 1. *Immunogenetics*, **30**, 169–74.

100 Rubio, N., Sharp, P. M., Rits, M., Zahedi, K., and Whitehead, A. S. (1993). Structure, expression, and evolution of guinea pig serum amyloid P component and C-reactive protein. *J. Biochem. (Tokyo)*, in press.

101 Robey, F. A., Jones, K. D., Tanata, T., and Liu, T.-Y. (1984). Binding of C-reactive protein to chromatin and nucleosome core particles. A possible physiological role of C-reactive protein. *J. Biol. Chem.*, **259**, 7311–6.

102 Pepys, M. B. and Butler, P. J. G. (1987). Serum amyloid P component is the major calcium-dependent specific DNA binding protein of the serum. *Biochem. Biophys. Res. Commun.*, **148**, 308–13.

103 Zahedi, K. and Whitehead, A. S. (1989). Acute phase induction of mouse serum amyloid P component (SAP): correlation with other parameters of inflammation. *J. Immunol.*, **143**, 2880–6.

104 Arcone, R., Gualandi, G., and Ciliberto, G. (1988). Identification of sequences responsible for acute phase induction of human C-reactive protein. *Nucleic Acids Res.*, **16**, 3195–207.

105 Ganter, U., Arcone, R., Toniatti, C., Morrone, G., and Ciliberto, G. (1989). Dual control of C-reactive protein gene expression by interleukin-1 and interleukin-6. *EMBO J.*, **8**, 3773–9.

106 Steel, D. M. and Whitehead, A. S. (1991). Heterogeneous modulation of acute phase reactant mRNA levels by interleukin-1β and interleukin-6 in the human hepatoma cell line PLC/PRF/5. *Biochem. J.*, **277**, 477–82.

107 Whitehead, A. S., Zahedi, K., Rits, M., Mortensen, R. F., and Lelias, J. M. (1990). Mouse C-reactive protein: generation of complementary DNA clones, structural analysis, and induction of mRNA during inflammation. *Biochem. J.*, **266**, 283–90.

108 Ciliberto, G., Arcone, R., Wagner, E. F., and Ruther, U. (1987). Inducible and tissue-specific expression of human C-reactive protein in transgenic mice. *EMBO J.*, **6**, 4017–22.

109 Benditt, E. P. and Eriksen, N. (1977). Amyloid protein SAA is associated with high density lipoprotein from human serum. *Proc. Natl. Acad. Sci. U.S.A.*, **74**, 4025–8.

110 Coetzee, G. A., Strachan, A. F., van der Westhuyzen, D. R., Hoppe, H. C., Jeenah, M. S., and DeBeer, F. C. (1986). Serum amyloid A-containing high density lipoprotein 3: density, size, and apolipoprotein composition. *J. Biol. Chem.*, **261**, 9644–51.

111 Betts, J. C., Edbrooke, M. R., Thakker, R. V., and Woo, P. (1991). The human acute phase serum amyloid A gene family: structure, evolution, and expression in hepatoma cells. *Scand. J. Immunol.*, **34**, 471–82.

112 Steel, D. M., Sellar, G. C., Uhlar, C. M., Simon, S., DeBeer, F. C., and Whitehead, A. S. (1993). A constitutively expressed serum amyloid A protein (C-SAA)

gene is closely linked to, and shares structural similarities with, an acute phase serum amyloid A protein (A-SAA) gene. *Genomics*, in press.

113 Sack Jr, G. H. and Talbot Jr, C. C. (1989). The human serum amyloid A (SAA)-encoding gene GSAA1. *Gene*, **84**, 509–15.

114 Kluve-Beckerman, B., Drumm, L., and Benson, M. D. (1991). Non-expression of the serum amyloid A three (SAA3) gene. *DNA Cell Biol.*, **10**, 651–61.

115 Whitehead, A. S., DeBeer, M. C., Steel, D. M., Rits, M., Lelias, J. M., Lane, W. S., and DeBeer, F. C. (1992). Identification of novel members of the serum amyloid A protein (SAA) superfamily as constitutive apolipoproteins of high density lipoprotein. *J. Biol. Chem.*, **267**, 3862–7.

116 Taylor, B. A. and Rowe, L. (1984). Genes for serum amyloid A proteins map to chromosome 7 in the mouse. *Mol. Gen. Genet.*, **195**, 491–9.

117 Lowell, C. A., Potter, D. A., Stearman, R. S., and Morrow, J. F. (1986). Structure of the murine amyloid A gene family. *J. Biol. Chem.*, **261**, 8442–52.

118 Stearman, R. S., Lowell, C. A., Peltzman, C. G., and Morrow, J. (1986). The sequence and structure of a new serum amyloid A gene. *Nucleic Acids Res.*, **14**, 797–809.

119 Woo, P., Sipe, J., Dinarello, C. A., and Colten, H. R. (1987). Structure of a human serum amyloid A gene and modulation of its expression in transfected L cells. *J. Biol. Chem.*, **262**, 15790–5.

120 Edbrooke, M. R., Burt, D. W., Cheshire, J. K., and Woo, P. (1989). Identification of *cis*-acting sequences responsible for phorbol ester induction of human SAA gene expression via a NFκB-like transcription factor. *Mol. Cell. Biol.*, **9**, 1908–16.

121 Steel, D. M., Rogers, J. T., DeBeer, F. C., DeBeer, M. C., and Whitehead, A. S. (1993). Post-transcriptional regulation of acute phase human serum amyloid A (A-SAA) synthesis *in vitro*: the roles of mRNA accumulation, poly(A) tail shortening, and translational efficiency. *Biochem. J.*, in press.

122 Macintyre, S. S., Kushner, I., and Samols, D. (1985). Secretion of C-reactive protein becomes more efficient during the course of the acute phase response. *J. Biol. Chem.*, **260**, 4169–73.

123 Rogers, J. T., Bridges, K. R., Durmowicz, G. P., Glass, J., Auron, P. E., and Munro, H. N. (1990). Translational control during the acute phase response. Ferritin synthesis in response to interleukin-1. *J. Biol. Chem.*, **265**, 14572–8.

124 Levin, M., Franklin, E. C., Frangione, B., and Pras, M. (1972). The amino acid sequence of a major non-immunoglobulin component of some amyloid fibrils. *J. Clin. Invest.*, **51**, 2773–6.

125 Husebekk, A., Skogen, B., Husby, G., and Marhaug, G. (1985). Transformation of amyloid precursor SAA to protein AA and incorporation in amyloid fibrils *in vitro*. *Scand. J. Immunol.*, **21**, 283–7.

126 Li, J. J. and McAdam, K. P. W. J. (1984). Human amyloid P component: an elastase inhibitor. *Scand. J. Immunol.*, **20**, 219–26.

127 Zahedi, K., Gonnerman, W. A., DeBeer, F. C., DeBeer, M. C., Sipe, J. D., and Whitehead, A. S. (1991). Major acute phase reactant synthesis during chronic inflammation in amyloid susceptible and resistant mouse strains. *Inflammation*, **15**, 1–15.

128 Hawkins, P. N., Myers, M. J., Lavender, J. P., and Pepys, M. B. (1988). Diagnostic radionucleotide imaging of amyloid: biological targeting by circulating human serum amyloid P component. *Lancet*, **i**, 1413–18.

129 Tall, A. R. (1990). Plasma high density lipoproteins. Metabolism and relationship to atherogenesis. *J. Clin. Invest.*, **86**, 379–84.
130 Fielding, C. J., Shore, V. G., and Fielding, P. E. (1972). A protein cofactor of lecithin-cholesterol acyltransferase. *Biochem. Biophys. Res. Commun.*, **46**, 1493–8.
131 Pincus, T. and Callahan, L. F. (1986). Taking mortality in rheumatoid arthritis seriously — predictive markers, socioeconomic status, and comorbidity. *J. Rheumatol.*, **13**, 841–5.
132 Mitchell, T. I., Coon, C. I., and Brinckerhoff, C. E. (1991). Serum amyloid A (SAA3) produced by rabbit synovial fibroblasts treated with phorbol esters or interleukin-1 induces synthesis of collagenase and is neutralized with specific antiserum. *J. Clin. Invest.*, **87**, 1177–85.

2 Interleukin-1

H. U. BEUSCHER AND M. RÖLLINGHOFF

1 Introduction

Interleukin-1 (IL-1) is the term for two related proteins, IL-1α and IL-1β, produced by activated macrophages and many other cells. Although both forms of IL-1 are distinct gene products, they are recognized by the same cell surface receptors and are similar in function. Historically, IL-1 was discovered as an endogenous pyrogen and later identified as a co-stimulator promoting the growth of lectin-stimulated thymocytes (1, 2). IL-1 is now considered to be a central mediator of host responses to infection and other forms of trauma. The many regulatory roles attributable to IL-1 include the control of cellular and humoral immune responses, inflammation, fever, acute phase responses, and haemopoiesis (3) (see Chapter 1). Its biological effects are not restricted to a particular cell lineage, but instead IL-1 is a multi-functional cytokine acting on a variety of cells both within the immune system and other cellular systems, as briefly illustrated in Figure 2.1 (see also Figure 1.1).

IL-1 forms, together with two other peptide hormones, namely IL-6 and TNFα, a group of cytokines that are expressed during infection and particularly in infection with Gram-negative bacteria. The biological properties of IL-1 share remarkable similarities to those of TNFα, most notably the

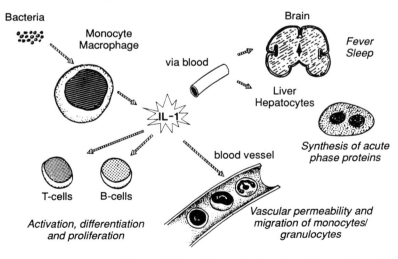

Fig. 2.1 Cellular targets and bio-activities of IL-1 after its release from activated monocytes and macrophages.

induction of fever, inflammation, and haemodynamic shock (4, 5). Nearly all responses to either IL-1 or TNFα can be enhanced when the two are administered together. IL-6, like IL-1 and TNFα, increases synthesis of acute phase proteins and causes fever. Thus, although this review focuses on IL-1, the reader should keep in mind that IL-1 is part of a cytokine network in which its expression and biological properties are influenced by IL-6 (Chapter 3) and TNFα (Chapter 4).

Much interest has focused on IL-1 as a mediator in disease. Elevated circulating levels of IL-1 correlate with a variety of clinical situations including septic shock (6). Moreover, a role of IL-1 as a mediator in chronic inflammation can be inferred from animal and human studies and is particularly emphasized in acute rheumatoid arthritis (7). Thus, IL-1 can be viewed as a mediator of host defence as well as of disease.

Because of the potent and profound biological effects of IL-1 it is not surprising that its activities are tightly regulated, most notably at the levels of transcription, translation, and secretion (8–10). Additional regulatory mechanisms are provided by the concomitant action of other cytokines, differences in the expression of IL-1 receptors on target cells, and the production of natural inhibitory proteins, as for example the recently identified IL-1 receptor antagonist (IL-1ra) (11). Moreover, understanding the exact mechanisms that regulate IL-1 activity *in vivo* requires consideration of additional parameters such as distinct micro-environment and anatomical compartmentalization.

The purpose of this chapter is to review our current knowledge of the structure, biosynthesis, and biological activities of IL-1 as it contributes to the host response against infection.

2   Structure and molecular properties of IL-1

Complementary DNA (cDNA) cloning, protein purification, and sequencing studies isolated two forms of IL-1, termed IL-1α (pI 5.0) and IL-1β (pI 7.0), which are present in several species including man and mouse (12, 13). The genes for IL-1α and IL-1β have been sequenced and were localized to the long arm of chromosome 2. The size of the human IL-1α and IL-1β gene is 10.5 kb and 7.8 kb, respectively. Each IL-1 gene contains seven exons but they share only 45 per cent homology in their nucleic acid sequence (14, 15).

The IL-1α mRNA is about 2.3 kb in length, whereas the reported size of the IL-1β mRNA ranges from 1.4 to 1.8 kb. Both IL-1 mRNAs are translated into polypeptides (271 amino acids for IL-1α and 269 amino acids for IL-1β) of approximately 31 kDa (12, 13). However, the predominant molecular weight of the two IL-1 proteins in culture supernatants from macrophages and in biological fluids is only about 17.5 kDa (16, 17). The data indicate that IL-1α and IL-1β are synthesized as precursor proteins which are subsequently modified to yield extracellular low molecular weight IL-1 polypeptides. Comparison of the N-terminal protein sequence data with respective cDNA sequences further revealed that, for both forms of IL-1, it is the carboxyl-terminal portion of the molecule that is present in culture supernatants as active IL-1. Receptor binding and full biological activity requires a minimum amino acid sequence spanning residues 128 to 267 in IL-1α, and residues 120 to 266 in IL-1β (18).

Human IL-1β has been crystallized and the structure analysed by nuclear magnetic resonance spectroscopy (19). According to these studies, IL-1β resembles a tetrahedron and is composed of 12 β-strands arranged in three pseudosymmetric topological units.

At the amino acid level, the sequence identity between the IL-1α and IL-1β precursor as well as the extracellular forms of IL-1 is only in the order of 25 to 30 per cent. Yet, their biological activities are similar, and both IL-1α and IL-1β competitively bind to a common receptor on various target cells (see Section 4). Moreover, the two forms of IL-1 are structurally of particular interest, in that neither IL-1α nor IL-1β contains a secretory signal peptide as would be expected for a protein destined for secretion.

3   Biosynthesis and secretion of IL-1

IL-1α and IL-1β arise by *de novo* RNA and protein synthesis. Although cells of the monocyte/macrophage lineage remain an important source for IL-1, IL-1 is now known to be produced by a large number of lymphoid and non-lymphoid cells. With the exception of skin keratinocytes, production of both forms of IL-1 is not constitutive, but is only transiently induced by various stimuli including other cytokines, complement components, immune-complexes, phorbol esters, bacteria, and several microbial products (for review see references 5, 20). The best studied of these is lipopolysaccharide (LPS), which stimulates IL-1 production at concentrations as low as 10 pg/ml.

3.1   Transcription and translation

The two forms of IL-1 appear to be under separate transcriptional control (21–24). In human monocytes both IL-1 genes are transcribed within 15 minutes after stimulation with LPS (8, 9, 21). However, stimulation of the cells with phorbol myristate acetate (PMA) induces IL-1β, but not IL-1α transcription (24). Furthermore, a differential expression of IL-1α and IL-1β has been observed in various cell types listed in Table 2.1.

The transcriptional activation mechanisms of the IL-1 genes are poorly defined. There is, however, evidence that activation of protein kinase C (PKC) is involved in signal transmission: PKC activating phorbol esters, (e.g. PMA) induce IL-1β expression in human monocytes, and LPS-induced expression of both IL-1α and IL-1β can be down-regulated by PKC inhibitors (9, 24).

Table 2.1 Differential mRNA expression of IL-1α and IL-1β

Cell type	mRNA	Reference
Human monocytes	IL-1α and IL-1β [a]	22
Human T lymphocytes	IL-1α	23
Human synovial macrophages	IL-1β	22

[a] 25- to 50-fold more β than α (5).

The production of IL-1 is also regulated at the level of mRNA stability and translation. Although the IL-1α gene is transcribed in cultured (aged) monocytes there are no detectable levels of IL-1α mRNA in such cells, indicating that the IL-1α mRNA is rapidly degraded. Moreover, adherence of monocytes to glass or plastic triggers IL-1 gene expression without translation into IL-1 proteins. The latter, however, can be induced by a second signal, provided by LPS or by the complement component C5a (see Chapter 8) (10). Accordingly, it appears that transcription and translation of IL-1 are separately regulated.

The cytokines inducing IL-1 production include IL-1 (α and β) itself, TNFα, granulocyte macrophage colony-stimulating factor (GM-CSF), and macrophage-CSF. Suppression of IL-1 production has been observed in the presence of IL-4, IL-6, IL-10, and transforming growth factor-β (TGFβ) (25–28). IFNγ has a dual role, it augments IL-1 production induced by LPS, but suppresses IL-1 production induced by IL-1 (29).

3.2   Processing of IL-1

IL-1α and IL-1β mRNAs are translated into precursor proteins (pro-IL-1α and pro-IL-1β) of 31 kDa which are cleaved by proteases either during or after secretion. IL-1α cannot be translocated across microsomal membranes (30). Immunoelectron microscopy as well as subcellular fractionation studies confirmed that neither form of IL-1 is detectable in the endoplasmic reticulum or in the Golgi apparatus (31, 32). This clearly relates to the apparent lack of a N-terminal signal peptide. Therefore, all indications favour IL-1α and IL-1β as being cytosolic proteins.

Association of IL-1 proteins with other cell organelles has been reported for lysosomes and mitochondria (32, 33). A number of studies suggest that IL-1α, but not IL-1β exists as a membrane protein on activated macrophages. Initially, membrane IL-1 was detected by measuring IL-1 activity on paraformaldehyde-fixed murine macrophages (34). Later it has been shown that most of the measured bio-activity was probably due to the leakage of IL-1α out of the fixed cells, indicating that fixation of the macrophages with paraformaldehyde is inadequate to prove the existence of a membrane form of IL-1 (35). However, IL-1α was detected on the membrane of monocytes and macrophages, using fluorescence labelling and cell surface iodination (36, 37).

The mechanism by which IL-1α may be anchored to the membrane remains to be determined. The IL-1α precursor is phosphorylated at serine residue 90 (38) and phosphorylated pro-IL-1α binds to membrane vesicles of monocytes in the presence of calcium (39). Thus, phosphorylation could serve as a mechanism, facilitating the interaction of pro-IL-1α with cell membranes. Alternatively, anchoring of pro-IL-1α to the membrane has been proposed via lectin-like binding because D-mannose dissociates the pro-IL-1α from the membrane (40).

It is unclear how IL-1 is transported out of the cells and how it is cleaved to its bio-active peptides. IL-1α can be released from intact macrophages by trypsin-like enzymes and it has been proposed that membrane IL-1 is a pre-requisite for secretion of IL-1α, since a calcium-activated neutral protease has been described to process pro-IL-1α (41). The secretion of IL-1β from macrophages occurs much earlier and faster than that of IL-1α (17, 42), suggesting that the secretion of the two forms of IL-1 is controlled by separate mechanism(s). Pro-IL-1β lacks biological activity (18); it is secreted unprocessed (17) and cleaved only later by various enzymes including elastase and plasmin. A monocyte-specific protease has been described that specifically cleaves pro-IL-1β at alanine position 117 (43). Incomplete processing of secreted pro-IL-1β may be due to spontaneous disulfide-mediated protein folding (44a).

Recently, cDNA has been cloned from a human monocytic cell line which encodes an enzyme which specifically hydrolyses the pro-form of IL-1β to the mature form. The enzyme has 404 amino acids and does not belong to any known family of proteases. The gene for the converting enzyme has been localized to chromosome 11 at the 11q23 band. This band has been identified as being frequently involved in rearrangements in human leukaemias and lymphomas and it has been suggested that this enzyme may have a functional role in regulating cell growth (44b).

4   The IL-1 receptors

The various biological activities of IL-1 are mediated by specific receptors on the surface of many cells (45–47). The binding of IL-1 is specific and saturable and occurs with high affinity; K_d in the order of 5×10^{-10} to 5×10^{-11} M. To date, two distinct single chain receptors have been identified: one of 80 kDa is designated IL-1 receptor type I (IL-1R type I) and is expressed on T cells, fibroblasts, and epithelial cells (45); the other of 68 kDa is called IL-1R type II and is expressed on B cells, neutrophils, and macrophages (46). Both types of IL-1R have been cloned and sequenced and belong to the immunoglobulin (Ig) superfamily (47). Besides being expressed on different cells, the two IL-1R differ with respect to their binding affinities and regulation of surface expression. Although IL-1α and IL-1β are equally recognized by the IL-1R type I, IL-1α binds better to the type I receptor whereas IL-1β does so to the type II receptor. In fact, there is evidence that IL-1β triggers B cells *in vivo* whereas IL-1α does not. In this context, it has been suggested that IL-1α may act as a competitive inhibitor of the immunostimulatory properties of IL-1β (48). The molecular mechanism by which a signal resulting from IL-1 binding to its receptor is transduced intracellularly is not completely understood (49).

5   Role of IL-1 in infection

Many of the biological properties of IL-1 attest to its having a fundamental role in both non-specific immunity and specific immunity in the host defence against infection.

When administered into animals, IL-1 induces a series of physiological changes mimicking the acute phase response to infection (50). These changes, including fever, increased synthesis of acute phase reactants in the liver, and reductions in plasma iron are thought to be beneficial for the host by increasing opsonization of micro-organisms and by inhibiting microbial growth. IL-1 induces gene expression of neutrophil and monocyte chemotactic cytokines, such as IL-8, IL-9, and macrophage inflammatory proteins which, in turn, stimulate neutrophil migration and degranulation *in vivo* (51). Also, IL-1 induces the expression of adhesion molecules which promote neutrophil and lymphocyte adherence to the vascular endothelium (52). These effects on endothelial cells are clinically important in that they limit the spread of infections and also allow leucocytes to pass and be retained at the site of inflammation. Thus, if synthesis and secretion of IL-1 represents a first line of defence against acute infection, its local and systemic effects may help to mobilize non-specific defence mechanisms.

To evaluate IL-1 for its capacity to mobilize anti-microbial resistance, animals have been treated with IL-1 in a variety of infectious disease models. When injected in a low dose, IL-1 appears to protect mice from lethal infections due to bacteria, and parasites (53, 54). In most cases, maximal enhancement of survival following acute infection was observed when IL-1 treatment preceded infection by at least 4 hours. The mechanism(s) by which IL-1 enhances anti-microbial resistance remains to be further elucidated. Although IL-1 treatment clearly induces neutrophilia (53) a decrease in the number of pathogens is not detectable in all models, suggesting that IL-1-induced protection is not only due to increased microbicidal mechanisms.

In Gram-negative bacterial infection detrimental and even lethal effects are mediated by TNFα (55), the receptor expression of which is down-regulated by IL-1 (56). Accordingly, IL-1-induced protection is likely to involve a desensitization due to the action of TNFα. In addition, there is evidence that IL-1-induced suppression of parasitaemia in murine cerebral malaria is at least partly mediated by IFNγ released by T cells (54).

Cell-mediated immunity plays a major role in host defence against intra-cellular pathogens. One of the cytokines required to enhance the anti-microbial activity of infected macrophages is IFNγ produced by activated T cells. All indications favour IL-1 as being an important component in the activation of a subset of T helper cells designated T_H2 cells. However, IL-1 only serves as a co-stimulator to induce IL-2 and IL-2R expression in the context of antigen presentation (for review see reference 57).

Extracellular pathogens are usually adequately dealt with by antibody-mediated mechanisms. IL-1 is a co-stimulator for B cell activation and Ig production and it particularly acts together with IL-4 and IL-6 (4), and thus contributes to the antibody-mediated anti-microbial defence.

5.1   Production of IL-1 at a local site of infection

To gain further insights into the action of IL-1 during infection several questions need to be answered. Firstly, which cells produce IL-1 (α and β) and when do they do so. Secondly, does the micro-environment affect the expression of IL-1 genes. Thirdly, do the IL-1 producing cells also synthesize TNFα and IL-6. Fourthly, which cells have receptors for IL-1 in normal and diseased tissue.

To investigate the induction of IL-1 at a local site of infection we have used the mouse model of yersiniosis (58). The advantages of this model of infection include the ability of *Yersinia enterocolitica* 08, an entero-pathogenic bacterium, to preferentially invade the Peyer's Patches of the distal ileum after oral infection. Figure 2.2 illustrates the localization of IL-1α and IL-1β producing cells by immunoperoxidase staining of adjacent tissue sections of Peyer's Patches prepared from mice after six days of infection. The labelling patterns reveal a clear distinction between cells recog-nized by the antiserum to either IL-1α (Figure 2.2a) or IL-1β (Figure 2.2b). IL-1α producing cells are mature macrophages while IL-1β producing cells are monocytes (Beuscher, unpublished). When comparing the kinetics of appearance of IL-1α and IL-1β immunoreactive cells, it is clear that the induction of IL-1α is delayed by at least 24 hours. In addition, production of IL-1α and IL-1β in inflamed Peyer's Patches does not originate from resident cells, but rather from monocytes migrating from the circulation into the tissue. We conclude from these results that the differential production of IL-1α and IL-1β is controlled by the differentiation of activated monocytes to activated tissue macrophages.

5.2   Production of IL-1 during sepsis

Elevated circulating levels of IL-1 and TNFα have been reported in patients and animals with sepsis due to a variety of micro-organisms, and the rela-tive amounts of both cytokines correlate with the degree of hypotension

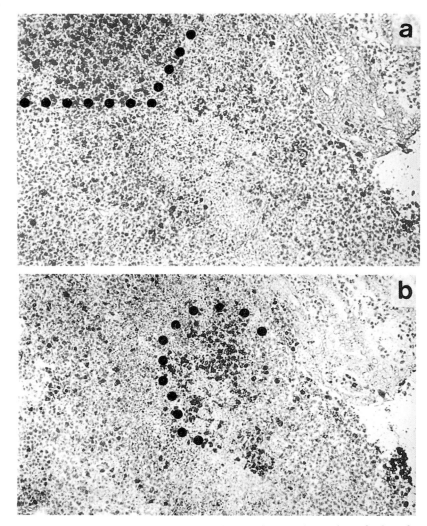

Fig. 2.2   Immunolocalization of IL-1α and IL-1β in Peyer's patches of mice after six days of infection with *Y. enterocolitica 08*. Consecutive frozen tissue sections of Peyer's patches were incubated with antiserum to either (a) murine IL-1α or (b) murine IL-1β. Visualization of binding was with horseradish peroxidase staining. IL-1α and IL-1β producing cells can be seen in different, non-overlapping tissue areas (*dotted lines*).

(6, 55). IL-1β, but not IL-1α reaches peak elevation two to four hours after injection of Gram-negative bacteria or LPS. When compared to IL-1β, TNFα levels rise more rapidly and reach peak levels at one hour and then decrease as do IL-1 levels. Antibodies to TNFα reduce IL-1β and IL-6 appearance during lethal bacteraemia (59), indicating that under these circumstances IL-1β and IL-6 are under the control of TNFα. These data emphasize the importance of IL-1 and TNFα for the development of the septic shock syndrome. Thus, substances that would allow a co-ordinated modulation of IL-1 and TNFα activities would be of potential benefit as therapeutic agents.

6 Modulation of IL-1 activity

There are several strategies for inhibiting IL-1 activity. As reviewed elsewhere (60), reduction or prevention of IL-1 synthesis by either corticosteroids or agents that block the lipoxygenase pathway of arachidonate metabolism (see Chapters 12 and 13) may provide an important approach to anti-inflammatory therapy. In addition, cytokines such as TGFβ, and IL-10 may also be useful to reduce IL-1 synthesis (see Section 2.3.1).

Inhibition of IL-1 already released into circulation, as for example during septic shock, requires a separate strategy. IL-1R blockade with antibodies to the IL-1R type I has been shown to attenuate the host inflammatory response and protect mice from LPS and IL-1-induced acute inflammation (61). In addition, administration of the extracellular domain of the IL-1R type I (soluble IL-1R protein) to animals seems to decrease inflammatory responses (62). Antibodies that specifically bind to IL-1 have not been tested so far, but antibodies to TNFα were shown to protect mice from endotoxaemia and *Escherichia coli* sepsis (55).

The existence of naturally occurring inhibitors of IL-1 activity has been firmly established *in vitro* and *in vivo*. These inhibitors can be divided into two groups, one of which consists of substances, e.g. α_2-macroglobulin and lipoproteins, that inhibit IL-1 activity (63), but they also interact with other proteins not related to IL-1. The second group consists of polypeptides that specifically inhibit IL-1 activity. A member of this group of IL-1 inhibitors has recently been cloned and termed IL-1R antagonist (IL-1ra) (64, 65). The cDNA sequence codes for a polypeptide of 17–3 kDa. Similar to the naturally occurring IL-1ra polypeptide (23 kDa) (11), the recombinant IL-1ra binds avidly only to IL-1R type I and appears to prevent signal transduction by directly blocking the binding of IL-1 without inducing a signal of its own. Comparison of the deduced protein sequences and intron-exon organization of the genes for IL-1α, IL-1β, and IL-1ra indicate that the three IL-1R ligands have a common evolutionary ancestor (66).

In animal models, administration of IL-1ra prevents death from endotoxin shock and reduces *E. coli*-induced hypotension (67, 68). In addition, IL-1ra blocks IL-1-induced PGE_2 synthesis from synovial cells and collagenase synthesis from chondrocytes (69). Figure 2.3 illustrates various strategies for the modulation of IL-1 activity.

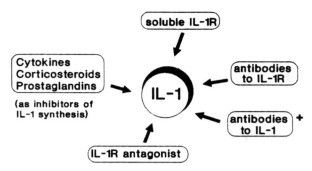

Fig. 2.3 Possibilities for inhibiting IL-1 activity. IL-1R is IL-1 receptor. [+]Thus far, no definitive experiments reported.

7   Summary

IL-1 is a multi-functional cytokine closely related to IL-6 and TNFα. IL-1 mediates inflammatory reactions, activates B and T cells, and stimulates haemopoiesis. In addition, IL-1 is a major inducer of IL-6 and TNFα, which reinforces the synergistic action of the three molecules.

Molecular cloning of IL-1 has led to the characterization of two distinct IL-1 proteins, i.e. IL-1α and IL-1β, which share a similar spectrum of activities. IL-1α and IL-1β appear to be differently expressed in certain cell types and also differ in their binding affinities to IL-1 receptors expressed on T and B cells, respectively. However, at present it is still difficult to understand the significance for the existence of the two forms of IL-1.

The recent availability of recombinant proteins that specifically inhibit IL-1 activity has led to a burst of studies on their potential therapeutic application and clinical assessment of their value is within reach.

Acknowledgements

The work from our laboratory quoted in this chapter was supported by the Deutsche Forschungsgemeinschaft through SFB 263 and by the Johannes and Frieda Marohn Stiftung.

References

1   Bennett, I. L. and Beeson, P. B. (1953). The effect of the injection of extracts and suspensions of infected rabbit tissues upon the body temperature of normal rabbits. *J. Exp. Med.*, **98**, 477–92.
2   Grey, I., Gershon, R. K., and Waksman, B. H. (1972). Potentiation of the T lymphocyte response to mitogens. I. The responding cell. *J. Exp. Med.*, **136**, 128–38.

3 Dinarello, C. A. (1991). Interleukin-1 and interleukin-1 antagonism. *Blood*, **77**, 1627–52.

4 Akira, S., Hirano, T., Toga, T., and Kishimoto, T. (1990). Biology of multifunctional cytokines: IL-6 and related molecules (IL-1 and TNF). *FASEB J.*, **4**, 2860–7.

5 Dinarello, C. A. (1991). The pro-inflammatory cytokines interleukin-1 and tumour necrosis factor and treatment of the septic shock syndrome. *J. Infect. Dis.*, **163**, 1177–84.

6 Cannon, J. G., Tompkins, R. G., Gelfand, J. A., *et al.* (1990). Circulating interleukin-1 and tumour necrosis factor in septic shock and experimental endotoxin fever. *J. Infect. Dis.*, **161**, 73–84.

7 Shore, A., Jaglal, S., and Keystone, E. C. (1986). Enhanced interleukin-1 generation by monocytes *in vitro* is temporarily linked to an early event in the onset or exarcerbation of rheumatoid arthritis. *Clin. Exp. Immunol.*, **167**, 1957–62.

8 Fenton, M. J., Clark, B. D., Collins, K. L., Webb, A. C., Rich, A., and Auron, P. E. (1987). Transcriptional regulation of the human pro-interleukin-1 beta gene. *J. Immunol.*, **138**, 3972–9.

9 Fenton, M. J., Vermeulen, M. W., Clark, B. D., Webb, A. C., and Auron, P. E. (1988). Human pro-IL-1 beta gene expression in monocytic cells is regulated by two distinct pathways. *J. Immunol.*, **140**, 2267–73.

10 Schindler, R., Gelfand, J. A., and Dinarello, C. A. (1990). Recombinant C5a stimulates transcription rather than translation of IL-1 and TNF; priming of mononuclear cells with recombinant C5a enhances cytokine synthesis induced by LPS, IL-1, or PMA. *Blood*, **76**, 1631–8.

11 Seckinger, P., Lowenthal, J. W., Williamson, K., Dayer, J. M., and MacDonald, H. R. (1987). A urine inhibitor of interleukin-1 activity that blocks ligand binding. *J. Immunol.*, **139**, 1546–9.

12 Auron, P. E., Webb, A. C., Rosenwasser, L. J., Mucci, S. F., Rinch, A., Wolff, S. M., and Dinarello, C. A. (1984). Nucleotide sequence of human monocyte interleukin-1 precursor cDNA. *Proc. Natl. Acad. Sci. U.S.A.*, **81**, 7907–11.

13 Lomedico, P. T., Gubler, R., Hellmann, C. P., Dukovich, M., Giri, J. G., Pan, Y. E., Collier, K., Semionow, R., Chua, A. O., and Mizel, S. B. (1984). Cloning and expression of murine interleukin-1 cDNA in *Escherichia coli*. *Nature* **312**, 458–62.

14 Furutani, Y., Notake, M., Fukui, T., Ohue, M., Nomura, H., Yamada, M., and Nakamura, S. (1986). Complete nucleotide sequence of the gene for human interleukin-1 alpha. *Nucleic Acids Res.*, **14**, 3167–79.

15 Webb, A. C., Collins, K. L., Auron, P. E., Eddy, R. L., Nakai, H., Byers, M. G., Haley, L. L., Henry, W. M., and Shows, T. B. (1986). Interleukin-1 gene (IL-1) assigned to long arm of human chromosome 2. *Lymphokine Res.*, **5**, 77–85.

16 Auron, P. E., Warner, S. J., Webb, A. C., Cannon, J. G., Bernheim, H.-A., McAdam, K. J., Rosenwasser, L. J., LoPreste, G., Mucci, S. F., and Dinarello, C. A. (1987). Studies on the molecular nature of human interleukin-1. *J. Immunol.*, **138**, 1447–56.

17 Beuscher, H. U., Günther, C., and Röllinghoff, M. (1990). IL-1 beta is secreted by activated murine macrophages as biologically inactive precursor. *J. Immunol.*, **144**, 2179–83.

18 Mosley, B., Dower, S. K., Gillis, S., and Cosman, D. (1987). Determination of the minimum polypeptide lengths of the functionally active sites of human interleukins-1α and 1β. *Proc. Natl. Acad. Sci. U.S.A.*, **84**, 4572–6.

19 Clore, G. M., Wingfield, P. T., and Gronenborn, A. M. (1991). High-resolution three-dimensional structure of interleukin-1β in solution by three- and four-dimensional nuclear magnetic resonance spectroscopy. *Biochemistry*, **30**, 2315–23.

20 Giovine, F. S. and Duff, G. W. (1990). Interleukin-1: the first interleukin. *Immunol. Today*, **11**, 13–20.

21 Turner, M., Chantry, D., Buchan, D., Barrett, K., and Feldman, M. (1989). Regulation of expression of human IL-1α and IL-1β genes. *J. Immunol.*, **143**, 3556–62.

22 Macnaul, K. L., Hutchinson, N. I., Parson, J. N., Bayne, E. K., and Tocci, M. J. (1990). Analysis of IL-1 and TNFα gene expression in human rheumatoid synoviocytes and normal monocytes by *in situ* hybridization. *J. Immunol.*, **145**, 4154–66.

23 Cerdan, C., Martin, Y., Brailly, H., Courcoul, M., Flavetta, S., Costello, R., and Olive, D. (1991). IL-1α is produced by T lymphocytes via the CD2 and CD28 pathways. *J. Immunol.*, **146**, 560–4.

24 Hurme, M. and Serkkola, E. (1991). Different activation signals are required for the expression of interleukin-1 α and β genes in human monocytes. *Scand. J. Immunol.*, **33**, 713–18.

25 Hart, P. H., Vitti, G. F., Burgess, D. R., Whitty, G. A., and Piccoli, D. S. (1989). Potential anti-inflammatory effects of interleukin-4: suppression of human monocyte tumour necrosis factor, interleukin-1, and prostaglandin E$_2$. *Proc. Natl. Acad. Sci. U.S.A.*, **86**, 3803–7.

26 Chantry, D., Turner, M., Abney, E., and Feldman, M. (1989). Modulation of cytokine production by transforming growth factor-beta. *J. Immunol.*, **142**, 4295–300.

27 Moore, K. W, Vieira, P., Fiorentino, D. F., Trounstine, M. L., Khan, T. A., and Mosman, T. R. (1990). Homology of cytokine synthesis inhibitor factor (IL-10) to the Epstein–Barr virus gene BCRFI. *Science*, **248**, 1230–4.

28 Schindler, R., Mancilla, J., Endres, S., Ghorbani, R., Clark, S. C., and Dinarello, C. A. (1990). Correlations and interactions in the production of interleukin-6 (IL-6), IL-1, and tumour necrosis factor (TNF) in human mononuclear cells: IL-6 suppresses IL-1 and TNF. *Blood*, **76**, 40–7.

29 Schindler, R. Ghezzi, P., and Dinarello, C. A. (1990). IL-1 induces IL-1. IV. IFNγ suppresses IL-1 but not lipopolysaccharide-induced transcription of IL-1. *J. Immunol.*, **144**, 2216–22.

30 Suttles, J., Giri, J. G., and Mizel, S. B. (1990). IL-1 secretion by macrophages. Enhancement of IL-1 secretion and processing by calcium ionophores. *J. Immunol.*, **144**, 175–82.

31 Singer, I. I., Scott, S., Hall, G., Limjuco, G., Chin, J., and Schmidt, J. A. (1988). Interleukin-1 beta is localized in the cytoplasmic ground substance but is largely absent from the Golgi apparatus and plasma membranes of stimulated human monocytes. *J. Exp. Med.*, **167**, 389–407.

32 Bakouche, O., Brown, D. C., and Lachman, L. B. (1987). Subcellular localization of human monocyte interleukin-1: evidence for an inactive precursor molecule and a possible mechanism for IL-1 release. *J. Immunol.*, **138**, 4249–55.

33 Beesley, J. E., Bomford, R., and Schmidt, J. A. (1990). Ultrastructural localization of IL-1 in human periperal blood monocytes, evidence for IL-1β in mitochondria. *Histochem. J.* **22**, 234–44.

34 Kurt-Jones, E. A., Beller, D. I., Mizel, S. B., and Unanue, E. R. (1985). Identification of a membrane-associated interleukin-1 in macrophages. *Proc. Natl. Acad. Sci. U.S.A.*, **82**, 1204–9.

35 Streck, H., Günther, C., Beuscher, H. U., and Röllinghoff, M. (1988). Studies on the release of cell-associated interleukin-1 by paraformaldehyde-treated murine macrophages. *Eur. J. Immunol.*, **18**, 1609–13.

36 Conlon, P. J., Grabstein, K. H., Alper, A., Prickett, K. S., Hopp, T. P., and Gillis, S. (1987). Localization of human mononuclear cell interleukin-1. *J. Immunol.*, **139**, 98–105.

37 Beuscher, H. U., Fallon, R. J., and Colten, H. R. (1987). Macrophage membrane interleukin-1 regulates the expression of acute phase proteins in human hepatoma Hep 3B cells. *J. Immunol.*, **139**, 1896–901.

38 Beuscher, H. U., Nickells, M. W., and Colten, H. R. (1988). The precursor of interleukin-1 alpha is phosphorylated at residue serine 90. *J. Biol. Chem.*, **263**, 4023–8.

39 Kobayashi, Y., Oppenheim, J. J., and Matsushima, K. (1990). Calcium dependent binding of phosporylated human pre-interleukin-1α to phospholipids. *J. Biochem.*, **107**, 666–70.

40 Brody, D. T. and Durum, S. K. (1989). Membrane IL-1: IL-1α precursor binds to the plasma membrane via lectin-like interaction. *J. Immunol.*, **143**, 1183–8.

41 Kobayashi, Y., Yamamoto, K., Saido, T., Kawasaki, H., Oppenheim, J. J., and Matsushima, K. (1990). Identification of calcium-activated neutral protease as a processing enzyme of human interleukin-1 alpha. *Proc. Natl. Acad. Sci. U.S.A.*, **87**, 5548–52.

42 Hazuda, D. J., Lee, J. C., and Young, P. R. (1988). The kinetics of interleukin-1 secretion from activated monocytes. Differences between interleukin-1 alpha and interleukin-1 beta. *J. Biol. Chem.*, **263**, 8473–79.

43 Black, R. A, Kronheim, S. R., Merriam, J. E., March, C. J., and Hopp, T. P. (1989). A pre-aspartate-specific protease from human leucocytes that cleaves pro-interleukin-1β *J. Biol. Chem.*, **264**, 5323–6.

44*a* Günther, C., Röllinghoff, M., and Beuscher, H. U. (1991). Formation of intrachain disulfide bonds gives rise to two different forms of the murine IL-1β precursor. *J. Immunol.*, **146**, 3025–31.

44*b* Cerreti, D. P., Kozlosky, C. J., Mosley, B., Nelson, N., van Ness, K., Greenstreet, T. A., March, C. J., Kronheim, S. R., Druck, T., Cannizzaro, L. A., Huebner, K., and Black, R. A. (1992). Molecular cloning of the interleukin-1 converting enzyme. *Science*, **256**, 97–100.

45 Sims, J. E., March, C. J., Cosman, D., Widmer, M. B., MacDonald, H. R., McMahan, C. J., Grubin, C. E., Wignall, J. M., Jackson, J. L., Call, S. M., Gillis, S., and Dower, S. R. (1988). cDNA expression cloning of the IL-1 receptor, a member of the immunoglobulin superfamily. *Science*, **241**, 585–9.

46 Bomsztyk, K., Sims, J. E., Stanton, T. H., Slack, F., McMahan, C. J., Valentine, M. A., and Dower, S. K. (1989). Evidence for different interleukin-1 receptors in murine B and T cell lines. *Proc. Natl. Acad. Sci. U.S.A.*, **86**, 8034–8.

47 Dower, S. K., McMahan, C., Flack, J., Grubin, C., Lupton, S., Moseley, B., and Sims, G. E. (1990). Molecular characterization of two types of interleukin-1 receptor coding peptides on murine and human cells. *J. Leukoc. Biol.*, **1**, 103–7 (suppl.).

48 Boraschi, D., Villa, L., Volpini, G., Boss'u, P., Censini, S., Ghlara, P., Scapigliat, G., Nencioni, L., Bartalini, M., and Matteucci, G. (1990). Differential activity of interleukin-1 alpha and interleukin-1 beta in the stimulation of the immune response *in vivo*. *Eur. J. Immunol.*, **20**, 317–21.

49   Mizel, S. B. (1990). Cyclic AMP and interleukin-1 signal transduction. *Immunol. Today*, **11**, 390–1.

50   Dinarello, C. A., Cannon, J. G., and Wolff, S. M. (1988). New concepts on the pathogenesis of fever. *Rev. Infect. Dis.* **10**, 168–89.

51   Oppenheim, J. J., Matsushima, K., Yoshimura, T., Leonard, E. J., and Neta, R. (1989). Relationship between interleukin-1 (IL-1), tumour necrosis factor (TNF), and a neutrophil attracting peptide (NAP-1). *Agents Actions*, **16**, 134–40.

52   Bevilacqua, M. P., Prober, M. S., Wheeler, M. E., Cotran, R. S., and Gibrone, M. A. (1985). Interleukin-1 acts on cultured human vascular endothelium to increase the adhesion of polymorphouclear leucocytes, monocytes, and related leucocyte cell lines. *J. Clin. Invest.*, **76**, 2003–11.

53   Zhan, Y. F., Stanley, E. R., and Cheer, C. (1991). Prophylaxis of treatment of experimental Brucellosis with interleukin-1. *Infect. Immun.*, **59**, 1790–4.

54   Curfs, J. H. A., van der Meer, J. W. M., Sauerwein, R. W., and Eling, W. M. C. (1990). Low dosages of interleukin-1 protect mice against lethal cerebral malaria. *J. Exp. Med.*, **172**, 1287–91.

55   Tracey, K. J., Fong, Y., Hesse, D. G., Manogue, K. R., Lee, A. T., Kuo, G. C., Lowry, S. F., and Cerami, A. (1987). Anti-cachectin/TNF monoclonal antibodies prevent septic shock during lethal bacteraemia. *Nature*, **330**, 662–4.

56   Holtmann, H. and Wallach, D. (1987). Down-regulation of the receptors for tumour necrosis factor by interleukin-1 and 4-beta-12-myristata-13-acetate. *J. Immunol.*, **139**, 1161–7.

57   Durum, S. K., Schmidt, J. A., and Oppenheim, J. J. (1985). Interleukin-1: an immunological perspective. *Annu. Rev. Immunol.*, **3**, 263–87.

58   Cornelis, G., Laroche, Y., Balligand, G., and Sory, M. P. (1987). *Yersinia enterocolitica*, a primary model for bacterial invasiveness. *Rev. Infect. Dis.*, **9**, 64–87.

59   Fong, Y., Tracey, K. J., Moldamer, L. L., Hesse, D. G., Manogue, K. B, Kennedy, J. S., Lee, A. T., Kuo, G. C., Allison, A. C., Lowry, A. C., and Cerami, A. (1989). Antibodies to cachectin/tumour necrosis factor reduce interleukin-1β and interleukin-6 appearance during lethal bacteraemia. *J. Exp. Med.*, **170**, 1627–33.

60   Dinarello, C. A. (1989). Strategies for anti-interleukin-1 therapies. *Int. J. Immun. Pharm.*, **2**, 203–11.

61   Gershenwald, J. E., Fong, Y., Fahey, T. J., Calvano, S. E., Chizzonite, R., Kilian, P. L., Lowry, S. F., and Moldawer, L. L. (1990). Interleukin-1 receptor blockade attenuates the host inflammatory response. *Proc. Natl. Acad. Sci. U.S.A.*, **87**, 4966–70.

62   Jacobs, C. A., Baker, P. E., Roux, E. R., Picha, K. S., Toivola, B., Waugh, S., and Kennedy, M. K. (1991). Experimental auto-immune encephalomyelitis is exacerbated by IL-1α and suppressed by soluble IL-1 receptor. *J. Immunol.*, **146**, 2983–9.

63   James, K. (1990). Interactions between cytokines and α_2 macroglobulin. *Immunol. Today*, **11**, 163–6.

64   Eisenberg, S. P., Evans, R. J., Arend, W. P., Verderber, E., Brewer, M. T., Hannum, C. H., and Thompson, R. C. (1990). Primary structure and functional expression from complementary DNA of a human interleukin-1 receptor antagonist. *Nature*, **343**, 341–6.

65   Zahedi, K., Seldin, M. F., Rits, M., Ezekowitz, R. A., and Whitehead, A. S. (1991). Mouse IL-1 receptor antagonist protein: molecular characterization, gene mapping, and expression of mRNA *in vitro* and *in vivo*. *J. Immunol.*, **146**, 4228–33.

66 Eisenberg, S. P., Brewer, M. T., Verderber, E., Heimdal, P., Brandhuber, B. J., and Thompson, R. C. (1991). Interleukin-1 receptor antagonist is a member of the interleukin-1 gene family: evolution of a cytokine control mechanism. *Proc. Natl. Acad. Sci. U.S.A.*, **88**, 5232–6.

67 Ohlsson, K., Bjork, P., Bregenfeldt, M., Hagemann, R., and Thompson, R. C. (1990). IL-1 receptor antagonist reduces mortality from endotoxin shock. *Nature*, **248**, 550–2.

68 Wakabayashi, G., Gelfand, J. A., Burke, F. F., Thompson, R. C., and Dinarello, C. A. (1991). A specific receptor antagonist for interleukin-1 prevents *Escherichia coli* induced shock in rabbits. *FASEB J.*, **5**, 338–43.

69 Arend, W. P, Welgus, H. G., Thompson, R. C., and Eisenberg, S. P. (1990). Biological properties of recombinant human monocyte-derived interleukin-1 receptor antagonist. *J. Clin. Invest.*, **85**, 1694–7.

3   Interleukin-6

P. C. HEINRICH AND S. ROSE-JOHN

1   Introduction

Interleukin-6 (IL-6) is a multi-functional cytokine showing different actions on many different cells (Figure 3.1). IL-6 has been reported to be involved in (i) the induction of immunoglobulin production in activated B cells (1, 2), (ii) the induction of proliferation of hybridoma/plasmacytoma/myeloma cells (3–6), (iii) in the induction of IL-2 production, cell growth, and cytotoxic T cell differentiation of T cells (7–9), (iv) the stimulation of multipotent colony formation in haematopoietic stem cells (10), (v) the regulation of acute phase proteins (11, 12), (vi) growth inhibition and induction of differentiation into macrophages of myeloid leukaemic cell lines (13), and (vii) the induction of neural differentiation (14).

IL-6 has previously been named (see Table 3.1) according to its different functions. Following the molecular cloning of the cDNAs encoding the 26 kDa protein (15), interferon β_2 (16), B cell stimulatory factor-2 (2), and hepatocyte

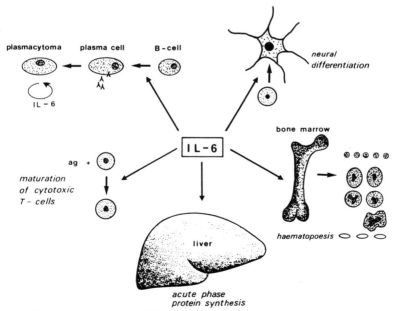

Fig. 3.1   Pleiotropic actions of IL-6.

Table 3.1   Interleukin-6 synonyms

Name	Abbreviation
Hepatocyte stimulating factor	HSF
B cell stimulatory factor-2	BSF-2
Interferon β_2	IFNβ_2
26 kDa protein	
Hybridoma–plasmacytoma growth factor	HPGF
Myeloid blood cell differentiation-inducing protein	MGI-2A

stimulating factor (11, 12), it was realized that all these molecules were identical (17) and it was agreed to name the molecule interleukin-6.

Many excellent reviews on IL-6 have appeared in the literature (18–24) and IL-6 is also discussed in Chapters 1, 2, and 4. In this chapter, we concentrate on structural aspects of IL-6 and its cell surface receptor in relation to function. IL-6 is clearly involved in induction of acute phase proteins and as such is an important control molecule in natural immunity. The involvement of IL-6 in clinical problems has been reviewed (25).

2   Biosynthesis of IL-6

2.1   Primary structure of IL-6

Although most mammalian cells are able to synthesize IL-6 (Table 3.2) after appropriate stimulation, the major IL-6 producing cells are monocytes/macrophages, fibroblasts, and endothelial cells. IL-6 is synthesized as a precursor with an amino-terminal extension of 28 amino acids (Figure 3.2).

Table 3.2   IL-6 producing cells

Cells	Major stimulator
Monocytes/macrophages	LPS
Fibroblasts	IL-1
Endothelial cells	IL-1
Chondrocytes	IL-1
Endometrial stromal cells	IL-1
Smooth muscle cells	IL-1
Astrocytes	IL-1

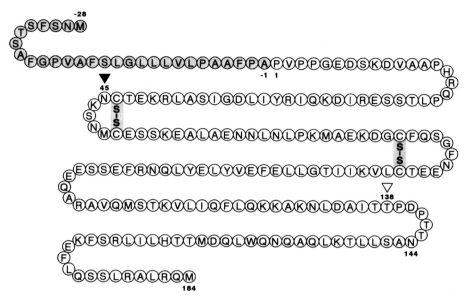

Fig. 3.2 Primary structure of human IL-6. Threonine 138 and asparagine 45 are glycosylated.

The mature protein consists of 184 amino acids and contains two sequential disulfide-bridges (26). IL-6 secreted by mammalian cells is N- and O-glycosylated (27–29) and it has been reported that IL-6 derived from fibroblasts and monocytes is phosphorylated at several serine residues (30).

2.2   Structure of the IL-6 gene

The gene for human IL-6 has been localized on chromosome 7 p21 (31, 32) and consists of five exons and four introns (33). The gene organization of IL-6 shows a distinct similarity with the G-CSF gene (33). Several *cis* acting elements have been characterized in the 5′ region of the gene and an IL-1-dependent nuclear factor has recently been cloned (34) (see also Chapters 1 and 4). Interestingly, this factor also seems to be involved in the regulation of several acute phase proteins in liver (34).

2.3   Regulation of expression of the IL-6 gene

Table 3.2 shows a list of the major IL-6 producing cells. In monocytes/ macrophages, IL-6 synthesis is mainly stimulated by lipopolysaccharide, whereas in most other cells control is by IL-1. A more extensive summary of IL-6 producing cells and their inhibitors can be found in reference 21.

2.4   Post-translational modification of IL-6

After removal of the signal peptide of 28 amino acids by the signal peptidase in the endoplasmic reticulum, IL-6 is N- and O-glycosylated along the secretory pathway. We have recently produced glycosylated IL-6 by expression of human IL-6 cDNA in mammalian cells (29). Analysis of the secreted IL-6 showed that less than 5 per cent of IL-6 is both N- and O-glycosylated, 60 per cent is O-glycosylated, and 35 per cent is non-glycosylated. The O-glycosylation site of IL-6 has been localized after desialylation and re-sialylation with an O-glycan-specific sialyltransferase in the presence of radioactively labelled CMP-sialic acid, cleavage by trypsin, and identification of the labelled tryptic peptides. We found that human IL-6 is O-glycosylated only at one site, threonine 138 (35). By an analogous approach we identified asparagine 45 as the N-glycosylation site of IL-6 (35). The structure of the O-linked oligosaccharide side chain is Gal-β1–3GalNAc carrying one or two sialic acid residues (35). Comparison of the biological activities of non-glycosylated and glycosylated IL-6 measured by induction of γ-fibrinogen in HepG2 cells, as well as in an IL-6-specific proliferation assay (B9 cells) showed glycosylated IL-6 to be three to four times more active than the non-glycosylated cytokine.

3   Structure of IL-6

No experimental data on the tertiary structure of human IL-6 are presently available. From the amino acid sequence of human IL-6, a secondary structure of the molecule has been predicted (36, 37): 58 per cent α-helix, 14 per cent β-structure, and 28 per cent turn and coil. The C-terminus of human IL-6 exhibits an α-helical structure (see below). A content of 67 per cent α-helix was determined from the circular dichroism spectrum of recombinant human IL-6 (36), verifying the high content of alpha helix predicted from the protein sequence.

Once the primary structure of human IL-6 had been deduced from the cDNA sequence, it has been possible to investigate which parts of the IL-6 molecule are indispensable for its biological function. Brakenhoff *et al.* (38) showed that 28 amino acids can be removed from the N-terminus without affecting the biological activity of IL-6. Removal of amino acids 29 and 30 resulted in an approximately 50-fold decrease of activity, whereas the deletion of amino acids 31 to 34 completely abolished the activity. The authors concluded from their study that the amino acids starting from 29 are important for the function of IL-6.

Experiments from our laboratory have shown that in contrast to the N-terminus the amino acids at the C-terminus of IL-6 are of particular importance for its biological function. Stepwise truncation of the C-terminal amino acids of human IL-6 resulted in a stepwise loss of biological activity

(Figure 3.3). Removal of methionine 184 led to an 80 per cent decrease of biological activity. No change was detected after deletion of glutamine 183, whereas biological activity was completely abrogated when methionine 184, glutamine 183, and arginine 182 were removed from the C-terminus of IL-6 (36, 39).

When point mutations were introduced into the full-length IL-6 molecule, evidence was obtained for the importance of a positive charge (Arg 182) and an α-helical structure in the C-terminus for biological activity of human IL-6 (40).

A first contribution to understanding the topography of IL-6 was achieved with a series of neutralizing monoclonal antibodies (37). Brakenhoff *et al.* (37) could show that a group of monoclonal antibodies did not recognize IL-6 when 21 amino acids from the N-terminus or 4–5 amino acids from the C-terminus were deleted. The authors concluded that the epitope recognized by these monoclonal antibodies consisted of parts of the N- and of the C-terminus of IL-6, indicating a juxtaposition of N- and C-termini in the correctly folded IL-6 molecule. These monoclonal antibodies also neutralized the biological activity of IL-6 indicating that the N- and C-termini are involved in the active site of the molecule. These antibody results are consistent with the data on deletion mutants. Interestingly, a C-terminal extension by 4–5 amino acids (41) or an N-terminal addition of several hundred amino acids (S. Rose-John, unpublished work) does not affect the biological activity of IL-6.

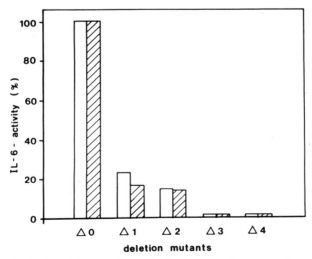

Fig. 3.3 Biological activity of C-terminal IL-6 deletion mutants. The biological activities of IL-6 mutants lacking 1(Δ1), 2(Δ2), 3(Δ3), and 4(Δ4) amino acids from the C-terminus were compared with full-length IL-6 (Δ0). *Open bars* show IL-6 induced-proliferation of B9 cells; *hatched bars* show induction of γ-fibrinogen synthesis by HepG2 cells.

It has been proposed that there is a family of alpha helical cytokines comprising growth hormone, prolactin, myelomonocytic growth factor, erythropoietin, granulocyte colony-stimulating factor, and IL-6 (42). Although there is no detectable homology in the amino acid sequence of the members of this family, secondary structure elements seem to appear at comparable positions within these molecules. Furthermore, similar gene organizations are found for the different members of this cytokine family. Since the crystal structure of growth hormone has been determined and shows a characteristic bundle of four anti-parallel α-helices (43), and since prolactin is a homologue of growth hormone, it is proposed, by analogy, that prolactin is similarly folded. Circular dichroism spectra suggested that erythropoietin, granulocyte colony-stimulating factor, and IL-6 are characterized by a high α-helical content comparable to that seen in the crystal structure of growth hormone. A model for the different members of the helical cytokine family (42) is shown in Figure 3.4. It should be noted that in the proposed model the N- and C-termini are in close proximity. This is in agreement with the experimental observations on the roles of N- and C-termini in determining the biological activity of IL-6 discussed above.

4   Plasma clearance, carrier proteins, and target cells for IL-6

When radiolabelled human IL-6 was intravenously injected into rats, a biphasic disappearance from the circulation was observed. A rapid initial

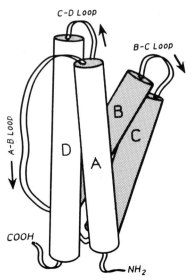

Fig. 3.4 Proposed model for the secondary and tertiary structure of cytokines of the helical cytokine family (taken from (42)).

elimination corresponding to a half-life of about three minutes and a second slower decrease from the circulation corresponding to a half-life of about 55 minutes has been estimated (44). Twenty minutes after intravenous injection, about 80 per cent of [^{125}I]IL-6 had disappeared from the circulation and was found in the liver. Autoradiography showed that [^{125}I]IL-6 was exclusively localized on the surface of parenchymal cells suggesting the existence of IL-6 receptors on hepatocytes. One hour after injection, [^{125}gI]IL-6 disappeared from the liver and accumulated in skin reaching 35 per cent of injected material after 5–8 hours (45) or was degraded in the bile (46).

In blood, IL-6 probably associates with a plasma protein resulting in a complex with β-γ-mobility (44). The binding protein has so far not been identified although α_2-macroglobulin has been reported as a carrier for IL-6 (47) but since an extremely small amount of IL-6 bound to human α_2-macroglobulin, it is very unlikely that α_2-macroglobulin is a major binding protein for IL-6 in plasma. A soluble IL-6 receptor has recently been isolated and characterized from urine of normal individuals (48). It is likely that the IL-6 plasma protein complex with β-γ-mobility (44) consists of IL-6 and this soluble IL-6 receptor.

5 The IL-6 receptor

5.1 The 80 kDa subunit

IL-6 confers its signal to target cells by binding to IL-6-specific cell surface receptors. A cDNA coding for an IL-6 receptor molecule has been cloned from the human natural killer-like cell line YT (49). The IL-6 receptor cDNA encodes a protein consisting of 468 amino acids including a signal peptide of 19 amino acids. The 90 amino acid long N-terminal part of the extracellular domain shows homology to the immunoglobulin superfamily. The cytoplasmic part of 82 amino acids lacks a tyrosine kinase domain unlike other growth factor receptors (Figure 3.5).

In view of the fact that the biological responses of various target cells of IL-6 differ, the question has been asked, whether different IL-6 receptors are expressed on various cells and tissues. Cloning of cDNA for the IL-6 receptor from human (50) and rat (51) liver revealed that liver cells and leucocytes express the same type of IL-6 receptor. Little is known about the regulation of the IL-6 receptor 80 kDa subunit. In the case of the hepatic IL-6 receptor, it has been shown that dexamethasone up-regulates mRNA as well as the functional surface receptor (52–54). Recent experiments have shown that the phorbol ester PMA also stimulates expression of the 80 kDa IL-6 receptor subunit in liver cells indicating a role of protein kinase C in regulation of IL-6 receptor expression (54*a*).

Various soluble IL-6 receptors have been produced by genetic engineering (55, 56, 56*a*). Surprisingly, soluble IL-6 receptor together with its ligand IL-6

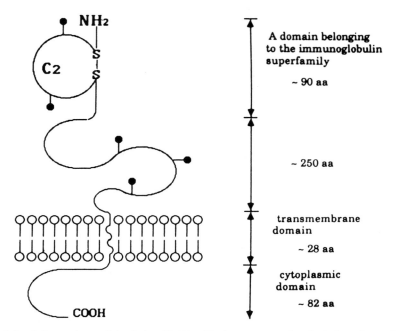

Fig. 3.5   Schematic model of the 80 kDa IL-6 receptor subunit (taken from (23)).

was able to produce an IL-6-specific signal on target cells indicating an agonistic action of the soluble receptor–ligand complex (Figure 3.6). This observation was completely unexpected since all known soluble cytokine receptors act as antagonists by competing with the membrane-bound receptors.

5.2   The 130 kDa subunit of the IL-6 receptor

Deletion of the cytoplasmic and transmembrane domains of the 80 kDa subunit of the IL-6 receptor showed that neither was required for IL-6 signalling (55). This finding led to the discovery of the second subunit needed for the signal transduction of IL-6, a protein of molecular weight 130 kDa (gp130). Taga and colleagues (55) clearly demonstrated an IL-6-triggered aggregation of the two subunits of the IL-6 receptor. The cDNA coding for gp130 has been cloned (56) and predicts a signal peptide of 22 amino acids, an extracellular region of 597 amino acids, a membrane spanning region of 22 amino acids, and a cytoplasmic domain of 277 amino acids. The extracellular domain of gp130 contains six fibronectin type III modules although the physiological significance of this is unclear. It should be noted that expression studies of gp130 revealed that gp130 mRNA is not only present in IL-6 responsive cells, but in all cells tested so far (56).

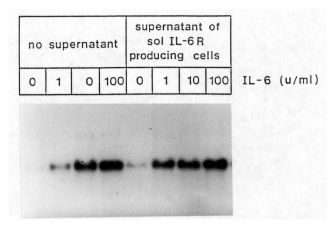

no supernatant				supernatant of sol IL-6 R producing cells				IL-6 (u/ml)
0	1	0	100	0	1	10	100	

Fig. 3.6 Induction by a soluble IL-6 receptor/IL-6 complex. HepG2 cells were treated with human IL-6 at increasing concentrations for 18 hours in the absence or presence of a soluble form of the 80 kDa human IL-6 receptor. As a measure of IL-6 responsiveness, production of α_1-antichymotrypsin mRNA was estimated by Northern blotting analysis. In the presence of soluble IL-6 receptor HepG2 cells become more sensitive to low concentrations of IL-6.

The number of IL-6 receptors found on different cells is generally low (between several hundreds and several thousands per cell). Two types of binding sites with dissociation constants of 10 to 30 pM, and 700 pM for high and low affinity binding, respectively, have been identified (49). It has been shown that a monoclonal antibody to gp130 completely blocked high affinity binding of IL-6 (56) suggesting that the 130 kDa subunit of the IL-6 receptor is involved in the formation of high affinity ligand binding sites. When gp130 was transfected into cells with very low levels of gp130, high affinity binding sites for IL-6 could be created (56). On the other hand, transfection of HepG2 cells with a cDNA coding for the 80 kDa subunit of the IL-6 receptor resulted in the induction of low affinity binding sites (Figure 3.7). This experiment clearly indicates that the 80 kDa IL-6 receptor subunit is responsible for the formation of low affinity IL-6 binding sites. Figure 3.8 schematically shows the interaction of the 80 kDa and 130 kDa IL-6 receptor subunits forming a high affinity binding site for the ligand IL-6.

6   Signal transduction

It has been shown that cAMP, cGMP, PKC, inositol phosphates, and changes in intracellular calcium concentrations are not likely to be involved in the transduction of the IL-6 signal in liver (21). In hepatoma cells we have measured that IL-6 after binding is internalized and degraded (Figure 3.9).

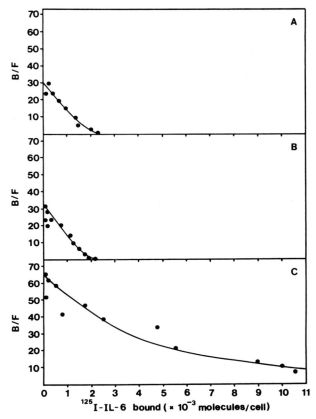

Fig. 3.7 Involvement of the 80 kDa IL-6 receptor subunit in the formation of low affinity IL-6 binding sites. HepG2 cells were transfected with cDNA for the 80 kDa subunit of the human IL-6 receptor under the transcriptional control of a mouse metallothionein promotor (50, 53). In the transfected cells IL-6 receptor expression can be up-regulated by $ZnCl_2$. Normal HepG2 cells (A), transfected HepG2 cells (B), and transfected HepG2 cells treated with $ZnCl_2$ (C) were incubated with $[^{125}I]IL$-6 at different concentrations at 4°C. Specific binding was measured and data were transformed using a Scatchard analysis (57).

It is clear from the figure that all bound IL-6 molecules are internalized. It remains to be elucidated, whether IL-6 internalization and signal transduction are functionally linked. Internalization after binding has been described for various cytokines (58, 59) but no connection to the biological response has yet been demonstrated. It has been demonstrated that the effect of TNF on fibroblasts (see Chapter 4) acts via IL-6 and that this effect is likely to involve cAMP.

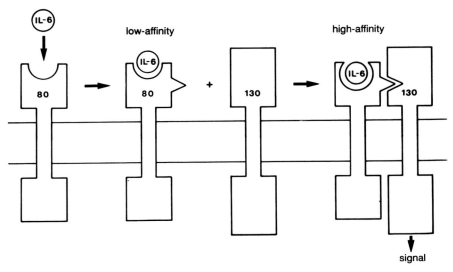

Fig. 3.8 3.8 IL-6-induced aggregation of the two IL-6 receptor subunits.

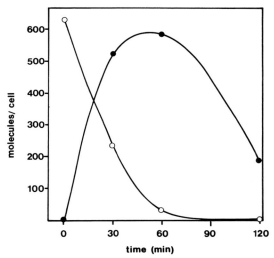

Fig. 3.9 Internalization of [^{125}I]IL-6 by human hepatoma cells. HepG2 cells were pre-loaded with [^{125}I]IL-6 at 4 °C. After a temperature shift to 37 °C surface-bound IL-6 (o) or internalized IL-6 (•) was measured.

7 A superfamily of cytokine receptors

Molecular cloning of the cDNAs coding for the receptors of IL-2 (75 kDa subunit), IL-3, IL-4, IL-5, IL-6 (80 and 130 kDa subunits), IL-7, growth hormone, prolactin, erythropoietin, granulocyte colony-stimulating factor, GM-CSF (both subunits), leukaemia inhibitory factor, and the comparison of the respective amino acid sequences led to the recognition of an absolute conservation of four cysteine residues and a Trp-Ser-X-Trp-Ser (WSXWS) motif. However, the overall sequence homology between the cytokine receptors mentioned is only about 20 per cent (60). In addition, Bazan proposes that seven consensus β-strands form an anti-parallel β-sandwich with a topology analogous to an immunoglobulin constant domain. The receptors listed above form a new family of cytokine receptors also designated as haematopoietic or haemopoietic receptor superfamily (Figure 3.10). The structural features of the members of this new cytokine receptor superfamily distinguish them from other receptor families such as the growth factor receptor tyrosine kinases (61), the immunoglobulin superfamily (62), the receptors related to the β-adrenergic receptors (63), and a newly emerging group that includes nerve growth factor receptor and tumour necrosis factor receptor (64).

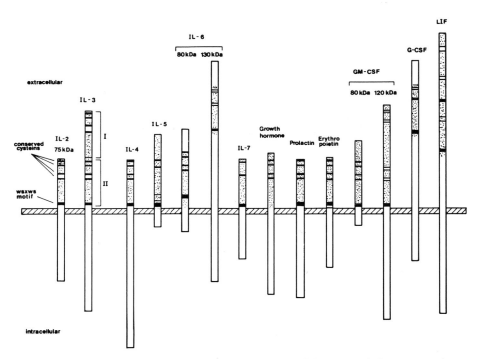

Fig. 3.10   Schematic representation of the structures of the presently known members of the cytokine receptor superfamily. *Horizontal bars* represent conserved cysteine residues. The *black boxes* represent the conserved Trp-Ser-X-Trp-Ser (WSXWS) motif. The *stippled areas* define the stretch of homology between the different receptors of the superfamily. G-CSF, granulocyte colony-stimulating factor; GM-CSF, granulocyte macrophage colony-stimulating factor; LIF, leukaemia inhibitory factor.

8　IL-6 is a growth and differentiation factor

Presently, the multiple actions of IL-6 can be divided into two main categories. The cytokine IL-6 can be involved in cell growth regulation and differentiation processes. In both instances, the regulation can be stimulatory or inhibitory. A pleiotropic spectrum of action is a common feature of many cytokines. Since *in vivo* cytokines are simultaneously released their combined action which might be synergistic or antagonistic has to be considered within the frame of a complex network. In spite of the many biological responses exerted by IL-6, it acts via one single type of surface-bound receptor. Therefore, the type of biological response is determined within the cell. Eventually, activation and/or inactivation of a set of transcription factors leads to the expression of the genes required for the respective biological response.

9　Summary

IL-6 is a multi-functional cytokine synthesized by and acting on many different cells. Its actions can be divided into two classes. The cytokine is involved in the regulation of proliferation and differentiation. In defence against infection and injury, the differentiation of liver cells to switch on synthesis of acute phase proteins is under control of IL-6. *In vitro* studies have shown that proliferative and differentiation activities of IL-6 reside in the same region of the IL-6 molecule. IL-6 is a single polypeptide chain of 184 amino acids. It is N- and O-glycosylated at asparagine 45 and threonine 138, respectively. Deletion analysis revealed that C- and N-terminus of IL-6 are important for its biological function. IL-6 exerts its action via a cell surface receptor. The IL-6 receptor consists of two subunits of molecular masses 80 and 130 kDa. The IL-6 receptor has been recognized as a member of a new cytokine receptor family, the haematopoietic receptor superfamily and one member of this receptor family (growth hormone receptor) has recently been crystallized as a dimer with a single molecule of ligand (65). It may be that cross-linking of receptors by ligand is an important aspect of the stimulatory response in this receptor family.

Acknowledgements

The authors thank M. Robbertz and Dr P. Freyer for their help with the artwork. The experimental work referred to in this review has been supported by the Deutsche Forschungsgemeinschaft, the Fonds der Chemischen Industrie and the Stiftung Volkswagenwerk.

References

1 Hirano, T., Taga, T., Nakano, N., Yasukawa, K., Kashiwamura, S., Shimizu, K., Nakajima, K., Pyun, K. H., and Kishimoto, T. (1985). Purification to homogeneity and characterization of human B cell differentiation factor (BCDF or BSFp-2). *Proc. Natl. Acad. Sci. U.S.A.*, **82**, 5490–4.
2 Hirano, T., Yasukawa, K., Harada, H., Taga, T., Watanabe, Y., Matsuda, T., Kashiwamura, S., Nakajima, K., Koyama, K., Iwamatu, A., Tsunasawa, S., Sakiyama, F., Matsui, H., Takahara, Y., Taniguchi, T., and Kishimoto, T. (1986). Complementary DNA for a novel human interleukin (BSF-2) that induces B lymphocytes to produce immunoglobulin. *Nature*, **324**, 73–6.
3 Van Snick, J., Cayphas, S., Vink, A., Uyttenhove, C., Coulie, P. G., Rubira, M. R., and Simpson, R. J. (1986). Purification and NH_2 terminal amino acid sequence of a T cell-derived lymphokine with growth factor activity for B cell hybridomas. *Proc. Natl. Acad. Sci. U.S.A.*, **83**, 9679–83.
4 Van Snick, J., Vink, A., Cayphas, S., and Uyttenhove, C. (1987). Interleukin-HP1, a T cell-derived hybridoma growth factor that supports the *in vitro* growth of murine plasmacytomas. *J. Exp. Med.*, **165**, 641–9.
5 Nordan, R. P. and Potter, M. (1986). A macrophage-derived factor required by plasmacytomas for survival and proliferation *in vitro*. *Science*, **233**, 566–9.
6 Kawanao, M., Hirano, T., Matsuda, T., Taga, T., Horii, Y., Iwato, K., Asaoku, H., Tang, B., Tanabe, O., Tanaka, H., Kuramoto, A., and Kishimoto, T. (1988). Autocrine generation and requirement of BSF-2/IL-6 for human multiple myelomas. *Nature*, **332**, 83–5.
7 Garman, R. D., Jacobs, K. A., Clark, S. C., and Raulet, D. H. (1987). B cell-stimulatory factor 2 (β_2-interferon) functions as a second signal for interleukin-2 production by mature murine T cells. *Proc. Natl. Acad. Sci. U.S.A.*, **84**, 7629–33.
8 Lotz, M., Jirik, F., Kabouridis, R., Tsoukas, C., Hirano, T., Kishimoto, T., and Carson, D. A. (1988). BSF-2/IL-6 is a co-stimulant for human thymocytes and T lymphocytes. *J. Exp. Med.*, **167**, 1253–8.
9 Okada, M., Kitahara, M., Kishimoto, S., Matsuda, T., Hirano, T., and Kishimoto, T. (1988). BSF-2/IL-6 functions as killer helper factor in the *in vitro* induction of cytotoxic T cells. *J. Immunol.*, **141**, 1543–9.
10 Ikebuchi, K., Wong, G. C., Clark, S. C., Ihle, J. N., Hirai, Y., and Ogawa, M. (1987). Interleukin-6 enhancement of interleukin-3-dependent proliferation of multipotential haemopoietic progenitors. *Proc. Natl. Acad. Sci. U.S.A.*, **84**, 9035–9.
11 Andus, T., Geiger, T., Hirano, T., Northoff, H., Ganter, U., Bauer, J., Kishimoto, T., and Heinrich, P. C. (1987). Recombinant human B cell stimulatory factor 2 (BSF-2/IFNβ_2) regulates β-fibrinogen and albumin mRNA levels in Fao-9 cells. *FEBS Lett.*, **221**, 18–22.
12 Gauldie, J., Richards, C., Harnish, D., Landsdorp, P., and Baumann, H. (1987). Interferon β_2/B cell stimulatory factor type 2 shares identity with monocyte-derived hepatocyte-stimulating factor and regulates the major acute phase protein response in liver cells. *Proc. Natl. Acad. Sci. U.S.A.*, **84**, 7251–5.
13 Miyaura, C., Onozaki, K., Akiyama, Y., Taniyama, T., Hirano, T., Kishimoto, T., and Suda, T. (1988). Recombinant human interleukin-6 (B cell stimulatory factor 2) is a potent inducer of differentiation of mouse myeloid leukaemia cells (M1) *FEBS Lett.*, **234**, 17–21.
14 Satoh, T., Nakamura, S., Taga, T., Matsuda, T., Hirano, T., Kishimoto, T., and Kaziro, Y. (1988). Induction of neural differentiation in PC12 cells by B cell stimulatory factor 2/interleukin-6. *Mol. Cell. Biol.*, **8**, 3546–9.

15 Haegeman, G., Content, J., Volckaert, G., Derynck, R., Tavernier, J., and Fiers, W. (1986). Structural analysis of the sequence coding for an inducible 26 kDa protein in human fibroblasts. *Eur. J. Biochem.*, **159**, 625–32.

16 Zilberstein, A., Ruggieri, R., Korn, J. H., and Revel, M. (1986). Structure and expression of cDNA and genes for human interferon-beta-2, a distinct species inducible by growth-stimulatory cytokines. *EMBO J.*, **5**, 2529–37.

17 Billiau, A. (1986). BSF-2 is not just a differentiation factor. *Nature*, **324**, 415.

18 Kishimoto, T. and Hirano, T. (1988). Molecular regulation of B lymphocyte response. *Ann. Rev. Immunol.*, **6**, 485–512.

19 Kishimoto, T. (1989). The biology of interleukin-6. *Blood*, **74**, 1–10.

20 Sehgal, P. B., Grieninger, G., and Tosata, G. (1989). Interleukin-6. *Ann. N. Y. Acad. Sci.*, **557**, 1–583, New York Academy of Sciences, New York.

21 Heinrich, P. C., Castell, J. V., and Andus, T. (1990). Interleukin-6 and the acute phase response. *Biochem. J.*, **265**, 621–36.

22 Van Snick, J. (1990). Interleukin-6: an overview. *Ann. Rev. Immunol.*, **8**, 253–79.

23 Hirano, T. and Kishimoto, T. (1990). Interleukin-6. In *Handbook of experimental pharmacology*, 95/1, Peptide growth factors and their receptors I, (ed. M. B. Sporn and A. B. Roberts), pp. 633–65. Springer-Verlag, Berlin.

24 Sehgal, P. B. (1990). Interleukin-6: a regulator of plasma protein gene expression in hepatic and non-hepatic tissues. *Mol. Biol. Med.*, **7**, 147–59.

25 Hirano, T. and Kishimoto, T. (1989). Interleukin-6: possible implications in human diseases. *Res. Clin. Lab.*, **19**, 1–10.

26 Clogston, C. L., Boonie, T. C., Crandall, B. C., Mendiaz, E. A., and Lu, H. S. (1989). Disulfide structures of human interleukin-6 are similar to those of human granulocyte colony-stimulating factor. *Arch. Biochem. Biophys.*, **272**, 144–51.

27 May, L. T., Ghrayeb, J., Santhanam, U., Tatter, S. B., Stoeger, Z., Helfgott, D. C., Chiorazzi, N., Grieninger, G., and Sehgal, P. B. (1988). Synthesis and secretion of multiple forms of β_2-interferon/B cell differentiation factor 2/hepatocyte stimulation factor by human fibroblasts and monocytes. *J. Biol. Chem.*, **263**, 7760–6.

28 Gross, V., Andus, T., Castell, J., Vom Berg, D., Heinrich, P. C., and Gerok, W. (1989). O- and N-glycosylation lead to different molecular weight forms of human monocyte interleukin-6. *FEBS Lett.*, **247**, 323–6.

29 Schiel, X., Rose-John, S., Dufhues, G., Schooltink, H., and Heinrich, P. C. (1990). Microheterogeneity of human interleukin-6 synthesized by transfected NIH/3T3 cells: comparison with human monocytes, fibroblasts, and endothelial cells. *Eur. J. Immunol.*, **20**, 883–7.

30 May, L. T., Santhanam, U., Tatter, S. B., Bhardwaj, N., Ghrayeb, J., and Sehgal, P. B. (1988). Phosphorylation of secreted forms of human β_2-interferon/hepatocyte stimulating factor/interleukin-6. *Eur. J. Immunol.*, **18**, 193–7.

31 Sehgal, P. B., Zilberstein, A., Ruggieri, R.-M., May, L. T., Ferguson-Smith, A., Slate, D. L., and Revel, M., and Ruddle, F. (1986). Human chromosome 7 carries the β_2-interferon gene. *Proc. Natl. Acad. Sci. U.S.A.*, **83**, 5219–22.

32 Bowcock, A. M., Kidd, J. R., Lathrop, M., Danshvar, L., May, L. T., Ray, A., Sehgal, P. B., Kidd, K. K., and Cavallisforza, L. L. (1988). The human 'beta-2 interferon/hepatocyte stimulating factor/interleukin-6' gene: DNA polymorphism studies and localization to chromosome 7p21. *Genomics*, **3**, 8–16.

33 Yasukawa, K., Hirano, T., Watanabe, Y., Muratani, K., Matsuda, T., Nakai, S., and Kishimoto, T. (1987). Structure and expression of human B cell stimulatory factor 2 (BSF-2/IL-6) gene. *EMBO J.*, **6**, 2939–45.

34 Akira, S., Isshiki, H., Sugita, T., Tanabe, O., Kinoshita, S., Nishio, Y., Nakajima, T., Hirano, T., and Kishimoto, T. (1990). A nuclear factor for IL-6 expression (NF-IL6) is a member of a C/EBP family. *EMBO J.*, **9**, 1897–906.

35   Heinrich, P. C., Dufhues, G., Flohe, S., Horn, F., Krause, E., Krüttgen, A., Legres, L, Lenz, D., Lütticken, C., Schooltink, H., Stoyan, T., Conradt, H. S., and Rose-John, S. (1991). Interleukin-6, its hepatic receptor and the acute phase response of the liver. In *42nd Mosbacher Colloquium on "Molecular Aspects of Inflammation"* (ed. H. Sies, L. Flohé, and G. Zimmer) pp. 129–45. Springer-Verlag, Berlin.

36   Krüttgen, A., Rose-John, S., Möller, C., Wroblowski, B., Wollmer, A., Müllberg, J., Hirano, T., Kishimoto, T., and Heinrich, P. C. (1990). Structure-function analysis of human interleukin-6. Evidence for the involvement of the carboxy-terminus in function. *FEBS Lett.*, **262**, 323–6.

37   Brakenhoff, J. P. J., Hart, M., de Groot, E. R., Di Padova, F., and Aarden, L. A. (1990). Structure-function analysis of human IL-6. Epitope mapping of neutralizing monoclonal antibodies with amino- and carboxyl-terminal deletion mutants. *J. Immunol.*, **145**, 561–8.

38   Brakenhoff, J. P. J., Hart, M., and Aarden, L. A. (1989). Analysis of human IL-6 mutants expressed in *Escherichia coli*. Biological activities are not affected by deletion of amino acids 1–28. *J. Immunol.*, **143**, 1175–82.

39   Krüttgen, A., Rose-John, S., Dufhues, G., Bender, S., Lütticken, C., Freyer, P., and Heinrich, P. C. (1990). The three carboxy-terminal amino acids of human interleukin-6 are essential for its biological activity. *FEBS Lett.*, **273**, 95–8.

40   Lütticken, C., Krüttgen, A., Möller, C., Heinrich, P. C., and Rose-John, S. (1991). Evidence for the importance of a positive charge and an α-helical structure of the C-terminus for biological activity of human IL-6. *FEBS Lett.*, **282**, 265–7.

41   Danley, D. E., Strick, C. A., James, L. C., Lanzetti, A. J., Otterness, I. G., Grenett, H. E., and Fuller, G. M. (1991). Identification and characterization of a C-terminally extended form of recombinant murine IL-6. *FEBS Lett.*, **283**, 135–9.

42   Bazan, F. (1990). Haemopoietic receptors and helical cytokines. *Immunol. Today*, **11**, 350–4.

43   Abdel-Meguid, S. S., Shieh, H. S., Smith, W. W., Dayringer, H. E., Violand, B. N., and Bentle, L. A. (1987). Three-dimensional structure of a genetically engineered variant of porcine growth hormone. *Proc. Natl. Acad. Sci. U.S.A.*, **84**, 6434–7.

44   Castell, J. V., Geiger, T., Gross, V., Andus, T., Walter, E., Hirano, T., Kishimoto, T., and Heinrich, P. C. (1988). Plasma clearance, organ distribution, and target cells of interleukin-6/hepatocyte stimulating factor in the rat. *Eur. J. Biochem.*, **177**, 357–61.

45   Castell, J. V., Klapproth, J., Gross, V., Walter, E., Andus, T., Snyers, L., Content, J., and Heinrich, P. C. (1990). Fate of IL-6 in the rat: involvement of skin in its catabolism. *Eur. J. Biochem.*, **189**, 113–8.

46   Sonne, O., Davidsen, O., Möller, B. K., and Munck Petersen, C. (1990). Cellular targets and receptors for interleukin-6. *In vivo* and *in vitro* uptake of IL-6 in liver and hepatocytes. *Eur. J. Clin. Invest.*, **20**, 366–70.

47   Matsuda, T., Hirano, T., Nagasawa, S., and Kishimoto, T. (1989). Identification of α_2-macroglobulin as a carrier protein for IL-6. *J. Immunol.*, **142**, 148–52.

48   Novick, D., Engelmann, H., Wallach, D., and Rubinstein, M. (1989). Soluble cytokine receptors are present in normal human urine. *J. Exp. Med.*, **170**, 1409–14.

49   Yamasaki, K., Taga, T., Hirata, Y., Yawata, H., Kawanishi, Y., Seed, B., Taniguchi, T., Hirano, T., and Kishimoto, T. (1988). Cloning and expression of the human interleukin-6 (BSF-2/IFNβ_2) receptor. *Science*, **241**, 825–8.

50   Schooltink, H., Stoyan, T., Lenz, D., Schmitz, H., Hirano, T., Kishimoto, T., Heinrich, P. C., and Rose-John, S. (1991). Structural and functional studies on the human hepatic IL-6-receptor: molecular cloning and over-expression in HepG2 cells. *Biochem. J.*, **277**, 659–4.

51 Baumann, M., Baumann, H., and Fey, G. H. (1990). Molecular cloning, characterization, and functional expression of the rat liver interleukin-6 receptor. *J. Biol. Chem.*, **265**, 19853–62.

52 Rose-John, S., Schooltink, H., Lenz, D., Hipp, E., Dufhues, G., Schmitz, H., Schiel, X., Hirano, T., Kishimoto, T., and Heinrich, P. C. (1990). Studies on the structure and regulation of the human hepatic interleukin-6 receptor. *Eur. J. Biochem.*, **190**, 79–83.

53 Rose-John, S., Hipp, E., Lenz, D., Legrès, L. G., Korr, H., Hirano, T., Kishimoto, T., and Heinrich, P. C. (1991). Structural and functional studies on the human interleukin-6 receptor. *J. Biol. Chem.*, **266**, 3841–6.

54 Snyers, L., De Wit, L., and Content, J. (1990). Glucocorticoid up-regulation of high affinity interleukin-6 receptors on human epithelial cells. *Proc. Natl. Acad. Sci. U.S.A.*, **87**, 2838–42.

54a Pietzko, D., Zohlnhöfer, D., Graeve, L., Fleischer, D., Stoyan, T., Schooltink, H., Rose-John, S., and Heinrich, P. C. (1993). The hepatic interleukin-6-receptor: studies on its structure and regulation by PMA/dexamethasone. *J. Biol. Chem.*, in press.

55 Taga, T., Hibi, M., Hirata, Y., Yamasaki, K., Yasukawa, K., Matsuda, T., Hirano, T., and Kishimoto, T. (1989). Interleukin-6 triggers the association of its receptor with a possible signal transducer, gp130. *Cell*, **58**, 573–81.

56 Hibi, M., Murakami, M., Saito, M., Hirano, T., Taga, T., and Kishimoto, T. (1990). Molecular cloning and expression of an IL-6 signal transducer, gp130. *Cell*, **63**, 1149–57.

56a Mackiewicz, A., Schooltink, H., Heinrich, P. C., and Rose-John, S. (1992). Complex of soluble human interleukin-6-receptor/interleukin-6 upregulates expression of acute-phase proteins. *J. Immunol.*, **149**, 2021–7.

57 Zohlnhöfer, D., Graeve, L., Rose-John, S., Schooltink, H., Dittrich, E., and Heinrich, P. C. (1992). The hepatic interleukin-6-receptor: down-regulation of the interleukin-6-binding subunit (gp80) by its ligand. *FEBS Lett.*, **306**, 219–22.

58 Mizel, B., Kilian, P. L., Lewis, J. C., Paganelli, K. A., and Chizzonite, R. A. (1987). The interleukin-1 receptor. Dynamics of interleukin-1 binding and internalization in T cells and fibroblasts. *J. Immunol.*, **138**, 2906–12.

59 Grenfell, St., Smithers, N., Miller, K., and Solari, R. (1989). Receptor-mediated endocytosis and nuclear transport of human interleukin-1α. *Biochem. J.*, **264**, 813–22.

60 Bazan, J. F. (1990). Structural design and molecular evolution of a cytokine receptor superfamily. *Proc. Natl. Acad. Sci. U.S.A.*, **87**, 6934–8.

61 Yarden, Y. and Ullrich, A. (1988). Growth factor receptor tyrosine kinases. *Annu. Rev. Biochem.*, **57**, 443–78.

62 Williams, A. F. and Barclay, A. N. (1988). The immunoglobulin superfamily-domains for cell surface recognition. *Annu. Rev. Immunol.*, **6**, 381–405.

63 O'Dowd, B. F., Lefkowitz, R. J., and Caron, M. G. (1989). Structure of the adrenergic and related receptors. *Annu. Rev. Neurosci.*, **12**, 67–83.

64 Schall, T. J., Lewis, M., Koller, K. J., Lee, A., Rice, G. C., Wong, H. W., Gatanaga, T., Granger, G. A., Lentz, R., Raab, H., Kohr, W. J., and Goeddel D. V. (1990). Molecular cloning and expression of a receptor for human tumour necrosis factor. *Cell*, **61**, 361–70.

65 De Vos, A., Ultsch, M., and Kossiakoff, A. A. (1992). Human growth hormone and the extracellular domain of its receptor: crystal structure of the complex. *Science*, **255**, 306–12.

4 Tumour necrosis factor

W. FIERS

1 Historical background

The name 'tumour necrosis factor' (TNF) was introduced by Lloyd Old and coworkers in 1975 to indicate a protein identified in serum which was able to cause haemorrhagic necrosis in methylcholanthrene-A (MethA)-induced, transplantable sarcoma tumours in mice (1). This was the culmination of over two centuries of clinical observations and experimentation. In the 18th century, a number of cases were reported where coincidental infection of a cancer patient led to regression of the tumour (2). Many examples were described where an induced infection was used successfully as a cancer treatment. Such observations led William B. Coley to use local administration of bacterial extracts, 'Coley's Toxins', for cancer therapy. Although largely anecdotal, the list of successful cases is very impressive. It may be noted that the treatments usually involved local administration (presumably local TNF production) and resulted in high fever (tumour cells are much more susceptible to TNF at higher temperatures). The Coley toxin preparations contained filtrates from *Streptococci* (isolated from erysipelas) and *Serratia marcescens*. Later more controlled studies were carried out in animal model systems. For example, in 1936 Shwartzman and Michailovsky (3) obtained haemorrhagic necrosis of a sarcoma in mice by parenteral injection of extracts from *Meningococci*. It should not be concluded that these effects were simply due to TNF. Under such conditions a variety of cytokines are induced but TNF is the key actor in the cast.

Not only lipopolysaccharide (LPS) derived from Gram-negative bacteria was active in these *in vivo* systems, also many studies were carried out using bacillus Calmette–Guérin (BCG). These may have been based on a belief held in the previous century, when some physicians were convinced of an inverse correlation between tuberculosis and cancer. BCG as well as *Corynebacterium parvum* (CP) and zymosan (yeast cell walls) are immuno-stimulants: they cause reticulo-endothelial hyperplasia and hepatosplenomegaly. As such, these treatments have a modest anti-tumour activity. But mice primed in this way for two to three weeks, become hypersensitive to LPS. This led to the key finding in 1975 (1) that mice primed with BCG and then treated with LPS, release within hours in their serum a factor which causes haemorrhagic tumour necrosis in MethA-sarcoma-bearing mice. This factor, a high molecular weight protein, was given the name tumour necrosis factor or TNF. The factor was shown to be cytotoxic for murine L cells and this provided a quantitative assay system. It could be determined that the TNF titre in the serum upon LPS injection is 100 to 1000-fold higher in BCG- or *C. parvum*-primed animals as compared to controls (4). Using this convenient *in vitro* assay, pure TNF protein was obtained from animals and cultured cell lines, partially sequenced, and on this basis TNF cDNA was cloned both from human and from a number of animal species (5; reviewed in 6).

Independent research led to the discovery of the same factor. Cerami and colleagues had been studying the severe wasting or cachexia which occurs in persistently infected animals, such as those carrying the parasite *Trypanosoma brucei* (7, 8). Their studies led to the identification of a serum factor named 'cachectin' which suppressed lipoprotein lipase expression in an adipocyte cell line. Cachectin was found to be identical to the previously cloned murine (m) TNF (7, 9).

A third route of research led to the discovery of lymphotoxin or TNFβ*. Activated lymphocytes are toxic to certain, even allotypic cell types (10) and it was found that toxicity was mediated by a protein, named lymphotoxin (11). A cytotoxic factor released by lymphocytes after mitogenic stimulation, e.g. by phytohaemagglutinin, had also been described (12, 13) and finally, in 1984, Aggarwal and colleagues isolated lymphotoxin (14) and cloned the gene (15).

The historical background of TNF has been covered by other reviews (2, 16–18).

2   Biosynthesis of TNF: cellular source and induction conditions

There were already strong indications in 1975 that in animals treated with endotoxin, macrophages were the cells responsible for *in vivo* TNF production (1). It was soon found that macrophages, monocytes, and monocytic cell lines could be used *in vitro* to synthesize TNF (19–21). Macrophages from peritoneal, hepatic, or bone marrow origin, and peripheral blood monocytes require activation, for example, by treatment with IFNγ, in order to become effective producers of TNF after induction by LPS. The induction of TNF (and IL-1) in human mononuclear cells can be considerably enhanced by C5a (see Chapter 8) (22). Transforming growth factor-β, in contrast, deactivates and leads to unresponsiveness to LPS (23) and glucocorticoids down-regulate TNF synthesis (24).

Murine myeloid cell lines can be induced by LPS to produce TNF (9, 20). Human (h) TNF can be obtained from the histiocytic lymphoma-derived cell line U937 by induction with phorbol ester and retinoic acid (25) and from HL-60 cells (a human pro-myelocytic cell line) induced with phorbol ester (5), or phorbol ester with calcium ionophore and LPS (26).

Although LPS is the most important stimulus for TNF synthesis, it is not the only one. Viruses, such as Sendai virus and influenza, can induce

---

* In order to avoid confusion, lymphotoxin will be used for TNFβ and TNF will be used for TNFα.

TNF, as do trypanosomal lysates, plasmodium lysates, muramyl dipeptide, teichoic acid, some plant polysaccharides, alginates, and certain Gram-positive organisms, such as *Staphylococci* (18, 27, 28). T lymphocytes can produce TNF when treated with mitogens or phorbol ester together with the calcium ionophore A23187 (29). Also NK cells, mast cells, and astrocytes have the potential to synthesize TNF (30–32). Neutrophils can be induced to synthesize TNF mRNA, but fail to translate it (33). Also in macrophages the intra-cellular TNF mRNA level may not be related to the amount of protein secreted: treatment with LPS increases gene transcription three-fold, intra-cellular TNF mRNA 100-fold, and TNF protein production 1000-fold (8).

Cells of non-haematopoietic origin can also produce TNF. For example, vascular smooth muscle cells have been shown to be inducible for TNF synthesis (34). When murine L cells, which are exquisitely sensitive to the cytotoxic action of TNF, are kept for a long time at increasing concentrations of TNF, resistant clones can be obtained. These are of two types. In one type of clone, showing complete and permanent resistance, the endogenous TNF gene has become expressed, and the cells secrete small amounts of TNF in the medium (35, 36). TNF mRNA has also been found, either constitutively produced or induced, in human, non-haematopoietic tumour cell lines (37, 38) and in human ovarian cancer specimens (39). Except for some types of tumour cells, there is no reason to believe that *in vivo* any cell type other than activated monocytes/macrophages is involved in TNF biosynthesis.

Unlike TNF, lymphotoxin is exclusively made by T lymphocyte subsets, both of CD4$^+$- and CD8$^+$-type, following antigenic stimulation in the context of Class II and Class I restriction, respectively (40, 41) and therefore can be considered as a specific defence response. Lymphotoxin synthesis can also be induced by IL-2 or IL-2 plus IFNγ, or some viruses such as vesicular stomatitis virus (VSV) or herpes simplex-2 (HSV2) (40).

T cell hybridomas and virus (HTLV-I)-transformed T cell lines produce lymphotoxin, either constitutively or upon T cell receptor (TCR) triggering or mitogenic stimulation. A particular T hybridoma (AC5–8) produced lymphotoxin on treatment with PMA or PMA plus concanavalin A, while induction with PMA plus the calcium ionophore A23187 led to synthesis of TNF (42). Some B lymphoblastoid cell lines, such as RPMI 1788, can produce lymphotoxin, either constitutively or upon PMA induction (40) but only T cells are likely to be important *in vivo* as a source of lymphotoxin.

3 Cloning and characterization of recombinant TNF and lymphotoxin

As referred to above, Aggarwal *et al.* (14) obtained pure, human lymphotoxin, and in this way they could establish a partial amino acid sequence. This provided the information needed to synthesize probes for selection of a human lymphotoxin cDNA clone (15). The library used for screening was derived from stimulated human peripheral blood lymphocytes. The lymphotoxin clone coded for a 34 amino acid signal peptide, followed by a 171 amino acid mature protein. The latter contains a single N-glycosylation site at residue 62, and this confirms previous evidence that human lymphotoxin is a glycoprotein. Purified, natural lymphotoxin is 60 to 70 kDa by gel filtration (it is a trimer, see below) and by SDS-PAGE after reduction, it shows a 25 kDa and a 20 kDa band, the latter being a biologically active degradation product, which lacks the first 23 amino acids. The mature protein produced in *Escherichia coli* is not glycosylated, but is fully biologically active. An improved bacterial expression system and purification protocol for recombinant lymphotoxin protein was later reported by Seow *et al.* (43). Murine lymphotoxin shows 74 per cent amino acid homology to human lymphotoxin. It has a 33 amino acid signal peptide followed by a 169 amino acid mature polypeptide. Like its human counterpart, it contains one potential N-glycosylation site (40).

Cloning of human lymphotoxin and hTNF (15) were reported independently but simultaneously by groups from the Genentech company. Other investigators obtained a similar hTNF cDNA clone (reviewed in 6). The first TNF cDNA may well have been cloned from rabbits by scientists of the Asahi Kasei company (44). The list of mammalian species from which the TNF gene has been isolated, characterized, and often expressed is rapidly growing (Figure 4.1).

TNF cDNA encodes a 76 amino acid pre-sequence (79 amino acids for mouse and several other species) followed by a 157 amino acid mature polypeptide (156 for mouse and some other species). In comparing these primary structures as listed in Figure 4.1, it is clear that the sequences are highly conserved. Moreover, the pre-sequence is almost as strongly maintained as the mature sequence (75.9 per cent and 79.6 per cent between man and mouse, respectively). This indicates that this pre-sequence fulfils a very important function biologically. There are two segments with very high sequence conservation, namely the N-terminal segment -76 to -63 (human numbering) and the region -44 to -26. The hydrophilicity plot reveals that the latter segment is fairly hydrophobic and presumably plays a role in the membrane insertion of the pre-polypeptide. The region between residues -14 and -1 is the most variable and may constitute a stem from which the mature TNF polypeptide is cleaved upon final processing. A serine-type protease may be responsible for this process (6, 45).

That the pre-sequence could not be considered an ordinary secretion signal was already suggested by experiments which showed that TNF mRNA added to an *in vitro* translation mixture supplemented with dog pancreas microsomes, could be translated to a full-length precursor form (26 kDa), but could not be further processed under conditions where classical secretion signals were readily clipped off (46). The cleavage before amino acid one does not occur efficiently in all cell types, and often polypeptides of slightly different lengths (e.g. 18.5 and 20 kDa) can be observed. Furthermore, Cseh and Beutler (47) reported an 18.5 kDa polypeptide, which carried an N-terminal amino acid extension and which was biologically inactive.

Proper maturation may sometimes be lacking, and this processing may respond to physiological control mechanisms. Decker *et al.* (48) showed that activated macrophages can exert TNF-mediated cytotoxicity by means of membrane-bound TNF. The preparations could even be fixed with formaldehyde and still they retained biological function (48, 49). Kriegler *et al.* (50) provided direct evidence for a 26 kDa integral, transmembrane form of the TNF molecule, corresponding to the unprocessed translation product of the mRNA. This 26 kDa membrane-bound form can be readily detected on macrophages stimulated with LPS or PMA. Macrophages with this membrane-bound TNF may be the source of local inflammatory/immune reactions without systemic release of potentially toxic TNF (6, 51). The mature part of the TNF is clearly on the outside of the cell, as not only is it functional, but also it can readily be iodinated using intact cells. A mutant TNF gene was constructed which codes for a non-secretable, membrane-bound TNF; transfectants kill target cells by direct cellular contact (52).

Mature TNF in solution is a compact trimer of 52 kDa. The trimeric structure was shown by chemical cross-linking followed by SDS-PAGE after reduction, by ultracentrifugation, and by X-ray small-angle scattering spectrometry (53–55). Each subunit contains a single disulfide bond, and the three subunits are non-covalently linked by secondary forces. The interaction is so strong that even at very high dilution there is no evidence whatsoever for dissociation, meaning that the trimer is also the biologically active form. Although not directly demonstrated, it appears that membrane-bound TNF must likewise have a trimeric structure. Only the rat and mouse sequences contain a potential N-glycosylation site, and there is evidence in mice that the natural protein is glycosylated. The mature TNF gene can readily be expressed in *Escherichia coli* and expression yields of over 30 per cent of the total bacterial protein have been achieved and remarkably, TNF remains soluble in a fully biologically active conformation. Also in the yeast *Pichia pastoris*, TNF yields of over 30 per cent of the total soluble protein have been reported (56).

Well-diffracting crystals of TNF have been obtained (55, 57), and the three-dimensional structure was solved by Jones *et al.* at 2.9 Å resolution (58), and by Eck and Sprang at 2.6 Å (59). The shape of the molecule resembles a triangular pyramid, in which each of the three subunits has a typical jelly roll β-structure. Each subunit consists of two β-pleated sheets, five antiparallel β-strands in each. The three subunits are arranged edge to face. The outside β-sheet is rich in hydrophilic residues, while the inner sheet is largely hydrophobic and contains the C-terminal segment, which is located close to the central axis of the trimer (Figure 4.2). The first four N-terminal amino acids do not reflect and form loose ends. The 3D-structure is reminiscent of

Figure (A) — Amino acid sequence alignment of nine mammalian species (MAN, PIG, COW, SHEEP, DOG, CAT, RABBIT, RAT, MOUSE). Residue positions are numbered −76, −70, −60, −50, −40, −30, −20, −10, 1 (arrow), 10, 20, 30, 40, 50. Boxes enclose conserved / identical residues; dashes (−) indicate gaps.

```
Position markers: -76      -70         -60         -50
MAN     Met Ser Thr Glu Ser Met Ile Val Arg Asp Val Glu Leu Ala Glu Leu Ala Leu Pro Lys Thr Gly Gly Pro Gln Gly
PIG     Met Ser Thr Glu Ser Met Ile Val Arg Asp Val Glu Leu Ala Glu Leu Ala Leu Ala Lys Ala Gly Gly Pro Gln Gly
COW     Met Ser Thr Glu Ser Met Ile Val Arg Asp Val Glu Leu Ala Glu Leu Val Leu Ser Glu Gly Gly Gly Pro Gln Gly
SHEEP   Met Ser Lys Lys Ser Met Ile Val Arg Asp Val Glu Leu Ala Glu Leu Ala Leu Pro Lys Ala Gly Gly Pro Gln Gly
DOG     Met Ser Thr Glu Ser Met Ile Val Arg Asp Val Glu Leu Ala Glu Leu Pro Leu Pro Lys Ala Gly Gly Pro Gln Gly
CAT     Met Ser Thr Glu Ser Met Ile Val Arg Asp Val Glu Leu Ala Glu Gly Ala Leu Pro Lys Ala Gly Gly Pro Arg Gly
RABBIT  Met Ser Thr Glu Ser Met Ile Val Arg Asp Val Glu Leu Ala Glu Glu Ala Leu Pro Asn Met Gly Gly Pro Gln Gly
RAT     Met Ser Thr Glu Ser Met Ile Leu Arg Asp Val Glu Leu Ala Glu Glu Ala Leu Pro Lys Lys Gly Gly Leu Lys Asn
MOUSE   Met Ser Thr Glu Ser Met Ile Leu Arg Asp Val Glu Leu Ala Asp Gln Ala Asn Pro Gln Met Gly Gly Phe Gln Asn
```

```
Position markers:            -40         -30             1 (→)          10
MAN     Ser Arg Arg Cys Phe Leu Ser Leu Ile Val Ala Ala Thr Phe Cys Leu His Glu Gly Pro Val Ala His Val Val
PIG     Ser Arg Arg Cys Leu Ser Leu Phe Leu Val Ala Ala Thr Phe Cys His Glu Gly Pro Val Ala His Val Val
COW     Ser Arg Ser Cys Leu Ser Leu Met Leu Val Ala Gly Thr Phe Cys His Glu Gly Pro Val Ala His Val Val
SHEEP   Ser Arg Ser Phe Leu Ser Leu Met Leu Val Ala Gly Thr Phe Cys His Glu Gly Pro Val Ala His Val Val
DOG     Ser Arg Arg Cys Phe Leu Ser Leu Met Leu Val Ala Gly Thr Phe Cys His Gly Gly Pro Val Ala His Val Val
CAT     Ser Gly Arg Cys Leu Ser Leu Met Leu Val Ala Gly Thr Phe Cys His Glu Gly Pro Arg Ala His Val Val
RABBIT  Ser Lys Arg Cys Leu Ser Leu Met Leu Val Ala Gly Thr Phe Cys Arg Gly Asn Arg Glu Val Ala His Val Val
RAT     Ser Arg Arg Cys Leu Ser Leu Met Leu Val Ala Gly Thr Phe Cys Gly Gly Pro Asn Lys Val Ala His Val Val
MOUSE   Ser Arg Arg Ser Leu Ser Leu Met Leu Val Ala Gly Thr Phe Cys Asn Gly Pro Gln Arg Asp Ala His Val Val
```

```
Position markers:            -10          1 (→)         10
MAN     Pro Phe -   Pro Arg Asp Leu Ser Val Leu Arg Ser Ser Thr Pro Ser Asp Lys Ile Gly Pro Gln Glu
PIG     Glu Phe -   Pro Ala Gly Leu Ala Ala Leu Ser -   Ser Gln Thr -   -   Ser Ser Ala -   -   -
COW     Glu Gln Val Pro Ser Gly Pro Gln Val Gln -   Thr Ala Arg Ala Ser Asn -   Leu Pro Val Ala Leu
SHEEP   Glu Ser -   Pro Ala Ala Pro Leu Gln Gln -   Thr Leu Arg Asn Ser -   Gln Ser Ala Met Gly Glu
DOG     Glu Ser -   Pro Ala Gly Leu Ile Ala Gln -   Thr Val Ser Pro Gln Leu Ser Leu Pro Asp Gly Val
CAT     Glu Leu -   Pro Leu Gly Leu Pro Gln -   -   Thr Leu Arg Asp Ser -   Gln Ser Ala Leu Gly Met
RABBIT  Glu Gln Ser Pro Asn Leu His Leu Asn -   Met Thr Leu Arg Val Ala Leu Ser Ser Pro Gly Arg Val
RAT     Glu Lys Phe Pro Asn Gly Leu Pro Thr Leu -   Ser Ala Gln -   Thr Leu Arg Asp Ser Arg Lys Val
MOUSE   Glu Lys Phe Pro Asn Gly Leu Pro Thr Leu -   Ser Ala Gln Asn -   Thr Leu Arg Asp Arg Lys Val
```

```
Position markers: 20          30              40              50
MAN     Ala Asn Pro Gln Ala Glu Gly Gln Leu Asn Arg Ser Leu Ala Asn Leu Glu Val Asp Leu Asp Arg Leu Ala Asn Gln Leu Ser Pro Ser
PIG     Ala Asn Val Lys Ala Glu Gly Gln Leu Gln Ser Gly Ala Ala Leu Leu Val Lys Asp Leu Lys Lys Leu Ala Asn Gln Val Pro Pro Thr
COW     Ala Asn Ile Asp Ser Pro Gly Arg Trp Leu Asp Tyr Met Ala Leu Leu Lys Glu Leu Leu Glu Glu Leu Ala Asn Ala Leu Val Pro Ala
SHEEP   Ala Ala Ile Leu Ala Pro Gly Gly Trp Leu Arg Trp Leu Ala Leu Leu Gly Lys Leu Leu Pro Leu Leu Ala Asn Leu Ile Pro Pro Thr
DOG     Ala Asn Pro Glu Pro Gly Gly Trp Leu Leu Asp Leu Leu Ala Leu Leu Thr Glu Leu Leu Glu Asp Leu Ala Asn Leu Val Pro Pro Ser
CAT     Ala Asn Pro Arg Gly Arg Gly Leu Trp Leu Arg Leu Leu Ala Leu Leu Thr Lys Leu Leu Thr Lys Leu Ala Asn Lys Val Pro Pro Ser
RABBIT  Ala Asn Gln Leu Ser Gln Gly Gln Leu Gly Gln Leu Leu Ala Leu Met Leu Lys Leu Leu Leu Lys Leu Ala Asn Leu Val Pro Ala
RAT     Ala His Ser Leu Ser Gln Gly Gln Leu Gly Met Leu Leu Ala Leu Leu Gly Asp Leu Leu Met Asp Leu Ala Asn Leu Val Pro Ala
MOUSE   Ala His Gln Leu Arg Gln Gly Gln Leu Gly Met Leu Leu Ala Leu Leu Gly Met Leu Lys Met Lys Leu Ala Asn Leu Val Pro Ala
```

(A)

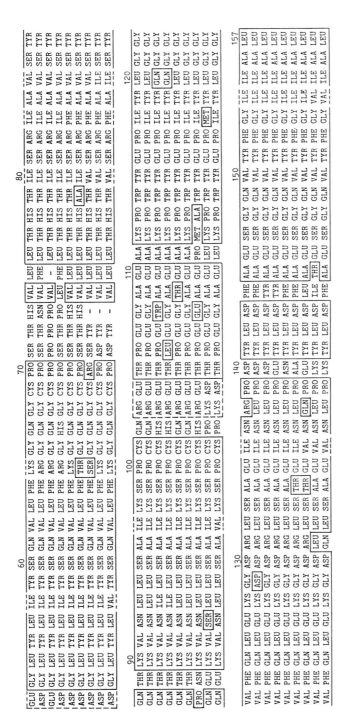

Fig. 4.1 Comparison of mammalian TNF polypeptide sequences. Identical residues in all sequences are boxed in with *solid lines*. Conservative changes are indicated with *dashed lines*. The *heavy arrow* indicates where the mature sequence is cleaved off. *Braces* above ASN indicate a glycosylation site. References: man (5, 25), pig (275, 276), cow (277), sheep (278), dog (the author's laboratory), cat (279), rabbit (280), rat (281), mouse (9, 282).

(B)

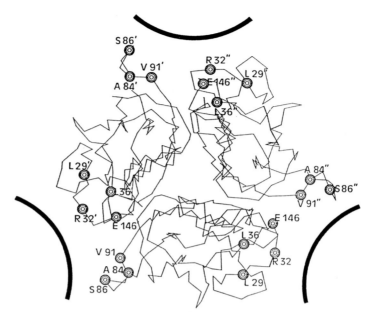

Fig. 4.2 Structure of the TNF molecule (top view) and location of the active sites. The backbone of the three subunits is shown (for details on the three-dimensional structure, see references 58 and 59). Also shown are a number of inactivating mutations, which are near the bottom of the molecule and which define the three receptor-binding sites responsible for clustering (single letter amino acid code is used). (Redrawn from reference 64.)

the arrangement of many viral capsids around three-fold symmetry axes, e.g. as found in picornaviruses, in influenza virus haemagglutinin, and in a number of icosahedral plant viruses, particularly satellite tobacco necrosis virus; up to 71 per cent of the TNF residues are structurally equivalent to residues in satellite tobacco necrosis virus capsid protein. It is a matter of conjecture, whether this represents convergent or divergent evolution!

An amino acid sequence comparison between hTNF and human lymphotoxin is given in Figure 4.3. Lymphotoxin has a classical signal sequence, and there is no evidence for a membrane-bound form. Human lymphotoxin and TNF are 28 per cent homologous in amino acid sequence, while murine lymphotoxin and TNF are 35 per cent homologous (40). The percentage of conserved residues is considerably higher. There are four regions of identical or highly conserved residues, and these four regions are on critical positions as they form the inner scaffold for the trimeric structure (59, 60). Therefore, there is little doubt that native lymphotoxin also has a fairly similar trimeric conformation.

TNF binds to specific receptors (Section 4.4) and there is no evidence for any additional function. Up to nine or ten residues can be removed from the

```
                                                                                          -76                 -70
                                                                                          Met Ser Thr Glu Ser Met Ile Arg Asp Val

          -60                                     -50                            -40
Glu Leu Ala Glu Glu Ala Leu Pro Lys Lys Thr Gly Gly Pro Gln Gly Ser Arg Arg Cys Leu Phe Leu Ser Leu Phe Ser Phe Leu Ile Val Ala Gly
                                                                                                                                Met
                                                                                                                                 ↓
        -30                           -20                           -10
Ala Thr Thr Leu Phe Cys Leu Leu His Phe Gly Val Ile Gly Pro Gln Arg Glu Glu Phe Pro Arg Asp Leu Ser Leu Ile Ser Pro Leu Ala Gln Ala
Thr Pro Pro Glu Arg Leu Phe Leu Pro Arg Val Cys Gly Thr Thr Leu His Leu Leu Leu Leu Gly Leu Leu Leu Val Leu Leu Pro Gly Ala Gln Gly

                                                                  1                                  10
 -   -   -   -   -   -   -   -   -   -   -   -   -   -   -   -   -  VAL ARG SER SER SER ARG THR PRO SER ASP LYS PRO VAL ALA HIS VAL
LEU PRO GLY VAL GLY LEU THR PRO SER ALA ALA GLN THR ALA ARG GLN HIS PRO LYS MET HIS LEU ALA HIS SER THR LEU LYS PRO ALA ALA HIS LEU

            20                            30                                                              40
VAL ALA ASN PRO GLN ALA GLU GLY GLN LEU GLN TRP LEU ASN ARG ARG ALA ASN  -   -   -  ALA LEU LEU ALA ASN GLY VAL GLU LEU ARG ASP ASN
ILE GLY ASP PRO SER LYS GLN ASN SER LEU LEU TRP  -   -   -  ARG ALA ASN THR ASP ARG ALA PHE LEU GLN ASP GLY PHE SER LEU SER ASN ASN

            50                            60                                  70
GLN LEU VAL VAL PRO SER GLU GLY LEU TYR LEU ILE TYR SER GLN VAL LEU PHE LYS GLY GLN GLY CYS  -  PRO  -   -   -  SER THR HIS VAL LEU
SER LEU LEU VAL PRO THR SER GLY ILE TYR PHE VAL TYR SER GLN VAL VAL PHE SER GLY LYS ALA TYR SER PRO LYS ALA THR SER SER PRO LEU TYR

                80                            90                                  100
LEU THR HIS THR ILE SER ARG ILE ALA VAL SER TYR GLN THR LYS VAL ASN LEU LEU SER ALA ILE LYS SER PRO CYS GLN ARG GLU THR PRO GLU GLY
LEU ALA HIS GLU VAL GLN LEU PHE SER SER GLN TYR PRO PHE HIS VAL PRO LEU LEU SER SER GLN LYS MET VAL TYR  -   -   -   -  PRO GLY LEU

    110                               120                                 130                                             140
ALA GLU ALA LYS PRO TRP TYR GLU PRO ILE TYR LEU GLY GLY VAL PHE GLN LEU GLU LYS GLY ASP ARG LEU SER ALA GLU ILE ASN ARG PRO ASP TYR
GLN GLU  -   -  PRO TRP LEU HIS SER MET TYR HIS GLY ALA ALA PHE GLN LEU THR GLN GLY ASP GLN LEU SER THR HIS THR ASP GLY ILE PRO HIS

                                150                   157
LEU ASP PHE ALA GLU SER GLY GLN VAL TYR PHE GLY ILE ILE ALA LEU
LEU VAL LEU SER PRO SER THR  -  VAL PHE PHE GLY ALA PHE ALA LEU
```

Fig. 4.3 Comparison between the amino acid sequence of human TNF (*top*) and lymphotoxin (*bottom*). The pre-sequence is 76 amino acids long in the case of TNF, and the signal sequence of lymphotoxin is 34 amino acids. The *heavy arrow* indicates where the cleavage occurs. The mature sequences are shown in capitals. *Boxes* indicate conserved residues (about 30 per cent) between the two sequences. Note that lymphotoxin contains a glycosylation site (indicated by an *anchor*), but no cysteine residues.

N-terminus, without loss of activity (61, 62). The C-terminus, however, cannot be shortened or significantly mutated, which is not surprising in view of its central location in the 3D-structure. Studies involving screening of a large collection of randomly obtained, single mutants have identified sites where loss or alteration of function was not due to a gross distortion of conformation of the molecule, but presumably a direct consequence of an involvement in the active site (63, 64). Some of these mutations are illustrated in Figure 4.2. They cluster in the lower half of the trimeric cone, in the cleft between two subunits. Each active site formed between two subunits corresponds to a receptor-binding domain, and consequently there are three such binding sites on a three-fold axis in the TNF molecule.

In the genomes of the mammalian species studied so far, there is only a single lymphotoxin gene and a single TNF gene per haploid set. Both the lymphotoxin gene and the TNF gene consist of four exons and three introns (65). These two genes are only 1100 nucleotides apart, and are localized in the middle of the MHC region between Class III and Class I genes, approximately 70 kb up-stream of the (mouse) H-2D locus on chromosome 17 in the mouse, and chromosome 6 in man (66–68).

4   Characterization of the TNF receptors and the soluble TNF-binding proteins

Early studies on the TNF receptor have shown that these are present on nearly all cell types studied, except for erythrocytes and unstimulated lymphocytes. The binding constant (K_d) is about 2×10^{-10} M and the number of receptors varies from about 200 to 10 000 per cell (57). The presence of the TNF receptor is a pre-requisite for a biological effect, but there is no correlation between the number of receptors and the magnitude of the response, or even the direction of the response. The number of TNF receptors on many cell lines can be increased two- to three-fold by treatment with IFNγ. This modest increase in receptor number, however, does not explain the dramatic increase in sensitivity towards TNF toxicity observed with many cell lines (69–71). Treatment of cells with TNF (or with lymphotoxin) leads to receptor down-modulation. Activation of protein kinase C, e.g. with phorbol ester, reduces the number of TNF receptors. It is not known whether the receptor itself or an accessory protein becomes phosphorylated (72). On the other hand, activation of the cyclic AMP-dependent protein kinase A may increase the receptor number up to seven-fold, at least in some cell lines (73). Much of this earlier work will have to be re-assessed in the light of the later dis-covery of two types of TNF receptor.

Cross-linking studies of radiolabelled TNF with its receptor on various cell lines led to the realization that two types of receptor exist, which also differed in their binding constant (74). Methods were developed to quantitate the receptor(s) in cell lysates, which allowed their purification, as well as the production of specific monoclonal antibodies (75–77). The latter reagents allowed unambiguous identification of two types of hTNF receptor, TNF-R55 and TNF-R75 (other names have been proposed, but only TNF-R55 and TNF-R75 will be used). Several adenocarcinoma cell lines, such as HEp-2, HeLa, and MCF7, contain exclusively or predominantly the smaller TNF-R55, while myeloid cell lines, such as HL-60 and U937, carry more of the larger TNF-R75. Therefore, the smaller receptor is also referred to as the epithelial cell-type and the larger as the myeloid cell-type. On the basis of a partial amino acid sequence, the hTNF-R55 was cloned (78, 79). The hTNF-R75 cDNA was first isolated by expression cloning (80). When transiently expressed in COS cells, both cDNA clones resulted in a single class of high affinity binding sites with K_d values of approximately 5×10^{-10} M for TNF-R55 and 1×10^{-10} M for TNF-R75 (Table 4.1). These values are about the same as obtained on the original cells, and therefore one can conclude that the TNF receptors themselves are sufficient for forming the high affinity ligand-binding site and that there is no need for an accessory protein. Both receptors also bind lymphotoxin, although with lower affinity.

Each receptor codes for a signal sequence, an extracellular domain, a transmembrane domain, and an intracellular, carboxy-terminal domain (Table 4.1). It was immediately apparent from the primary amino acid sequences that the two extracellular domains are related to each other, while the intracellular domains show no homology whatsoever, neither between each other, nor between the intracellular domain of any other known receptor. Each extracellular domain contains four conserved, cysteine-rich repeats, about 38 to 42 amino acids in length. Each repeat contains six cysteines characteristically located (except for two repeats of TNF-R75, which only contain four cysteines). Most or all of the cysteines are fixed in cystine-bridges. In the case of TNF-R75, the four repeat regions are connected to the transmembrane region by a stalk, and this explains the larger size of this receptor.

There is a striking homology between the extracellular domain of the two TNF receptors, and the extracellular domain of nerve growth factor, the cysteine-rich core region showing an amino acid sequence identity of about 34 per cent. Other members of this receptor family are the B cell antigen CD40, the murine 4–1BB T cell antigen, the T2 open reading frame from Shope fibroma virus, and the OX40 antigen present on activated CD4$^+$ rat T cells. More recently, the human *Fas* antigen has been cloned and again the extracellular domain was shown to be homologous to TNF-R (81); the ligand for the latter antigen is not known, but at least some of its functions are connected to those of the TNF-R (see below). Grouping these various extracellular domains into a family, however, does not provide any clues as to their mechanism of action.

The intracellular domains do not contain any obvious kinase site or phosphorylation site. They are fairly rich in serine, and, for example, that of the TNF-R75 contains six serines in a row.

Table 4.1 Characteristics of the TNF receptors

	Human TNF-R		Murine TNF-R	
	p55	p75	p55	p75
Binding constant (K$_d$)	$3.2–5 \times 10^{-10}$ M	$0.7–1 \times 10^{-10}$ M	2×10^{-10} M	5×10^{-10} M[a]
Specificity hTNF	yes	yes	yes	no
mTNF	yes	yes	yes	yes
Size (No. aa)				
Signal	29	22	29	22
Extracellular	182	235	183	235
Transmembrane	21	30	23	29
Intracellular	223	174	219	188
Total	455	461	454	474
Glycosylation				
Potential N-glycosylation sites	3	2	3	2
O-glycosylation	no	yes		
mRNA size	~3 kb	4.5 kb	~2.3–2.6 kb and ~5 kb	~3.2–3.6 kb and ~4.1–4.5 kb

[a] Possibly two or more affinity classes (83).

On the basis of homology to the hTNF receptor clones, the mTNF-R cDNAs have also been obtained (82–84). The mTNF-R55 and the mTNF-R75 are 64 per cent and 62 per cent identical to their human counterparts, respectively. Again, the two extracellular domains are homologous, having 20 per cent identity, and there is no relationship between the intracellular domains. Although mTNF binds to both receptors, hTNF only binds to mTNF-R55, and not to mTNF-R75. This finding explains earlier results regarding some species-specific effects (see below). Unlike the TNF/lymphotoxin genes, TNF receptors are not linked in the genome; TNF-R55 maps on the murine chromosome 6, and TNF-R75 on the murine chromosome 4 (83).

A number of groups have discovered soluble TNF-binding proteins (BP) in urine from febrile patients (85), in serum and urine from patients with renal insufficiency (86), in normal urine (87), and in serum ultra-filtrates from patients with advanced stages of cancer (88). These BP could be assayed on the basis of their interference with TNF action on target cells. Two BPs have been purified and characterized, both of about 27 to 30 kDa. Partial amino acid sequence determination, and especially reactivity with polyclonal and monoclonal sera, showed that the two BP, BP-I and BP-II, correspond to truncated forms of the extracellular domain of TNF-R55 and TNF-R75, respectively (89–92). As there are no separate messengers for these TNF-BPs, it was concluded that they arise by proteolytic cleavage from surface-bound TNF receptors. At the amino-terminus, eleven residues and four residues are missing from BP-I and BP-II, respectively. The cleavage at the C-terminus of BP-I is after residue 171 (93), while the C-terminal cleavage site for TNF-BP-II may be heterogeneous.

Extracellular domain shedding seems to be a normal physiological process, as many cells which synthesize TNF-Rs either constitutively or after transfection, release some TNF-BP in the medium. A major source of TNF-BP in circulation may be the neutrophils, as it has been shown that physiological agents as well as pharmacological agonists (e.g. the calcium ionophore A23187) induce a very fast shedding of the TNF receptors with a 50 per cent value reached in only two minutes (94). The physiological consequences of these circulating TNF-BPs in various pathophysiological situations may bring many surprises. It may be that normal serum contains TNF-BP in 100-fold molar excess over the (undetectable) TNF level (95). In certain diseases the serum concentration of TNF-BP may increase up to 100-fold (96). TNF-BPs modulate the availability of biologically active TNF. There is inhibition by competitive binding of the ligand, but TNF may be stabilized as a complex with binding protein acting as a reservoir of free and biologically active TNF (97).

Cancer patients who are treated with TNF in a continuous 24 hour infusion protocol, show an increase in circulatory TNF reaching a peak level at about two to three hours, which then decreases again. The reason for the decrease while the infusion is continuing, is unclear (98). One possibility is the disappearance of measurable TNF by binding to TNF-BP. In patients receiving an intravenous infusion of TNF (in combination with IFNγ) there was a rapid appearance of circulating TNF-BP, with peak levels at 30 to 60 minutes (99). IFNγ alone did not lead to release of TNF-BP.

5   Mechanism of action of TNF

5.1   Triggering of the TNF receptor and immediate/early events

TNF reacts with receptors present on nearly all cell types. The receptor is metabolically labile, with a half-life of 30 minutes (100) to two hours (101). After binding, the ligand–receptor complexes are internalized. The response of the cell correlates with the number of internalized complexes, and, although the number of receptors on the cell is low, this is usually not a limiting factor (101). The internalized receptor is subsequently degraded, as there is no recycling. The time course of events after TNF binds with its receptor can be followed by electron microscopy using gold particle-labelled TNF (102). The TNF-R complexes are internalized via clathrin-coated pits (maximum reached at five minutes), move to endosomes (maximum at 15 minutes), and then to multivesicle bodies (maximum at 30 minutes), and finally end up in the secondary lysosomes, where they are degraded. Somewhere along this pathway, the intracellular signal must have been transmitted. The only argument that internalization is necessary for signal transduction, is based on inhibition by chloroquine (103), but this could also be due to a direct effect on the membrane. Presumably the trigger is a direct result from clustering of receptor molecules brought about by the ligand binding. We have seen in Section 4.3 that each TNF molecule contains three receptor-binding sites formed in the cleft region between the subunits (64). The main argument in support of a clustering mechanism comes from the observation that monoclonal antibodies can mimic the TNF action (104). The fact that a pentameric IgM monoclonal antibody is considerably more active in mimicking TNF action as compared to the bivalent IgG, is further support for a clustering mechanism. It should be noted that so far only monoclonal antibodies against TNF-R55 have been shown to mimic TNF action; whether this is also true for the TNF-R75 remains to be determined.

Some events following treatment of susceptible cells with TNF occur very rapidly. For example, Bouchelouche *et al.* (105) observed a fast, but very transient increase in cytosolic calcium ion concentration; at the maximum there was a five-fold increase, but within one minute the concentration was back to normal. Whether this event is part of a major signalling pathway or is an irrelevant side activity is not known. It may be noted that the cytotoxic activity of TNF seems to be independent of intracellular calcium ion concentration (106). The rapid activation of neutrophils by TNF (see below) is physiologically important and may be correlated with a transient calcium release. The latter might be due to a short pulse of phospholipase C (PLC) activation, as in L-M cells a transient increase in inositol triphosphate was also observed, which is known to be a major secondary messenger for Ca^{2+} release (105). In 3T3 fibroblasts, however, the Ca^{2+} burst seems to come from the medium and no inositol phosphate release was detectable.

Within 20 seconds of TNF addition, phosphorylation of a 26 to 28 kDa protein can be observed, as well as of some other proteins (107, 108). Again, a rapid, transient increase in cytosolic calcium may be responsible for this reaction, as the same proteins can become phosphorylated by activation of PLC or by calcium ionophores. Presumably, this 28 kDa protein is identical to the mRNA cap-binding protein (109). Considering that phosphorylation of this protein does not occur in all cell types susceptible to TNF, it is questionable whether these early protein phosphorylations are part of a main line of signalling events, or are only bystander effects.

TNF treatment of primary FS4 fibroblasts, which causes a mitogenic rather than a toxic stimulus, results in a rapid increase in cyclic AMP, reaching a maximum at three to five minutes. This leads to activation of protein kinase A (110).

Another event which starts early, is the activation of the nuclear transcription factor NFκB. The latter plays a key role in TNF-induced gene activation and will be discussed in Section 4.5.3.

5.2 Cytotoxic action on transformed cell lines

Although the pleiotropic actions of TNF on a wide variety of cell types cannot be over-emphasized, nevertheless much attention, especially regarding the mechanism of action, has been paid to the cytotoxic activity of TNF on malignant cell lines. Although this may not be the major activity of TNF *in vivo*, it is the hallmark of this cytokine. The biological activity of TNF is usually assayed on the basis of its cytotoxicity. The classical cell line for testing TNF is the fibrosarcoma L929 or the cell clone WEHI 164 cl 13 (16, 111). Cells can die in at least two ways, either by apoptosis or by necrosis/ lysis. In the case of these cell lines, TNF leads to rapid lysis. In order to measure the titre of a TNF solution, dilutions are added to cell monolayers in microtitre plates. After a few days, the remaining cells which escaped lysis, can be quantitated by staining with crystal violet, followed by colorimetric measurement of the dye. Alternatively, the number of remaining cells can be quantitated with the substrate 3-(4,5-dimethylthiazol-2-yl)-2,5-diphenyltetrazolium bromide (MTT). This reagent needs functional mitochondria for colour development (112).

TNF cytotoxicity does not require new protein synthesis. On the contrary, the cytotoxic activity of TNF is enhanced 50 to 100-fold in the presence of transcription or translation inhibitors, such as actinomycin-D or cycloheximide, respectively (16). This enhancement by blocking new protein synthesis is generally interpreted as follows. Upon interaction with its receptor, TNF induces in the target cell not only nucleus-independent processes, which lead to cytotoxic reactions, but also results in transcriptional activation, followed by synthesis of new proteins (see below). Among the latter are also 'protective proteins', which either protect the cell from the damage caused by the toxic products, or repair the damage, or directly prevent the further synthesis of these toxic products (Figure 4.4). Hence, inhibition of protein synthesis prevents this auto-protection and enhances the sensitivity of the cell (113). Many cell lines are quite resistant to TNF, but become sensitive when also treated with actinomycin-D (70). Treatment of cells with IFN (which does require protein synthesis for toxicity), renders many cells much more sensitive to TNF (69, 70). Possibly, IFN also interferes with the induction or synthesis of these 'protective proteins'.

But which reaction is really responsible for cell killing? There are various arguments pointing to reactive oxygen species as primary suspects; for example, TNF cytotoxicity is decreased in anaerobic conditions (114). Mitochondria of TNF-treated cells look swollen and have fewer cristae. Glucose uptake and anaerobic respiration to lactate is increased presumably to compensate for reduced mitochondrial respiration (115). Another finding implicating mitochondrial involvement in response to TNF, was the observation (117) that, at least in some cells, TNF induces manganese superoxide dismutase (MnSOD), and this mitochondrial protein may function as a 'protective enzyme'. Over-expression of MnSOD conferred resistance to TNF, while a decrease, by means of antisense RNA, enhanced the sensitivity (118). Remarkably, many cancer cells are deficient in MnSOD (119). It is not clear how MnSOD might have a protective role. Peroxides, which are produced by this enzyme, may react with molecular oxygen forming the highly reactive hydroxyl radical ($OH^{\bullet}$). This reaction requires Fe^{2+} or Cu^{2+}. These hydroxyl radicals are extremely reactive and may be the real culprits responsible for cellular damage. Evidence that $OH^{\bullet}$ is formed in TNF-treated cells comes, on the one hand, from the observation that certain chelating agents, such as o-phenanthroline and 2,2'-bipyridine, are highly protective against TNF cytotoxicity (16, 120). Hydroxyl radical production was detected after 18 hours by the formation of methane gas from dimethyl sulfoxide, an insensitive assay which may account for the delay. Oxygen and hydroxyl radicals can damage proteins, lipids, and DNA. TNF leads to lipid peroxidation as measured by the formation of malonyldialdehyde. This was only detectable some 20 hours after the start of TNF treatment, but the delay may be due to the low sensitivity of the detection method (114). Also damage to DNA in TNF-treated cells can be detected by the formation of thymine glycols; cells with a lower glutathione content, and therefore with a lower scavenging capacity against reactive oxygen species, are more susceptible to TNF cytotoxicity (116).

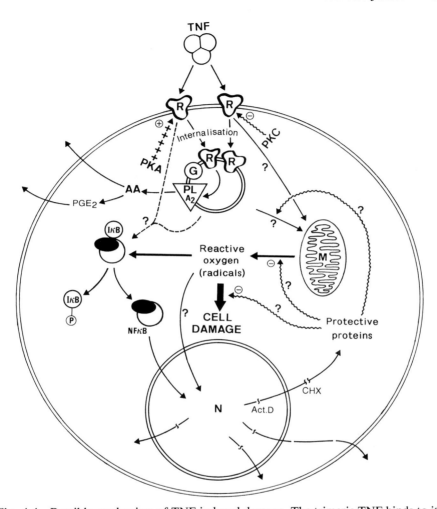

Fig. 4.4 Possible mechanism of TNF-induced damage. The trimeric TNF binds to its receptors (R) and causes them to cluster, followed by internalization. The number of receptors is positively regulated by protein kinase A and negatively by protein kinase C. Involvement of a G protein (inhibitable by pertussis toxin) and a phospholipase A_2 (releasing arachidonic acid or prostaglandins) is indicated. A signal goes to the mitochondria and perturbs the electron flow between complex I/II and complex III. Reactive oxygen species are formed, including hydroxyl radicals which lead to cytotoxicity. The reactive oxygen from mitochondria and other sources may also be responsible for activation of the transcription factor NFκB which, upon release from the Iκ regulatory element, moves to the nucleus and switches on a specific set of genes. Many cells are resistant to TNF toxicity, because TNF itself induces the synthesis of protective proteins. These may act either by preventing the mitochondrial perturbation or by detoxifying the oxidative reactions. In the presence of RNA synthesis inhibitors (actinomycin, Act.D) or protein synthesis inhibitors (cycloheximide, CHX), the protective proteins are not formed and the cell is much more sensitive to TNF-induced cytotoxicity.

Using digitonin-permeabilized cells, Lancaster *et al.* (121) could show directly that the mitochondrial electron transfer was impaired in TNF-treated cells. This inhibition was detectable after one and a half to two hours, which preceded cell lysis by at least five hours. Using a series of specific inhibitors, we could show that the electron transport flow in mitochondria is perverted at the entry of the complex III level (ubiquinone → cytochrome b → cytochrome c_1). As a result, the electrons reduce molecular oxygen with formation of superoxide. Cells can be completely protected from TNF cytotoxicity by blocking both the complex I and complex II-derived flow of electrons (coming from NADH and succinate, respectively) (122).

In some cell lines, TNF activates PKC with a maximum reached at six minutes (123) but it is doubtful whether PKC plays a major role in the TNF-induced signal transduction (124).

Treatment of sensitive target cells with TNF leads to release of arachidonic acid into the medium, and this is already significant from one hour onwards (57, 103, 114, 125). As arachidonic acid is mainly present in the 2-position of phospholipids (see Chapters 12 and 13), this TNF-induced release suggests activation of a phospholipase A_2. Using various combinations of cell lines, inhibitors (such as quinacrine and steroids), and some activators, Suffys *et al.* (125) observed a very good correlation between cytotoxicity and TNF-induced release of arachidonic acid. It is not clear whether this activation of phospholipase A_2 activity is a cause or a consequence of the cytotoxic events. It could be part of a signal transduction pathway, leading to a block in the mitochondrial electron flow, as discussed above. But it is equally possible that perturbations, such as lipid peroxidation, activate an endogenous phospholipase A_2. Also, peroxidized phospholipids may be preferred substrates for phospholipases (126).

Signal transduction from cross-linked receptors to the putative interference with the mitochondrial electron transport system, is completely unknown. However, a number of observations provide possible hints for essential components of the system. Pertussis toxin, which inactivates certain G proteins, protects, at least partially, against TNF toxicity (103, 127), suggesting that a G protein may directly or indirectly play a role. Possibly, a G protein may be involved in phospholipase A_2 activation (see Chapter 13).

A second observation is that a protease may be involved in the cell killing process. Inhibitors of serine-type proteases protect cells from TNF-induced lysis (128–130). Finally, a dramatic synergism between TNF and lithium ions has been observed (131). As one of the best documented effects of Li^+ is the inhibition of dephosphorylation of some inositol phosphates, these results suggest an involvement of inositol phosphate turnover in TNF-mediated cytotoxicity. How this is to be reconciled with the apparent lack of an effect of phospholipase C is unknown at present and is under investigation. Palombella and Vilček (132) argue that in diploid 3T3 cells phospholipase activity is part of essential, early signal transduction events.

Some cells killed by TNF are not lysed, but instead follow the typical pathway leading to apoptosis (133). Characteristics of apoptosis include chromatin condensation, swelling of cytoplasmic compartments, damage to mitochondria, blebbing of the cell surface, cross-linking of proteins by transglutaminase activity, and above all degradation of the nuclear DNA into nucleosome size fragments. The latter reaction is due to a nuclease which enters the nucleus and is activated by magnesium and calcium ions (134–137). ADP ribosylation of particular proteins is observed from four hours onwards after exposure to TNF (138). This enzymatic process is often indicative of DNA damage. Inhibitors of ADP ribosylation also prevent TNF-mediated cytotoxicity, suggesting an important role of this process, either in signal transduction or in mediating the toxic reactions.

The cytotoxic effects discussed above can all be mediated by interaction of TNF with TNF-R55. Under appropriate conditions TNF is cytotoxic for Hep-2 cells, which carry only TNF-R55. Also, prototype target cells, such as L929 and WEHI 164, are equally killed by mTNF as by hTNF, although hTNF does not act on mTNF-R75. Although TNF-R75 is not essential for cytolytic activity, it is not excluded that it does play a helping role (104).

There is a relationship between the TNF receptor and the *Fas*-antigen. In TNF-sensitive cells, the *Fas*-antigen seems to be associated with a TNF receptor, as they undergo simultaneous down-modulation. Cross-linking of the *Fas*-determinant leads to apoptotic death. When the human *Fas*-antigen was transfected into prototype murine target cell L929, the cells were killed in a typical apoptotic process upon treatment with anti-*Fas*-antibody (81).

Lymphotoxin binds with lower affinity to the same receptors as TNF, and would be expected to transmit the same signals, although more weakly. However it was observed by Browning and Ribolini (139) that different tumour cell lines varied considerably in their relative sensitivity towards TNF cytotoxicity as compared to lymphotoxin. These results cannot be explained in terms of one or the other of the two TNF receptors, and therefore it seems more likely that the TNF-R molecules are associated with accessory proteins, and that not all signals generated by TNF are also exerted by lymphotoxin, or *vice versa*. Alternatively, perhaps a third type of receptor may exist.

5.3   Gene induction by TNF

TNF induces the synthesis of a wide variety of proteins (a non-exhaustive list is given in Table 4.2). In nearly all cases where this has been studied in detail, the induction was due to transcriptional activation. Which genes are switched on, depends on the cell type; but even in the same cell, different genes become activated with divergent kinetics and degree of induction. Some proteins may require co-inducers, whilst the expression of a few other genes is down-modulated, including *c-myc*, thrombomodulin, tissue plasminogen activator, and protein S/protein C.

Table 4.2 Proteins induced by TNF[a]

Location of product	Protein
Nucleus	*c-fos*
	c-jun
	IRF-1
Cytosol	Metallothionine
	2′–5′ oligo-A synthetase
	Cytochrome P245 heavy chain
	Ferritin light chain
Mitochondria	Mn superoxide dismutase
Cell surface	Tissue factor
	ELAM-1
	ICAM-1
	IL-2 receptor-α
	EGF receptor
	Class I MHC
	Class II MHC
	Membrane IL-1
	CD11/CD18
Secreted	IL-1α and IL-1β
	IL-6
	IL-8
	gro
	IFNβ
	GM-CSF
	M-CSF
	G-CSF
	PDGF
	Plasminogen activator inhibitor 1 and 2
	Collagenase
	Stromelysin

[a] Reviewed in references 133, 176, and 283.

Gene induction usually means activation or transport into the nucleus of transcription factors. TNF rapidly induces the transcription factors *c-fos* and *c-jun*, which leads to active AP-1 (140). The two genes seem to be induced by a different pathway. The former, *c-fos*, seems to be dependent on a lipoxygenase product (Chapter 13) formed from released arachidonic acid (141).

The most important mediator of transcriptional activation by TNF is the transcription factor NFκB. It has been shown to be responsible (usually in association with other factors, like AP-1) for TNF induction of, amongst others, MHC genes, the IL-2 receptor-α gene, and the IL-6 gene. The induction of the latter has been studied extensively. On the one hand, TNF, and also IL-1, are the main physiological inducers of IL-6, and, on the other hand, IL-6 is a major secondary mediator of TNF and IL-1 effects *in vivo*. NFκB is a heterodimer consisting of a p50 and a p65 protein. This dimer is present in the cytosol in an inactive form, bound to the inhibitor Iκ. Upon activation, it is released from Iκ and moves to the nucleus, where it binds to a specific sequence motif (5′-GGGACTTTCC-3′), present in the up-stream region of the promoters of responsive genes (Figure 4.4) (142, 143). It was first observed in the case of an MHC Class I gene that TNF inducibility indeed corresponds to an up-stream motif recognized by the transcription factor NFκB, and that the latter became activated upon TNF treatment of the cells (144). The essential role of the NFκB-responsive element in the promoter region of the IL-6 gene for inducibility by TNF, has been documented by several studies (145–147). Both TNF and lymphotoxin can activate NFκB within two to four minutes after binding to the cell, even when only 20–25 per cent of the receptors are occupied (148). Triggering of either TNF-R55 or TNF-R75 leads to NFκB activation (149). The half-life of active NFκB is less than 30 minutes, and hence, upon prolonged activation in the absence of protein synthesis, depletion occurs (150). Remarkably, synthesis of the NFκB p50 precursor is itself induced by TNF (151). Also dissection of the IL-2 receptor-α gene promoter led to the identification of the NFκB-responsive element as the key to TNF inducibility (152).

How does TNF activate the transcription factor NFκB (or dissociate it from the Iκ-binding factor)? It was previously believed that NFκB activation was due to phosphorylation of the Iκ protein (142). This hypothesis is mainly based on *in vitro* experiments, and may perhaps not reflect physiological conditions. Neither protein kinase A, nor protein kinase C, nor several other kinases seem to be involved in TNF-induced NFκB activation (153, 154). An alternative activation pathway was proposed by Schreck *et al.* (155), namely that reactive oxygen intermediates can directly activate NFκB (or via an oxidation-sensitive kinase). This activation by, for example, hydrogen peroxide, could be blocked by reactive oxygen scavengers, such as N-acetyl-L-cysteine. As N-acetyl-L-cysteine and some other thiol-based inhibitors could also block the activation of NFκB induced either by phorbol ester or by TNF or IL-1, it was concluded that activation by the latter cytokines occurred likewise via reactive oxygen intermediates. This supports the evidence that TNF specifically and rapidly leads to production of reactive oxygen intermediates by perturbation of the electron flow in mitochondria. In L929 cells, the pathways leading to cytotoxicity and to IL-6 induction are largely superimposable, as shown by the action of various agents which inhibit or increase both effects in parallel (Figure 4.4) (156). Nevertheless, several important questions remain to be resolved. Is all reactive oxygen from mitochondria, or are there also more direct sources, such as NADPH oxidase? Also, how exactly do reactive oxygen species lead to release of NFκB from Iκ? This is not clear. It is unknown whether the wide variety of effects by TNF in different cell types can all be mediated by NFκB and/or AP-1, or whether modulation of additional transcription factors is involved.

6   TNF action on normal cells

6.1   Endothelial cells

Receptors for TNF are present on nearly all cells, and it is therefore not unexpected that TNF exerts a wide range of effects on primary cells or non-transformed cell lines. The response usually involves activation of a set of genes, and which ones are induced depends on the cell type. A few examples of particular interest are given below. When TNF is injected in an experimental animal or in a patient, or naturally released into the circulation, then the primary target is the endothelial cell bed. In general, TNF increases the immune modulatory, the inflammatory, and the thrombogenic capacity of the endothelial system. The immune properties of the endothelial cells are increased as a result of TNF-induced MHC Class I expression. TNF treatment leads to the surface expression of membrane-bound IL-1, as well as adhesion molecules, such as ELAM-1, ICAM-1, ICAM-2, and VCAM-1 (157–159). This results in the binding of granulocytes, lymphocytes, and monocytes to the inflamed regions of the vascular system. Also platelet activating factor (PAF) is produced (see Chapter 13) (160). TNF treatment of an endothelial cell layer causes morphological changes, and these effects may be why TNF leads to increased vascular permeability and extravasation of immune cells.

TNF not only induces the appearance of adhesion molecules on the endothelial cell surface which contribute to the inflammatory reaction, there is also synthesis of proteins, which lead to a pro-coagulant climate (see Chapters 10, 11). Induction of pro-coagulant activity occurs on the surface, while the activated protein C/protein S complex is inhibited, and there is an increased production of plasminogen activator inhibitor. Vasodilator compounds are synthesized (e.g. PGI$_2$ and NO), which may be implicated in TNF-induced hypotension (161) (see Section 4.7).

Nearly all effects of TNF on endothelial cells can be mimicked by IL-1 treatment. The latter cytokine clearly reacts with different receptors, but the secondary messenger profile may well be the same.

In the absence of endothelial growth factor, TNF kills endothelial cells by induction of apoptosis (162). On the other hand, under appropriate conditions, TNF has a strong angiogenic effect (163).

6.2   Neutrophils

TNF stimulates the adherence of leucocytes to the endothelial bed. This is due not only to induction of synthesis of adhesion molecules on the endothelial cell, but also to a rapid, direct action of TNF on neutrophils. This pheno-menon is protein synthesis-independent, and is complete within five minutes (164, 165). The neutrophil adherence is based, at least in part, on an increased surface expression of the complement iC3b receptor glycoprotein CR3. It may be physiologically significant that this rapid activation occurs with TNF, but not with IL-1. This is one of the rare examples of an activity carried out by TNF, and which cannot be mirrored by IL-1. TNF or lymphotoxin, as well as IFNγ, can also activate phagocytosis by neutrophils. The combination of TNF plus IFN enhances specific antibody-dependent cellular cytotoxicity (166). Furthermore, the respiratory burst, superoxide anion release, polarization, and aggregation are increased by TNF treatment (167).

6.3   Lymphocytes

Resting T cells have virtually no TNF receptors. But upon stimulation either by antigen or by mitogen, rapid synthesis of TNF receptors ensues, and the cells proliferate in response to TNF (168, 169). This involves co-induction of high affinity IL-2 receptors, and synthesis of IL-2. The experimental set-up is very similar to the classical assay system for IL-1: thymocytes are stimulated with phytohaemagglutinin and they respond, in a dose-dependent manner, to IL-1-induced proliferation driven by IL-2 receptor induction and IL-2 synthesis.

Although with considerably lower specific activity, TNF can replace IL-1 in this system. Remarkably, mTNF, but not hTNF, is active (170), showing that the observed murine T cell proliferation is driven by the p75 receptor (see Section 4.4 and Table 4.1). The first clear species-specific activity was also observed with a T cell, namely a rat/mouse thymoma, PC60, which could be differen-tiated to a cytotoxic T cell by addition of IL-1 and IL-2. The IL-1 induces IL-2 receptors, and can be replaced by mTNF, but not by hTNF (171). CT6 cells are another example; this is a murine T cell line, which proliferates in response to IL-1. However, the latter cytokine can be replaced by mTNF, but again not by hTNF (172). These systems indicate a role for the murine p75 receptor.

TNF can exert an IL-1-like effect on B lymphocytes. Human B cells, stimulated with Cowan I *Staphylococcus aureus*, and in the presence of IL-2, respond to TNF by proliferation and by differentiation into immunoglobulin-secreting cells (173) and there was a considerable increase in the number of TNF receptors upon activation (174).

6.4   Fibroblasts

TNF stimulates the synthesis of collagenase and PGE_2 (175), and MHC Class I expression (157) in dermal fibroblasts. Surprisingly, TNF has a growth-promoting activity on normal, diploid fibroblasts (176, 177); this growth-enhancing activity is not seen at low confluency, but TNF becomes clearly mitogenic at high cell densities. The mitogenic activity is synergistic with insulin, but less than additive with epidermal growth factor (178). In fibroblasts, as in many other cell types, TNF rapidly induces IL-6 and also membrane-bound IL-1 (179–181). The IL-6 induction seems to involve cAMP as a second messenger (presumably in addition to activated NFκB). cAMP rapidly accumulates upon TNF treatment of FS4 fibroblastoid cells, reaching a peak level in five minutes (110, 182).

Various irritants in experimental animals or patients can lead to fibrotic tissue formation, and TNF may well play a major role—in the form of a fibroblast mitogen—in these pathologies. Indeed, Piguet *et al.* have shown that silica-induced, pulmonary fibrosis can be prevented almost completely by pre-treatment with antibody against TNF (183).

6.5   Adipose tissue

One of the first recognized properties of TNF, then called cachectin, was the suppression of lipoprotein lipase expression in cultured fat cells (184). Furthermore, TNF also suppresses adipocyte differentiation and down-regulates the expression of a variety of adipose-specific genes (8). The treatment of cultured adipocytes with TNF also reverses the morphologic differentiation. *In vivo*, TNF leads to resorption of brown fat and to elevation of plasma triglycerides. TNF also inhibits *de novo* synthesis of fatty acids. This inhibition of the differentiated functions of the adipocyte occurs at the transcriptional level. Despite these profound effects, TNF is not toxic for murine fat cells.

These activities of TNF on murine adipocytes have not been confirmed for other species. No reduction of lipoprotein lipase was observed in rat or in human adipocytes (185). There was a decrease in lipoprotein lipase activity, however, when human adipose tissue still containing vascular, endothelial cells was treated with TNF, suggesting that another or secondary factor may be involved (186).

6.6   Muscle cells

TNF causes a drop in transmembrane potential and an increase in glucose transport (8). There is a rapid stimulation of glycogenolysis, a rise in fructose-2,6-biphosphate, and an increased release of lactate (187). Treatment of vascular, smooth muscle cells with TNF leads to synthesis and secretion of IL-1. There is also induction of (2'-5')-oligoadenylate synthetase, as well as release of prostaglandins (34).

7   *In vivo* effects of TNF—the cytokine network

In both mice and humans, the half-life of TNF in the circulation is about 6 to 30 minutes (188, 189). Clearance of injected TNF tends to fall with increasing doses. This may be due to saturation of a clearance mechanism or to the existence of more than one clearance system (190). When TNF was administered to cancer patients as a continuous infusion over 24 hours, a maximum level in the serum was obtained at three hours, which subsequently declined despite continuous infusion at a constant dose rate (98). Many explanations are possible, including sequestration of TNF by shed, soluble receptors. Enhanced capillary leakage may also occur in the course of the treatment.

The first endogenous pyrogen to be identified was IL-1. However, when TNF is injected intravenously in rabbits, it is, on an equal weight basis, as pyrogenic as IL-1 (191). Both cytokines apparently exert their effect by synthesis of prostaglandins, as the pyrogenic action can be blocked by cyclo-oxygenase inhibitors, such as indomethacin. When TNF was injected intravenously in rabbits, it produced a biphasic fever. The first wave is believed to correspond to a direct action, while the second fever peak (three hours later) might have been due to endogenous IL-1 induced by TNF (191). Studies in rats, however, have indicated that TNF is considerably less pyrogenic than IL-6, and certainly as compared with IL-1, either when injected peripherally or directly into cerebral ventricles (192). At higher dose levels, TNF causes hypothermia, followed by death. Again, these effects are presumably mediated by prostaglandins and can be largely prevented by pre-treatment with indomethacin (193).

When TNF is administered on a daily basis to experimental animals, it has an anorectic effect. For one or two days, the animals stop eating and drinking, and have increased diarrhoea (194, 195). This anorectic effect is thought to operate at the level of the hypothalamus/pituitary. When one continues to inject TNF daily, the animals recover weight and become tolerant to the anorectic effect.

TNF causes hypotension in experimental animals (196), and in clinical trials, hypotension is often the toxic effect which limits the dose (190, 197). Hypotension may be due to TNF-induced synthesis of nitric oxide (endothelial-derived relaxing factor), as the effect can be inhibited by NO synthetase inhibitors (198, 199).

An important action of TNF, perhaps indirectly, on the hypothalamus/pituitary is the release of adrenocorticotropic hormone (ACTH), which in turn results in an increase of glucocorticoid levels in circulation (185). Presumably, this is part of a feedback control mechanism, as the steroids interfere with TNF synthesis and with its action on most, but not all cells.

TNF administration leads to hypertriglyceridaemia. There is an increase of lactate in circulation and acidosis. High doses of TNF cause first hyperglycaemia, followed by a severe hypoglycaemia leading to death. Several of the biochemical and physiological parameters are mediated by prostaglandins, as they can largely be prevented by pre-treatment with indomethacin (193). A metabolite of prostaglandin PGE_2 has also been readily detected in the serum of TNF-treated animals.

TNF is part of a complex, interconnected cytokine defence network. When injected *in vivo*, TNF induces or facilitates the synthesis of a number of other mediators. One important cytokine induced by TNF is IL-1. IL-1, like TNF, is also a very pleiotropic factor, which is involved in a wide variety of immune and inflammatory phenomena (see Chapter 2). Although TNF and IL-1 have an almost overlapping spectrum of activities (17), the biological effects of the two cytokines are not identical. For example, IL-1, but not TNF, is a growth factor for bone marrow stem cells and has a very pronounced radioprotective effect. On the other hand, TNF, especially in combination with IFN, is toxic for many tumour cells, while this is only rarely so for IL-1. Also, granulocytes become activated within minutes after treatment with TNF, but do not respond to IL-1.

Upon a single, intravenous bolus injection, mTNF is considerably more lethal for C57/BL6 mice than hTNF, with LD_{50} values of approximately 10 μg/mouse and 500 μg/mouse, respectively (176, 200–202). Since hTNF does not bind to the mTNF-R75 (see Table 4.1), at least one cell type carrying the larger TNF-R must fulfil a key role in the toxicity steps leading to death.

In contrast, a single injection of IL-1 is not lethal, even at quite high concentrations. However, co-administration of mTNF or hTNF with IL-1 leads to a highly synergistic toxicity (200, 203, 204), suggesting that IL-1 sensitizes the animal to the toxic effect of TNF. When mice are treated with IL-1 12 hours before TNF, they become much more resistant to a normally lethal challenge with mTNF (205, 206). This protection can also be induced with low doses of TNF itself. The protective effect of IL-1 or TNF pre-treatment may operate via the liver.

Galactosamine is a specific hepatotoxic agent that exerts its activities by impairing macromolecular synthesis in hepatocytes through a depletion of UTP. Galactosamine-treated mice are extremely sensitive to the toxic action of LPS, and are more than 100-fold more sensitive to TNF (207). In this sensitive system, pre-treatment of mice with even a small concentration of IL-1 was protective against a challenge with a combination of TNF and galactosamine (206). These results indicate that the liver plays an important role in protection of the organism against TNF toxicity. The nature of this (presumably inducible) protective system is not known at present.

TNF and IL-1 are the main physiological inducers of IL-6. Following a live *E. coli* infection of mice treated with anti-TNF antibodies, a considerable reduction in subsequent IL-6 titre was observed, suggesting that TNF is the predominant natural inducer under these conditions (208). IL-6 is a key factor in a variety of immune, inflammatory, and cell differentiation phenomena. Many cells respond to TNF or IL-1 treatment by production of IL-6, including macrophages, lymphocytes, endothelial cells, fibroblasts, and epithelial cells. Even when an immune response or an inflammation is locally restricted, the IL-6 produced as a result of this reaction, circulates through the body and sets in motion a variety of secondary responses. It co-operates with colony-stimulating factors in the bone marrow, it acts on T and B lymphocytes, it causes differentiation of myeloid cells, it acts on the hypothalamus (induction of CRF followed by ACTH synthesis in the pituitary) and causes fever, and it stimulates nerve cells (see Figure 3.1). But the major action of IL-6 is on the liver, where synthesis of acute phase proteins is induced. The roles of these acute phase proteins are discussed in Chapter 1, but are likely to protect the host's tissue from excessive damage at an infection/inflammation site. The IL-6/ACTH-mediated induction of glucocorticoids also protects cells from the deleterious action of TNF, and is involved in synthesis of at least some acute phase proteins (Chapters 1, 3 and reviews 209–213).

When TNF is administered to cancer patients by continuous infusion, a peak level of TNF in the serum is reached after three hours, and this is followed by increasing IL-6 levels reaching a maximum three hours later (214). Likewise, after intravenous injection of hTNF or IL-1 in mice, a peak serum concentration of IL-6 is obtained about three hours later, and this subsequently decreases to background levels at about six hours (215). When mTNF was injected, there was a similar steep increase in IL-6 level up to three hours, but it stayed high, even after eight hours (215). The treatment with mTNF, but not hTNF, is lethal. Furthermore, when hTNF is combined with a sensitizing agent, such as IL-1 or the glucocorticoid antagonist RU486, then lethality ensues. Under these conditions, this toxicity is correlated with the inability to shut off synthesis of IL-6 (216). Possibly, IL-6 is part of a defence system, acting through synthesis of protective factors including acute phase proteins and glucocorticoids. Too much IL-6 may be deleterious for the organism, as shown by the results of Starnes *et al.* (208), who could protect mice from TNF-induced lethality by administration of antibodies to IL-6.

8 The role of TNF in infection

'What is tumour necrosis factor really for?' This question was asked and answered by Playfair and colleagues in 1984 (217). They noted that TNF is highly conserved in evolution and must provide a selective advantage. They proposed that its role is in protection from parasitic, bacterial, and viral diseases, and this hypothesis has subsequently been amply verified. However, quite often an over-reaction and an over-production of TNF, possibly in concert with other over-produced cytokines, might bring dire consequences to the host.

8.1 Parasitic infections

In Section 4.1 it was described that TNF was independently discovered as 'cachectin' in the serum of trypanosome-infected animals. Since recombinant TNF became available, many studies have appeared documenting its protective role *in vivo* against parasitic diseases. TNF has been shown to limit infection by *Plasmodium* spp., *Leishmania major*, *Trypanosoma cruzi*, *Toxoplasma gondii, Schistosoma mansoni*, and others (218, 219). Various mechanisms have been invoked to explain the protective effect of TNF *in vivo*. Except perhaps in the case of *Trypanosoma musculi* (220), there is little or no evidence that TNF can directly affect the parasite. TNF can prime neutrophils, such that upon triggering they produce a much enhanced burst of toxic peroxide. TNF enhances the antigen-dependent cytotoxicity of eosinophils. Further putative mechanisms involve activation of macrophages, NK cells, or mast cells.

Over-production of TNF can be detrimental to the host. This was shown by Grau *et al.* in an experimental model of cerebral malaria in mice (221); passive immunization with TNF antibodies protected the animals. Cerebral malaria is also the major cause of *Plasmodium falciparum*-induced mortality in man. The underlying basis of the pathology could possibly be the adherence of parasitized erythrocytes to TNF-induced inflammatory receptor molecules on the endothelial system in the brain. Patients with cerebral malaria have remarkably high TNF levels, and it is believed that an anti-TNF treatment may be beneficial in this stage of the disease (222).

8.2   Bacterial infection and septic shock

We have seen in Section 4.1 that the induction of TNF by LPS was the apex of two centuries of observations and experimental studies regarding a linkage between bacterial infection and tumour regression. But it was soon realized that TNF is also responsible for many of the pathological effects seen after injection of a high concentration of LPS (188). There is a close similarity in symptoms, such as increase in serum prostaglandin concentration, hypothermia, increased and decreased blood glucose level, diarrhoea, metabolic acidosis, cyanosis, and finally death (223). A number of these pathological effects are mediated by released prostaglandins and can be prevented by indomethacin pre-treatment (193). However, such a protocol of indomethacin/ TNF becomes highly toxic when given on a daily basis (W. Fiers, unpublished results). That TNF is the main executor of many deleterious endotoxin effects, was directly shown by Beutler *et al.* (224). They treated mice with TNF antibodies and could in this way protect them from the lethal effect of an LPS challenge. Passive immunization of baboons with a monoclonal antibody against hTNF protected the animals against an infusion with live *E. coli*, which led in the control animals to septic shock with cardiovascular collapse and acute organ failure (225). That TNF might be involved in fatal human septic shock, was reported by Waage *et al.* (226). In a retrospective study involving patients with meningococcal septicaemia, they found a correlation between degree of septic shock and TNF level; all patients with serum concentrations in excess of 440 U/ml had died. However, it is evident that a bacterial infection or LPS injection does not only induce TNF, but a whole array of interacting cytokines. The level of IL-6 in serum from septic shock patients was 10 000 times higher than the level of TNF. Also, 87 per cent of meningitis patients had elevated IL-6 serum levels, while only 23 per cent had measurable TNF (227). As mentioned already, anti-IL-6 antibodies can also protect against a normally lethal dose of *E. coli* (208). Furthermore, IL-1 receptor antagonist significantly protects against endotoxin-induced septic shock in rabbits, indicating that IL-1 also plays an important role (228). Nevertheless, TNF is presumably the key mediator. When a panel of cytokine levels was studied in adult patients with Gram-negative septic shock, it was found that admission levels of TNF and IL-1, but not IL-6, IFNα, or IFNγ, were correlated with outcome (229). The outcome could mainly be predicted from the evolution of the serum TNF levels; after ten days, the median TNF concentration remained high in the non-survivors, while it was undetectable in survivors. But these authors also caution that other parameters than admission TNF level contribute more significantly to the prediction of outcome (222).

It would be wrong to conclude, however, that induction of TNF as a result of a bacterial infection has only deleterious, even fatal effects. C$_3$H/HeJ mice, which do not produce TNF in response to LPS, are a thousand-fold more susceptible to a lethal infection with *E. coli* than congenic, LPS-sensitive C$_3$H/HeN mice. Protection could be restored by administration of IL-1 and TNF (230). Also in a number of other studies involving either free-living or facultative intracellular bacteria, TNF was shown to play a role in limiting the severity of infection, for example in the case of *Listeria monocytogenes*, *Legionella pneumophila*, *Streptococcus pneumoniae*, *Klebsiella pneumoniae*, *Salmonella typhimurium*, *Chlamydia trachomatis*, and others. Various mechanisms are involved in these protective processes, including selective killing of cells harbouring intracellular forms, activation of monocytes and granulocytes, and stimulation of specific immune responses (219).

8.3 Viral infections

TNF can protect both against RNA viruses (EMC and VSV) as well as DNA viruses (adenovirus-2, *herpes simplex*-2); it induces 2'-5' oligo-A synthetase (Table 4.2) and acts synergistically with IFNγ in protecting cells against viruses (231, 232). As TNF kills selectively virus-infected cells, it may clear the organism from an infection when relatively few cells contain replicating virus. But when the infection has spread, the action of TNF can be detrimental, leading to rapid death (233).

The virus which attracts most attention, is the human immunodeficiency virus (HIV). TNF selectively kills cells chronically infected with HIV (234). However, this activity is not necessarily protective, as *in vitro* TNF increases the virus yield from HIV-infected cells. As mentioned in Section 5.3, this enhancement could be due to the activation of the cellular transcription factor NFκB, which is a positive regulatory element for the HIV-LTR promoter. Patients who had enrolled in a trial of TNF therapy for Kaposi sarcoma, showed evidence of rising levels of circulating HIV antigen (235). As HIV induces TNF (and IL-1) and as TNF in turn activates latently infected cells, this may constitute a vicious circle for the patients (reviewed in 219), which possibly could be broken by anti-TNF therapy. It is still not clear whether in the sera of AIDS patients there is an increased TNF level (236), or whether this is only observed in relation to opportunistic infections (185).

9 Role of TNF in (auto-)immune responses, inflammation, and other pathophysiological phenomena

In an animal model of acute graft-versus-host disease, the histological changes could be prevented by injection of anti-TNF antibody (237). Also the mortality was reduced from 100 per cent to 30 per cent. In a retrospective study, it was shown that bone marrow transplantation patients with elevated serum TNF often developed major complications (238). In an experimental model system for heart transplantation in rats, evidence was obtained for synthesis of TNF in the rejected organ, while protection was achieved when TNF antibodies were given at the time of the transplantation (239). Renal allograft rejection has been correlated with raised TNF serum levels (240).

As part of the immune suppression therapy during the follow-up, OKT$_3$ antibody is often administered to renal transplantation patients. Ironically, however, this OKT$_3$ leads to release of TNF, which is the cause of significant patient distress (241). Presumably, this is due to T cells, which by their CD3 antigen interact with OKT$_3$ molecules bound via their Fc part to Fc receptors on monocytes; the resulting cross-linking then induces TNF synthesis.

In a rat model for ischaemia/reperfusion, there was clear evidence for synthesis of TNF, which reached a peak level about three hours post-reperfusion (239). The pathology of the liver, and also of the lung, was considerably improved by treatment with anti-TNF antibody. Furthermore, the adult respiratory distress syndrome (ARDS) may be linked to an ischaemic event and has a TNF component. In severe forms of ARDS, TNF, IL-1 and elastase in the broncho-alveolar fluid significantly increased during the first day of development of the clinical picture, and these levels subsequently decreased (222).

A TNF involvement is also suspected in a number of other auto-immune and inflammatory conditions. In the case of rheumatoid arthritis, TNF is often present in the synovial fluid, and sometimes even in the serum (242). TNF elicits secretion of collagenase from synovial cells and fibroblasts (175), and stimulates chondrocytes to degrade proteoglycan, while interfering with *de novo* synthesis (243). It may also be noted that IL-6 levels in the circulation are often elevated in patients with rheumatoid arthritis.

It is quite possible that TNF plays a role in demyelination and oligoden-drocyte toxicity in multiple sclerosis (244). It has also been suggested that TNF may be involved in type I diabetes; TNF plus IFNγ, but not either cytokine alone, induced HLA Class II expression on human β-islet cells and such an expression often marks a target for auto-immune responses (245). A careful study with non-obese, diabetic mice, however, did not reveal any contribution of TNF, at least in this model for auto-immune diabetes (246).

Patients with active psoriasis often have increased IL-6 levels in the psoriatic plaques, and even in their plasma (247, 248). The IL-6 may directly contribute to proliferation of the keratinocytes. Furthermore, patients with manic depression are usually treated chronically with lithium salt, and it is known that they often develop psoriasis or experience an exacerbation of this disease (249, 250). Considering that Li$^+$ has a remarkably strong synergy with TNF in induction of IL-6, this combination was tested by injection into the skin. Indeed, TNF plus Li$^+$ resulted in local IL-6 synthesis to levels far beyond those obtained with either agent alone. As this effect was only seen with TNF, and not with other cytokines, it seems quite possible that a low endogenous level of TNF (possibly induced), together with lithium salt, is a powerful trigger leading to IL-6-mediated psoriasis (251).

10   TNF and cancer

10.1   Role in cachexia

We have seen in Section 4.1 that TNF was independently discovered under the name 'cachectin' as a factor present in the serum of severely cachectic, trypanosome-infected animals. This factor was identified and purified on the basis of its inhibition of lipoprotein lipase activity. In view of its many proper-ties, it was proposed that TNF was a central mediator of wasting, both in chronic infectious diseases as well as in cancer patients (188). Cancer cachexia is so common that 50 per cent of the cancer patients have symptoms and signs of cachexia at the time of initial diagnosis (252). The characteristics of cachexia are weight loss, asthenia, anaemia, and loss of body protein and lipid. Various experimental lines of evidence indicate that cachexia is due to an unfavourable reaction of the host to the tumour. In experimental animals, removal of the tumour allows surviving animals to regain all weight which they had lost. When TNF is injected daily in mice and rats (253), there is a transient anorectic effect and no cachexia. In cancer cachexia, however, the state of anorexia persists.

There is good evidence from parabiotic experiments (two animals coupled so that they share a proportion of the circulation) that cancer-induced cachexia is due to factor(s) present in the serum (254). A number of tumour-derived factors have been shown to cause anorexia, such as serotonin and bombesin (the latter is often produced by small cell lung cancer). The question is whether TNF, for example induced by the host in response to its tumour, could be responsible for the cachectic effects. Mice treated on a daily basis with TNF, show anorexia for one or two days, but thereafter a state of tolerance sets in (255). By escalating the dose, Tracey *et al.* (256) could overcome the tolerance, and under these conditions TNF-induced cachexia was evident.

Chinese hamster ovary (CHO) cells, transfected to produce TNF constitutively, have been raised as a tumour in nude mice. This resulted in weight loss, lipid depletion, and earlier death as compared to animals bearing a tumour derived from non-transfected cells (257). These cells may have synthesized other factors in addition, which in concert with TNF could have been responsible for the observed phenomena. Also, TNF production levels of these CHO transfectants were very high, as compared, for example, with tumour cells which spontaneously had started to produce TNF. The TNF-CHO tumour-bearing animals had nanogram levels of TNF in their serum. On the other hand, although TNF assays have become very sensitive, no clear evidence has been found for enhanced, biologically active TNF levels in the sera of cachectic cancer patients.

Using TNF gene-transfected fibrosarcoma cells for tumour formation in nude mice, Vanhaesebroeck *et al.* (258) did not observe cachexia although there was a clear inverse correlation between the level of TNF expression and the rate of tumour growth.

In several studies, attempts were made to block the putative cachexia-inducing activity of TNF made in response to a tumour by passive immunization, but the results so far have been inconclusive (252). When the afore-mentioned, TNF-secreting CHO cells were injected in the brain, they caused an anorectic effect not seen in mice carrying the control tumour (259). This anorexia might have been induced directly at the level of the hypothalamus. When the same TNF-secreting cells were used to raise a tumour intramuscularly, there was no profound anorexia, but instead (after a much longer time) a more classical cachexia was observed (namely depletion of both protein and lipid, as well as anaemia). This observation that the outcome depends on the location of the tumour, suggests that factors released in response to a tumour, act as secondary mediators, which then would be responsible for the cachexia. TNF may play a key role in this induction, but possibly it may not be the only or even the major inducer.

10.2   Anti-cancer studies in animal model systems

In Section 4.1 it was described how, historically, anti-tumour activity has been studied, first with live bacteria, then with bacterial extracts, followed by purified LPS, and finally with recombinant TNF. The prototype assay system used for these studies involved a methylcholanthrene-A (MethA)-induced sarcoma in syngenic mice. This MethA tumour which is exquisitely sensitive to TNF. A single injection of 2 μg of TNF intraperitoneally or intravenously leads to a dramatic haemorrhagic necrosis and often to complete curing. TNF has to be injected seven to ten days after tumour inoculation. A newly formed, well developed vascular system with capillaries may be needed. The anti-tumour activity is undoubtedly indirect, as *in vitro* the MethA sarcoma cells are completely resistant to TNF, even in the presence of IFN. Intravascular coagulation in the tumour may be responsible for the therapeutic effect since the anti-coagulant, dicoumarol, inhibited the TNF action (260). An immune component may also be involved, as the haemorrhagic necrosis does not occur in a syngenic nude mouse system, or in mice depleted for T lymphocytes (261). Mice which had rejected the MethA sarcoma, became resistant to a re-challenge with the same tumour, but not to other, unrelated sarcomas (262). However, in contra-distinction to most human tumours, the MethA sarcoma is fairly immunogenic, and therefore the activation of a host immunity might perhaps not be generally applicable.

Williamson *et al.* reported in 1983 (69) that many malignant cells become selectively killed by the combination of TNF together with IFN and these results were amply confirmed and extended when the recombinant cytokines became available. *In vitro*, some malignant cells respond to TNF, but many more become susceptible to the cytotoxic action when IFN is also added. Under the same conditions, normal diploid cells are not affected (70, 177). The selective, direct effect of TNF and IFNγ could also be shown in organ culture; using pieces of heart tissue, challenged with B16 melanoma cells. After seven days treatment with the two cytokines, all malignant cells had disappeared, while the healthy tissue was unaffected (263).

The first *in vivo* study with syngenic tumours treated with homologous TNF and IFNγ was published by Brouckaert *et al.* (264). The tumour cells used were B16BL6, which are sensitive *in vitro* to the combination of TNF plus IFNγ, but not to TNF alone. A clear species specificity effect was observed. In the case of murine TNF, complete tumour regression could be obtained, with injection of the mTNF either paralesionally or intraperitoneally. With hTNF treatment, in contrast, complete regression was only obtained in combination with IFNγ a result reminiscent of the *in vitro* observations and suggesting direct anti-malignant cell activity. In the case of mTNF treatment, host-mediated effects were also involved. These must have been triggered by the species-specific mTNF receptor p75. In both series of experiments, however, the toxicity was very high, and only 20 to 30 per cent of the animals survived (most of which were cured). In a study involving a colon carcinoma-type, transplantable tumour in rats, a milder regimen of mTNF and recombinant IFNγ was used; a 50 per cent response rate was observed and all animals survived the treatment (265). An effective anti-tumour response was also reported for mice carrying a Friend erythroleukaemia tumour, although these cells are not responsive to TNF *in vitro*. Again this points to host-mediated effects (266).

For an effective anti-cancer therapy, it is necessary either to enhance anti-tumour efficacy, or lower general toxicity to increase the therapeutic index.

For some tumour cells there is a dramatic synergy between TNF and lithium chloride. This is also true *in vivo*, which is fortunate, because LiCl does not contribute to toxicity. Animals carrying tumours susceptible to the two agents, gave complete and lasting remissions when treated perilesionally with TNF plus LiCl with no lethality (131).

Experimental animals treated daily with low concentrations of LPS, become tolerant towards a normally lethal dose of LPS. Patton *et al.* (253) showed that daily treatment of rats with TNF also led to a state of tolerance. Under these conditions, some toxic effects were abrogated. Other effects, such as hypertriglyceridaemia and prostaglandin synthesis by splenocytes, still occurred in response to TNF (194, 267). Tolerized rats are resistant to a normally lethal dose of TNF, and are even protected against a lethal challenge with LPS (268). However, MethA sarcoma-bearing mice, which were rendered tolerant to TNF toxicity by daily injection of a sublethal, escalating dose of hTNF, no longer responded when a treatment dose was given (268). Takahashi *et al.*, in contrast, studied mice bearing a syngenic B16BL6 tumour (195). After tolerization for five to six days, a high, normally toxic, dose of TNF plus IFNγ could be administered perilesionally. The treatment was effective, the survival was 80 per cent and most animals were cured. The different outcomes of these studies are due to direct effects on the malignant cells by the combination of TNF plus IFNγ (195) rather than host-mediated effects (268).

Another system for studying anti-tumour responses involves xenografts derived from human cancer tissue carried in nude mice. Nearly all subcutaneous human tumour xenografts responded to hTNF therapy administered intratumorally. But only one out of seven regressed after intraperitoneal injections (269). In the case of human ovarian carcinoma xenografts growing intraperitoneally in nude mice, local intraperitoneal therapy with TNF and/or IFNγ was highly effective (depending on the tumour type) (270). TNF treatment induced the infiltration of inflammatory cells into the peritoneum and promoted the adhesion of tumour cells and their establishment as nodules below the mesothelial surface (271). We have mentioned in Section 4.2 that some tumour cells may synthesize TNF and may lead to tumour encapsulation (258), or to enhanced metastatic potential (272) depending on the tissue.

The interpretation of studies involving human xenografts in nude mice is complex, as these animals lack T lymphocytes. In addition, injected hTNF interacts with the TNF-R55 and TNF-R75 receptors on the tumour cells, but does not trigger the murine p75 receptor, which is suspected to have very important pathophysiological consequences (Section 4.5).

10.3   Clinical trials with TNF in human cancer patients

Many clinical trials have been initiated with TNF. In most of the phase I studies, TNF was injected intravenously, either as a bolus or by continuous infusion. Not unexpectedly, rather extensive, systemic toxicity was observed.

Fatigue, fever, chills, anorexia, headache, diarrhoea, nausea, and vomiting were noted, but were not dose-related. Similar effects had been observed after administration of other cytokines, such as interferons. The commoner, more serious and more specific dose-limiting toxicities were hypotension, hepato-toxicity, and thrombocytopaenia, in that order (190). In no case was there evidence for acceleration of cachexia.

In most studies, the maximum tolerated dose was only about 200 $\mu g/m^2$, except for a few studies, involving continuous infusion, where dose levels up to 500 $\mu g/m^2$ could be given. In neither phase I studies nor in limited phase II studies was there more than a very occasional response to the treatment. A few studies with the combination of TNF and IFNγ have been completed and the recommended dose was about 100 $\mu g/mv$ of hTNF and 200 $\mu g/mv$ of IFNγ (273). From recent animal experiments, the limitation of hypotension by NO synthesis blockers, or protection by tolerization would seem useful in humans and the doses used in the successful animal model studies, would indicate that much higher TNF levels are needed in humans in order to be effective. Indeed, in a limited number of studies where TNF could be injected in the tumour, a much higher success rate was achieved. Overall, for a number of different carcinomas, a response rate (complete and partial remission combined) of 42 per cent was obtained (190). In a study involving patients with refractory malignant ascites, TNF was administered by intra-peritoneal infusions; 22 out of 29 patients responded with a complete (viz. 16) or partial (viz. 6) resolution of their ascites (274).

There is still much scope for improvement. Adjuvant therapy can be developed, treatment protocols can be improved, and there are many indica-tions for useful synergistic activities, either with other cytokines or with other cancer drugs.

11 Summary

The gestation, birth, and explosive growth of our knowledge regarding (recom-binant) TNF have not been easy. The system is complex. Besides TNF, there is lymphotoxin which acts on the same receptors, but not always to the same extent. There are two TNF receptors with very different intracellular domains, and it is not yet known whether their purpose is cell specificity or signal specificity. The extracellular domains can easily be released in circulation, and the diagnostic potential which this represents, has still to be evaluated. TNF, in most of its activities, is indistinguishable from IL-1. Yet TNF, but not IL-1 is selectively toxic for many tumour cells. Especially the combination of treatment with TNF plus IFNγ exhibits this specificity for malignant cells. The exact role of IFN in this is unclear. The mechanism of TNF action on susceptible cells is slowly being elucidated. Mitochondria-derived, reactive oxygen species are involved. Why this is so toxic for many malignant cells, and not for normal cells, has still to be explained in detail, but the underlying molecular mechanisms certainly will require a better understanding of tumour cell biochemistry. Nearly all cells have TNF receptors, and their triggering usually results in activation of a particular set of genes. The pathway leading to this gene activation, is largely superimposable on that resulting in cytotoxicity.

Now that very sensitive tools are available to measure TNF and lymphotoxin, and their receptors, both at the protein and at the mRNA level, the involvement of these cytokines in an ever growing list of infectious and pathophysiological disease situations becomes more and more apparent. The TNF gene has presumably been conserved and improved in evolution, because its product protects the organism from some viral, bacterial, and parasitic infections. Over-production or lack of feedback controls can have dire consequences, such as in fatal cerebral malaria and septic shock. More and more, auto-immunity pathologies have been shown or are suspected to have TNF as one of its key components. These include rheumatoid arthritis, multiple sclerosis, psoriasis, ischaemia/reperfusion, and diabetes mellitus. The development of specific TNF inhibitors will open new approaches to treat these diseases.

Much hope had been placed in TNF as a selective anti-tumour agent. This optimism, however, rapidly evaporated when the many toxic effects of TNF became known. But the pendulum should not swing too far in the other direction. TNF, in combination with IFN, is still the most effective, natural, anti-malignant cell cytotoxic combination. Experiments in animal tumour model systems have shown that it is possible to develop appropriate protocols which enhance the anti-tumour activity of this pair of cytokines and reduce the toxic effects. Clinical trials in cancer patients have so far often used the most toxic approach, namely intravenous administration. Only in the case of direct intra-tumour therapy have promising clinical results been obtained. But pre-clinical research has taught us that there is much scope for improvement, and TNF may still find its place in the arsenal of effective anti-tumour agents. Possibly, by the end of this century, we may be able to achieve in a rational way, using well characterized molecules, the same successful anti-tumour therapies which were obtained by William B. Coley some hundred years ago.

References

1 Carswell, E. A., Old, L. J., Kassel, R. L., Green, S., Fiore, N., and Williamson, B. (1975). An endotoxin-induced serum factor that causes necrosis of tumours. *Proc. Natl. Acad. Sci. U.S.A.*, **72**, 3666–70.
2 Nauts, H. C. (1989). Bacteria and cancer—antagonisms and benefits. *Cancer Surveys*, **8**, 713–23.

3   Shwartzman, G. and Michailovsky, N. (1936). Phenomenon of local skin reactivity to bacterial filtrates in the treatment of mouse sarcoma. *Proc. Soc. Exp. Biol. Med.*, **34**, 323–5.

4   Gifford, G. E. and Flick, D. A. (1987). The natural production and release of TNF. In *Tumour necrosis factor and related cytotoxins* (Ciba Foundation Symposium 131) (ed. G. Bock. and J. Marsh), pp. 109–23. John Wiley and Sons, Chichester.

5   Pennica, D., Nedwin, G. E., Hayflick, J. S., Seeburg, P. H., Derynck, R., Palladino, M. A., Kohr, W. J., Aggarwal, B. B., and Goeddel, D. V. (1984). Human tumour necrosis factor: precursor structure, expression, and homology to lymphotoxin. *Nature*, **312**, 724–9.

6   Fiers, W. (1992). Precursor structures and structure/function analysis of TNF and lymphotoxin. In *Tumour necrosis factors: structure, function, and mechanism of action* (ed. B. B. Aggarwal and J. Vilček), pp. 79–92. Marcel Dekker, New York.

7   Beutler, B., Greenwald, D., Hulmes, J. D., Chang, M., Pan, Y. C., Mathison, J., Ulevitch, R., and Cerami, A. (1985). Identity of tumour necrosis factor and the macrophage-secreted factor cachectin. *Nature*, **316**, 552–4.

8   Beutler, B. and Cerami, A. (1988). Tumour necrosis, cachexia, shock, and inflammation: a common mediator. *Annu. Rev. Biochem.*, **57**, 505–18.

9   Fransen, L., Müller, R., Marmenout, A., Tavernier, J., Van der Heyden, J., Kawashima, E., Chollet, A., Tizard, R., Van Heuverswyn, H., Van Vliet, A., Ruysschaert, M. R., and Fiers, W. (1985). Molecular cloning of mouse tumour necrosis factor cDNA and its eukaryotic expression. *Nucleic Acids Res.*, **13**, 4417–29.

10 Rosenau, W. and Moon, H. D. (1961). Lysis of homologous cells by sensitized lymphocytes in tissue culture. *J. Natl. Canc. Inst.*, **27**, 471–83.

11 Ruddle, N. H. and Waksman, B. H. (1968). Cytotoxicity mediated by soluble antigen and lymphocytes in delayed hypersensitivity. III. Analysis of mechanism. *J. Exp. Med.*, **128**, 1267–79.

12 Granger, G. A. and Williams, T. W. (1968). Lymphocyte cytotoxicity *in vitro*: activation and release of a cytotoxic factor. *Nature*, **218**, 1253.

13 Granger, G. A., Yamamoto, R. S., Fair, D. S., and Hiserodt, J. C. (1978). The human lymphotoxin system: I. Physical-chemical heterogeneity of lymphotoxin molecules released by mitogen activated human lymphocytes *in vitro*. *Cell. Immunol.*, **38**, 388–402.

14 Aggarwal, B. B., Moffat, B., and Harkins, R. N. (1984). Human lymphotoxin. Production by a lymphoblastoid cell line, purification, and initial characterization. *J. Biol. Chem.*, **259**, 686–91.

15 Gray, P. W., Aggarwal, B. B., Benton, C. V., Bringman, T. S., Henzel, W. J., Jarrett, J. A., Leung, D. W., Moffat, B., Ng, P., Svedersky, L. P., Palladino, M. A., and Nedwin, G. E. (1984). Cloning and expression of cDNA for human lymphotoxin, a lymphokine with tumour necrosis activity. *Nature*, **312**, 721–4.

16 Ruff, M. R. and Gifford, G. E. (1981). Tumour necrosis factor. In *Lymphokines* Vol. 2. (ed. E. Pick), pp. 235–72. Academic Press, New York.

17 Old, L. J. (1990). Tumor necrosis factor. In *Tumour necrosis factor: structure, mechanism of action, role in disease and therapy* (ed. B. Bonavida and G. Granger), pp. 1–30. Karger, Basel.

18 Gifford, G. E. and Duckworth, D. H. (1991). Introduction to TNF and related lymphokines. *Biotherapy*, **3**, 103–11.

19   Matthews, N. (1978). Tumour necrosis factor from the rabbit. II. Production by monocytes. *Br. J. Cancer*, **38**, 310–15.

20   Männel, D. N., Moore, R. N., and Mergenhagen, S. E. (1980). Macrophages as a source of tumouricidal activity (tumour-necrotizing factor). *Infect. Immun.*, **30**, 523–30.

21   Matthews, N. (1981). Production of an anti-tumour cytotoxin by human monocytes. *Immunology*, **44**, 135–42.

22   Okusawa, S., Yancey, K. B., Van der Meer, J. W., Endres, S., Lonnemann, G., Hefter, K., Frank, M. M., Burke, J. F., Dinarello, C. A., and Gelfand, J. A. (1988). C5a stimulates secretion of tumour necrosis factor from human mononuclear cells *in vitro*. Comparison with secretion of interleukin-1β and interleukin-1α. *J. Exp. Med.*, **168**, 443–8.

23   Espevik, T., Figari, I. S., Shalaby, M. R., Lackides, G. A., Lewis, G. D., Shepard, H. M., and Palladino Jr, M. A. (1987). Inhibition of cytokine production by cyclosporin A and transforming growth factor-β. *J. Exp. Med.*, **166**, 571–6.

24   Libert, C., Van Bladel, S., Brouckaert, P., and Fiers, W. (1991). The influence of modulating substances on tumour necrosis factor and interleukin-6 levels after injection of murine tumour necrosis factor or lipopolysaccharide in mice. *J. Immunother.*, **10**, 227–35.

25   Marmenout, A., Fransen, L., Tavernier, J., Van der Heyden, J., Tizard, R., Kawashima, E., Shaw, A., Johnson, M. J., Semon, D., Müller, R., Ruysschaert, M. R., Van Vliet, A., and Fiers, W. (1985). Molecular cloning and expression of human tumour necrosis factor and comparison with mouse tumour necrosis factor. *Eur. J. Biochem.*, **152**, 515–22.

26   Wang, A. M., Creasey, A. A., Ladner, M. B., Lin, L. S., Strickler, J., Van Arsdell, J. N., Yamamoto, R., and Mark, D. F. (1985). Molecular cloning of the complementary DNA for human tumour necrosis factor. *Science*, **228**, 149–54.

27   Aderka, D., Holtmann, H., Toker, L., Hahr, T., and Wallach, D. (1986). Tumour necrosis factor induction by Sendai virus. *J. Immunol.*, **136**, 2938–42.

28   Otterlei, M., Østgaard, K., Skjåk-Bræk, G., Smidsrød, O., Soon-Shiong, P., and Espevik, T. (1991). Induction of cytokine production from human monocytes stimulated with alginate. *J. Immunother.*, **10**, 286–91.

29   Cuturi, M. C., Murphy, M., Costa-Giomi, M. P., Weinmann, R., Perussia, B., and Trinchieri, G. (1987). Independent regulation of tumour necrosis factor and lymphotoxin production by human peripheral blood lymphocytes. *J. Exp. Med.*, **165**, 1581–94.

30   Degliantoni, G., Murphy, M., Kobayashi, M., Francis, M. K., Perussia, B., and Trinchieri, G. (1985). Natural killer (NK) cell-derived haematopoietic colony-inhibiting activity and NK cytotoxic factor. Relationship with tumour necrosis factor and synergism with immune interferon. *J. Exp. Med.*, **162**, 1512–30.

31   Lieberman, A. P., Pitha, P. M., Shin, H. S., and Shin, M. L. (1989). Production of tumour necrosis factor and other cytokines by astrocytes stimulated with lipopolysaccharide or a neurotropic virus. *Proc. Natl. Acad. Sci. U.S.A.*, **86**, 6348–52.

32   Gordon, J. R. and Galli, S. J. (1990). Mast cells as a source of both pre-formed and immunologically inducible TNFα/cachectin. *Nature*, **346**, 274–6.

33   Lindemann, A., Riedel, D., Oster, W., Ziegler-Heitbrock, H. W., Mertelsmann, R., and Herrmann, F. (1989). Granulocyte macrophage colony-stimulating

factor induces cytokine secretion by human polymorphonuclear leucocytes. *J. Clin. Invest.*, **83**, 1308–12.

34 Warner, S. J. C. and Libby, P. (1989). Human vascular smooth muscle cells. Target for and source of tumour necrosis factor. *J. Immunol.*, **142**, 100–9.

35 Rubin, B. Y., Anderson, S. I., Sullivan, S. A., Williamson, B. D., Carswell, E. A., and Old, L. J. (1986). Non-haematopoietic cells selected for resistance to tumour necrosis factor produce tumour necrosis factor. *J. Exp. Med.*, **164**, 1350–5.

36 Vanhaesebroeck, B., Van Bladel, S., Lenaerts, A., Suffys, P., Beyaert, R., Lucas, R., Van Roy, F., and Fiers, W. (1991). Two discrete types of tumour necrosis factor-resistant cells derived from the same cell line. *Cancer Res.*, **51**, 2469–77.

37 Spriggs, D., Imamura, K., Rodriguez, C., Horiguchi, J., and Kufe, D. W. (1987). Induction of tumour necrosis factor expression and resistance in a human breast tumour cell line. *Proc. Natl. Acad. Sci. U.S.A.*, **84**, 6563–6.

38 Krönke, M., Hensel, G., Schlüter, C., Scheurich, P., Schütze, S., and Pfizenmaier, K. (1988). Tumour necrosis factor and lymphotoxin gene expression in human tumour cell lines. *Cancer Res.*, **48**, 5417–21.

39 Naylor, M. S., Malik, S. T. A., Stamp, G. W. H., Jobling, T., and Balkwill, F. R. (1990). *In situ* detection of tumour necrosis factor in human ovarian cancer specimens. *Eur. J. Cancer*, **26**, 1027–30.

40 Paul, N. L. and Ruddle, N. H. (1988). Lymphotoxin. *Annu. Rev. Immunol.*, **6**, 407–38.

41 Cherwinski, H. M., Schumacher, J. H., Brown, K. D., and Mosmann, T. R. (1987). Two types of mouse helper T cell clone. III. Further differences in lymphokine synthesis between T_H1 and T_H2 clones revealed by RNA hybridization, functionally monospecific bio-assays, and monoclonal antibodies. *J. Exp. Med.*, **166**, 1229–44.

42 Kobayashi, Y., Asada, M., and Osawa, T. (1987). Production of lymphotoxin and tumour necrosis factor by a T cell hybridoma. *Immunology*, **60**, 213–17.

43 Seow, H. F., Goh, C. R., Krishnan, L., and Porter, A. G. (1989). Bacterial expression, facile purification, and properties of recombinant human lymphotoxin (tumour necrosis factor beta). *Bio/Technology*, **7**, 363–8.

44 Itoh, H. A novel physiologically active polypeptide. *European Patent N° 0148311*, filed on July 5, 1984.

45 Scuderi, P. (1989). Suppression of human leucocyte tumour necrosis factor secretion by the serine protease inhibitor *p*-toluenesulfonyl-L-arginine methyl ester (TAME). *J. Immunol.*, **143**, 168–73.

46 Müller, R., Marmenout, A., and Fiers, W. (1986). Synthesis and maturation of recombinant human tumour necrosis factor in eukaryotic systems. *FEBS Lett.*, **197**, 99–104.

47 Cseh, K. and Beutler, B. (1989). Alternative cleavage of the cachectin/tumour necrosis factor pro-peptide results in a larger, inactive form of secreted protein. *J. Biol. Chem.*, **264**, 16256–60.

48 Decker, T., Lohmann-Matthes, M. L., and Gifford, G. E. (1987). Cell-associated tumour necrosis factor (TNF) as a killing mechanism of activated cytotoxic macrophages. *J. Immunol.*, **138**, 957–62.

49 Espevik, T. and Nissen-Meyer, J. (1987). Tumour necrosis factor-like activity on paraformaldehyde-fixed monocyte monolayers. *Immunology*, **61**, 443–8.

50 Kriegler, M., Perez, C., DeFay, K., Albert, I., and Lu, S. D. (1988). A novel form of TNF/cachectin is a cell surface cytotoxic transmembrane protein: ramifications for the complex physiology of TNF. *Cell*, **53**, 45–53.

51 Luettig, B., Decker, T., and Lohmann-Matthes, M. L. (1989). Evidence for the existence of two forms of membrane tumour necrosis factor: an integral protein and a molecule attached to its receptor. *J. Immunol.*, **143**, 4034–8.

52 Perez, C., Albert, I., DeFay, K., Zachariades, N., Gooding, L., and Riegler, M. (1990). A non-secretable cell surface mutant of tumour necrosis factor (TNF) kills by cell-to-cell contact. *Cell*, **63**, 251–8.

53 Arakawa, T. and Yphantis, D. A. (1987). Molecular weight of recombinant human tumour necrosis factor-α. *J. Biol. Chem.*, **262**, 7484–5.

54 Wingfield, P., Pain, R. H., and Craig, S. (1987). Tumour necrosis factor is a compact trimer. *FEBS Lett.*, **211**, 179–84.

55 Lewit-Bentley, A., Fourme, R., Kahn, R., Prangé, T., Vachette, P., Tavernier, J., Hauquier, G., and Fiers, W. (1988). Structure of tumour necrosis factor by X-ray solution scattering and preliminary studies by single crystal X-ray diffraction. *J. Mol. Biol.*, **199**, 389–92.

56 Sreekrishna, K., Nelles, L., Potenz, R., Cruze, J., Mazzaferro, P., Fish, W., Fuke, M., Holden, K., Phelps, D., Wood, P., and Parker, K. (1989). High-level expression, purification, and characterization of recombinant human tumour necrosis factor synthesized in the methylotrophic yeast *Pichia pastoris*. *Biochemistry*, **28**, 4117–25.

57 Fiers, W., Brouckaert, P., Devos, R., Fransen L., Leroux-Roels, G., Remaut, E., Suffys, P., Tavernier, J., Van der Heyden, J., and Van Roy, F. (1986). Lymphokines and monokines in anti-cancer therapy. In *Molecular biology of Homo sapiens* (Cold Spring Harbor Symposia on Quantitative Biology, Vol. 51), pp. 587–95. Cold Spring Harbor Laboratory, Cold Spring Harbor, NY.

58 Jones, E. Y., Stuart, D. I., and Walker, N. P. C. (1989). Structure of tumour necrosis factor. *Nature*, **338**, 225–8.

59 Eck, M. J. and Sprang, S. R. (1989). The structure of tumour necrosis factor-α at 2.6 Å resolution. Implications for receptor binding. *J. Biol. Chem.*, **264**, 17595–605.

60 Tavernier, J., Van Ostade, X., Hauquier, G., Prangé, T., Lasters, I., De Maeyer, M., Lewit-Bentley, A., and Fourme, R. (1989). Conserved residues of tumour necrosis factor and lymphotoxin constitute the framework of the trimeric structure. *FEBS Lett.*, **257**, 315–18.

61 Mark, D. F., Wang, A., and Levenson, C. (1987). Site-specific mutagenesis to modify the human tumour necrosis factor gene. *Methods Enzymol.*, **154**, 403–14.

62 Creasey, A. A., Doyle, L. V., Reynolds, M. T., Jung, T., Lin, L. S., and Vitt, C. R. (1987). Biological effects of recombinant human tumour necrosis factor and its novel muteins on tumour and normal cell lines. *Cancer Res.*, **47**, 145–9.

63 Yamagishi, J., Kawashima, H., Matsuo, N., Ohue, M., Yamayoshi, M., Fukui, T., Kotani, H., Furuta, R., Nakano, K., and Yamada, M. (1990). Mutational analysis of structure-activity relationships in human tumour necrosis factor alpha. *Protein Engin.*, **3**, 713–9.

64 Van Ostade, X., Tavernier, J., Prangé, T., and Fiers, W. (1991). Localization of the active site of human tumour necrosis factor (hTNF) by mutational analysis. *EMBO J.*, **10**, 827–36.

65 Nedwin, G. E., Naylor, S. L., Sakaguchi, A. Y., Smith, D., Jarrett-Nedwin, J., Pennica, D., Goeddel, D. V., and Gray, P. W. (1985). Human lymphotoxin and tumour necrosis factor genes: structure, homology, and chromosomal localization. *Nucleic Acids Res.*, **13**, 6361–73.

66 Spies, T., Morton, C. C., Nedospasov, S. A., Fiers, W., Pious, D., and Strominger, J. L. (1986). Genes for the tumour necrosis factors α and β are linked to the human major histocompatibility complex. *Proc. Natl. Acad. Sci. U.S.A.*, **83**, 8699–702.

67 Nedospasov, S. A., Hirt, B., Shakhov, A. N., Dobrynin, V. N., Kawashima, E., Accolla, R. S., and Jongeneel, C. V. (1986). The genes for tumour necrosis factor (TNF-alpha) and lymphotoxin (TNF-beta) are tandemly arranged on chromosome 17 of the mouse. *Nucleic Acids Res.*, **14**, 7713–25.

68 Müller, U., Jongeneel, C. V., Nedospasov, S. A., Fischer Lindahl, K., and Steinmetz, M. (1987). Tumour necrosis factor and lymphotoxin genes map close to H-2D in the mouse major histocompatibility complex. *Nature*, **325**, 265–7.

69 Williamson, B. D., Carswell, E. A., Rubin, B. Y., Prendergast, J. S., and Old, L. J. (1983). Human tumour necrosis factor produced by human B cell lines: synergistic cytotoxic interaction with human interferon. *Proc. Natl. Acad. Sci. U.S.A.*, **80**, 5397–401.

70 Fransen, L., Van der Heyden, J., Ruysschaert, R., and Fiers, W. (1986). Recombinant tumour necrosis factor: its effect and its synergism with interferon-γ on a variety of normal and transformed human cell lines. *Eur. J. Cancer Clin. Oncol.*, **22**, 419–26.

71 Tsujimoto, M., Feinman, R., and Vilček, J. (1986). Differential effects of type I IFN and IFN-γ on the binding of tumour necrosis factor to receptors in two human cell lines. *J. Immunol.*, **137**, 2272–6.

72 Unglaub, R., Maxeiner, B., Thoma, B., Pfizenmaier, K., and Scheurich, P. (1987). Down-regulation of tumour necrosis factor (TNF) sensitivity via modulation of TNF binding capacity by protein kinase C activators. *J. Exp. Med.*, **166**, 1788–97.

73 Scheurich, P., Kobrich, G., and Pfizenmaier, K. (1989). Antagonistic control of tumour necrosis factor receptors by protein kinases A and C. Enhancement of TNF receptor synthesis by protein kinase A and transmodulation of receptors by protein kinase *C. J. Exp. Med.*, **170**, 947–58.

74 Hohmann, H. P., Remy, R., Brockhaus, M., and Van Loon, A. P. G. M. (1989). Two different cell types have different major receptors for human tumour necrosis factor (TNFα). *J. Biol. Chem.*, **264**, 14927–34.

75 Stauber, G. B., Aiyer, R. A., and Aggarwal, B. B. (1988). Human tumour necrosis factor-α receptor. Purification by immunoaffinity chromatography and initial characterization. *J. Biol. Chem.*, **263**, 19098–104.

76 Brockhaus, M., Schoenfeld, H.-J., Schlaeger, E.-J., Hunziker, W., Lesslauer, W., and Loetscher, H. (1990). Identification of two types of tumour necrosis factor receptors on human cell lines by monoclonal antibodies. *Proc. Natl. Acad. Sci. U.S.A.*, **87**, 3127–31.

77 Loetscher, H., Schlaeger, E. J., Lahm, H.-W., Pan, Y.-C. E., Lesslauer, W., and Brockhaus, M. (1990). Purification and partial amino acid sequence analysis of two distinct tumour necrosis factor receptors from HL-60 cells. *J. Biol. Chem.*, **265**, 20131–8.

78 Loetscher, H., Pan, Y. E., Lahm, H. W., Gentz, R., Brockhaus, M., Tabuchi, H., and Lesslauer, W. (1990). Molecular cloning and expression of the human 55 kDa tumour necrosis factor receptor. *Cell*, **61**, 351–9.

79 Schall, T. J., Lewis, M., Koller, K. J., Lee, A., Rice, G. C., Wong, G. H. W., Gatanaga, T., Granger, G. A., Lentz, R., Raab, H., Kohr, W. J., and Goeddel,

D. V. (1990). Molecular cloning and expression of a receptor for human tumour necrosis factor. *Cell*, **61**, 361–70.

80   Smith, C. A., Davis, T., Anderson, D., Solam, L., Beckmann, M. P., Jerzy, R., Dower, S. K., Cosman, D., and Goodwin, R. G. (1990). A receptor for tumour necrosis factor defines an unusual family of cellular and viral proteins. *Science*, **248**, 1019–23.

81   Itoh, N., Yonehara, S., Ishii, A., Yonehara, M., Mizushima, S., Sameshima, M., Hase, A., Seto, Y., and Nagata, S. (1991). The polypeptide encoded by the cDNA for human cell surface antigen *Fas* can mediate apoptosis. *Cell*, **66**, 233–43.

82   Lewis, M., Tartaglia, L. A., Lee, A., Bennett, G. L., Rice, G. C., Wong, G. H. W., Chen, E. Y., and Goeddel, D. V. (1991). Cloning and expression of cDNAs for two distinct murine tumour necrosis factor receptors demonstrate one receptor is species specific. *Proc. Natl. Acad. Sci. U.S.A.*, **88**, 2830–4.

83   Goodwin, R. G., Anderson, D., Jerzy, R., Davis, T., Brannan, C. I., Copeland, N. G., Jenkins, N. A., and Smith, C. A. (1991). Molecular cloning and expression of the type I and type II murine receptors for tumour necrosis factor. *Mol. Cell. Biol.*, **11**, 3020–6.

84   Barrett, K., Taylor-Fishwick, D. A., Cope, A. P., Kissonerghis, A. M., Gray, P. W., Feldmann, M., and Foxwell, B. M. J. (1991). Cloning, expression, and cross-linking analysis of the murine p55 tumour necrosis factor receptor. *Eur. J. Immunol.*, **21**, 1649–56.

85   Seckinger, P., Isaaz, S., and Dayer, J. M. (1988). A human inhibitor of tumour necrosis factor alpha. *J. Exp. Med.*, **167**, 1511–16.

86   Peetre, C., Thysell, H., Grubb, A., and Olsson, I. (1988). A tumour necrosis factor binding protein is present in human biological fluids. *Eur. J. Haematol.*, **41**, 414–19.

87   Engelmann, H., Aderka, D., Rubinstein, M., Rotman, D., and Wallach, D. (1989). A tumour necrosis factor-binding protein purified to homogeneity from human urine protects cells from tumour necrosis factor toxicity. *J. Biol. Chem.*, **264**, 11974–80.

88   Gatanaga, T., Hwang, C., Kohr, W., Cappuccini, F., Lucci III, J. A., Jeffes, E. W. B., Lentz, R., Tomich, J., and Yamamoto, R. S. (1990). Purification and characterization of an inhibitor (soluble tumour necrosis factor receptor) for tumour necrosis factor and lymphotoxin obtained from the serum ultrafiltrates of human cancer patients. *Proc. Natl. Acad. Sci. U.S.A.*, **87**, 8781–4.

89   Olsson, I., Lantz, M., Nilsson, E., Peetre, C., Thysell, H., Grubb, A., and Adolf, G. (1989). Isolation and characterization of a tumour necrosis factor binding protein from urine. *Eur. J. Haematol.*, **42**, 270–5.

90   Engelmann, H., Novick, D., and Wallach, D. (1990). Two tumour necrosis factor-binding proteins purified from human urine. Evidence for immunological cross-reactivity with cell surface tumour necrosis factor receptors. *J. Biol. Chem.*, **265**, 1531–6.

91   Seckinger, P., Zhang, J. H., Hauptmann, B., and Dayer, J. M. (1990). Characterization of a tumour necrosis factor-α (TNFα) inhibitor: evidence of immunological cross-reactivity with the TNF receptor. *Proc. Natl. Acad. Sci. U.S.A.*, **87**, 5188–92.

92   Lantz, M., Gullberg, U., Nilsson, E., and Olsson, I. (1990). Characterization *in vitro* of a human tumour necrosis factor-binding protein: a soluble form of a tumour necrosis factor receptor. *J. Clin. Invest.*, **86**, 1396–402.

93 Nophar, Y., Kemper, O., Brakebusch, C., Engelmann, H., Zwang, R., Aderka, D., Holtmann, H., and Wallach, D. (1990). Soluble forms of tumour necrosis factor receptors (TNF-Rs). The cDNA for the type I TNF-R, cloned using amino acid sequence data of its soluble form, encodes both the cell surface and a soluble form of the receptor. *EMBO J.*, 9, 3269–78.

94 Porteu, F. and Nathan, C. (1990). Shedding of tumour necrosis factor receptors by activated human neutrophils. *J. Exp. Med.*, **172**, 599–607.

95 Loetscher, H., Steinmetz, M., and Lesslauer, W. (1991). Tumour necrosis factor: receptors and inhibitors. *Cancer Cells*, **3**, 221–6.

96 Wallach, D., Engelmann, H., Nophar, Y., Aderka, D., Kemper, O., Holtmann, H., and Brakebusch, C. (1990). Soluble and cell surface TNF receptors. *Third International Conference on tumour necrosis factor and related cytokines*. Makuhari (Chiba, Japan). Abstract N° I3–4.

97 Aderka, D., Engelmann, H., Maor, Y., Brakebusch, C., and Wallach, D. (1992). Stabilization of the bio-activity of tumour necrosis factor (TNF) by its soluble receptors. *J. Exp. Med.*, **175**, 323–9.

98 Spriggs, D. R., Sherman, M. L., Michie, H., Arthur, K. A., Imamura, K., Wilmore, D., Frei III, E., and Kufe, D. W. (1988). Recombinant human tumour necrosis factor administered as a 24 hour intravenous infusion. A phase I and pharmacologic study. *J. Natl. Cancer Inst.*, **80**, 1039–44.

99 Lantz, M., Malik, S., Slevin, M. L., and Olsson, I. (1990). Infusion of tumour necrosis factor (TNF) causes an increase in circulating TNF-binding protein in humans. **Cytokine**, **2**, 402–6.

100 Baglioni, C., Ruggiero, V., Latham, K., and Johnson, S. E. (1987). Cytocidal activity of tumour necrosis factor: protection by protease inhibitors. In *Tumour necrosis factor and related cytotoxins* (Ciba Foundation Symposium 131) (ed. G. Bock and J. Marsh), pp. 52–63. John Wiley and Sons, Chichester.

101 Scheurich, P., Thoma, B., Unglaub, R., and Pfizenmaier, K. (1988). Control of TNF sensitivity via regulation of TNF receptor expression. In *Tumor necrosis factor/cachectin and related cytokines* (ed. B. Bonavida, G. E. Gifford, H. Kirchner, and L. J. Old), pp. 38–44. Karger, Basel.

102 Mosselmans, R., Hepburn, A., Dumont, J. E., Fiers, W., and Galand, P. (1988). Endocytic pathway of recombinant murine tumour necrosis factor in L-929 cells. *J. Immunol.*, **141**, 3096–100.

103 Suffys, P., Beyaert, R., Van Roy, F., and Fiers, W. (1987). Reduced tumour necrosis factor-induced cytotoxicity by inhibitors of the arachidonic acid metabolism. *Biochem. Biophys. Res. Commun.*, **149**, 735–43.

104 Espevik, T., Brockhaus, M., Loetscher, H., Nonstad, U., and Shalaby, R. (1990). Characterization of binding and biological effects of monoclonal antibodies against a human tumour necrosis factor receptor. *J. Exp. Med.*, **171**, 415–26.

105 Bouchelouche, P. N., Bendtzen, K., Bak, S., and Nielsen, O. H. (1990). Recombinant human tumour necrosis factor increases cytosolic free calcium in murine fibroblasts and stimulates inositol phosphate formation in L-M and arachidonic acid release in 3T3 cells. *Cell. Sign.*, **2**, 479–87.

106 Hasegawa, Y. and Bonavida, B. (1989). Calcium-independent pathway of tumour necrosis factor-mediated lysis of target cells. *J. Immunol.*, **142**, 2670–6.

107 Hepburn, A., Demolle, D., Boeynaems, J. M., Fiers, W., and Dumont, G. E. (1988). Rapid phosphorylation of a 27 kDa protein induced by tumour necrosis factor. *FEBS Lett.*, **227**, 175–8.

108   Schütze, S., Scheurich, P., Pfizenmaier, K., and Krönke, M. (1989). Tumour necrosis factor signal transduction: tissue-specific serine phosphorylation of a 26 kDa cytosolic protein. *J. Biol. Chem.*, **264**, 3562–7.

109   Marino, M. W., Pfeffer, L. M., Guidon Jr, P. T., and Donner, D. B. (1989). Tumour necrosis factor induces phosphorylation of a 28 kDa mRNA cap-binding protein in human cervical carcinoma cells. *Proc. Natl. Acad. Sci. U.S.A.*, **86**, 8417–21.

110   Zhang, Y., Lin, J.-X., Yip, Y. K., and Vilček, J. (1988). Enhancement of cAMP levels and of protein kinase activity by tumour necrosis factor and interleukin-1 in human fibroblasts: role in the induction of interleukin-6. *Proc. Natl. Acad. Sci. U.S.A.*, **85**, 6802–5.

111   Espevik, T. and Nissen-Meyer, J. (1986). A highly sensitive cell line, WEHI 164 clone 13, for measuring cytotoxic factor/tumour necrosis factor from human monocytes. *J. Immunol. Methods*, **95**, 99–105.

112   Tada, H., Shiho, O., Kuroshima, K., Koyama, M., and Tsukamoto, K. (1986). An improved colorimetric assay for interleukin-2. *J. Immunol. Methods*, **93**, 157–65.

113   Wallach, D. (1984). Preparations of lymphotoxin induce resistance to their own cytotoxic effect. *J. Immunol.*, **132**, 2464–9.

114   Matthews, N., Neale, M. L., Jackson, S. K., and Stark, J. M. (1987). Tumour cell killing by tumour necrosis factor: inhibition by anaerobic conditions, free-radical scavengers, and inhibitors of arachidonate metabolism. *Immunology*, **62**, 153–5.

115   Matthews, N. (1983). Anti-tumour cytotoxin produced by human monocytes: studies on its mode of action. *Br. J. Cancer*, **48**, 405–10.

116   Zimmerman, R. J., Chan, A., and Leadon, S. A. (1989). Oxidative damage in murine tumour cells treated *in vitro* by recombinant human tumour necrosis factor. *Cancer Res.*, **49**, 1644–8.

117   Wong, G. H. W., and Goeddel, D. V. (1988). Induction of manganous superoxide dismutase by tumour necrosis factor: possible protective mechanism. *Science*, **241**, 941–4.

118   Wong, G. H. W., Elwell, J. H., Oberley, L. W., and Goeddel, D. V. (1989). Manganous superoxide dismutase is essential for cellular resistance to cytotoxicity of tumour necrosis factor. *Cell*, **58**, 923–31.

119   Oberley, L. W. and Buettner, G. R. (1979). Role of superoxide dismutase in cancer: a review. *Cancer Res.*, **39**, 1141–9.

120   Yamauchi, N., Kuriyama, H., Watanabe, N., Neda, H., Maeda, M., and Niitsu, Y. (1989). Intracellular hydroxyl radical production induced by recombinant human tumour necrosis factor and its implication in the killing of tumour cells *in vitro*. *Cancer Res.*, **49**, 1671–5.

121   Lancaster Jr, J. R., Laster, S. M., and Gooding, L. R. (1989). Inhibition of target cell mitochondrial electron transfer by tumour necrosis factor. *FEBS Lett.*, **248**, 169–74.

122   Schulze-Osthoff, K., Bakker, A. C., Vanhaesebroeck, B., Beyaert, R., Jacob, W. A., and Fiers, W. (1992). Cytotoxic activity of tumour necrosis factor is mediated by early damage of mitochondrial functions. Evidence for the involvement of mitochondrial radical generation. *J. Biol. Chem.*, **267**, 5317–23.

123   Schütze, S., Nottrott, S., Pfizenmaier, K., and Krönke, M. (1990). Tumour necrosis factor signal transduction. Cell-type-specific activation and translocation of protein kinase C. *J. Immunol.*, **144**, 2604–8.

124 Beyaert, R., Schulze-Osthoff, K., Van Roy, F., and Fiers, W. (1991). Lithium chloride potentiates tumour necrosis factor-induced and interleukin-1-induced cytokine and cytokine receptor expression. *Cytokine*, **3**, 284–91.

125 Suffys, P., Beyaert, R., De Valck, D., Vanhaesebroeck, B., Van Roy, F., and Fiers, W. (1991). Tumour necrosis factor-mediated cytotoxicity is correlated with phospholipase A_2 activity, but not with arachidonic acid release per se. *Eur. J. Biochem.*, **195**, 465–75.

126 Van Kuijk, F. J. G. M., Sevanian, A., Handelman, G. J., and Dratz, E. A. (1987). A new role for phospholipase A_2: protection of membranes from lipid peroxidation damage. *Trends Biochem. Sci.*, **12**, 31–4.

127 Hepburn, A., Boeynaems, J. M., Fiers, W., and Dumont, J. E. (1987). Modulation of tumour necrosis factor-α cytotoxicity in L929 cells by bacterial toxins, hydrocortisone, and inhibitors of arachidonic acid metabolism. *Biochem. Biophys. Res. Commun.*, **149**, 815–22.

128 Ruggiero, V., Johnson, S. E., and Baglioni, C. (1987). Protection from tumour necrosis factor cytotoxicity by protease inhibitors. *Cell. Immunol.*, **107**, 317–25.

129 Beyaert, R., Suffys, P., Van Roy, F., and Fiers, W. (1987). Inhibition of TNF cytotoxicity by protease inhibitors. *Immunobiology*, **175**, 3.

130 Suffys, P., Beyaert, R., Van Roy, F., and Fiers, W. (1988). Involvement of a serine protease in tumour necrosis factor-mediated cytotoxicity. *Eur. J. Biochem.*, **178**, 257–65.

131 Beyaert, R., Vanhaesebroeck, B., Suffys, P., Van Roy, F., and Fiers, W. (1989). Lithium chloride potentiates tumour necrosis factor-mediated cytotoxicity *in vitro* and *in vivo*. *Proc. Natl. Acad. Sci. U.S.A.*, **86**, 9494–8.

132 Palombella, V. J. and Vilček, J. (1989). Mitogenic and cytotoxic actions of tumour necrosis factor in BALB/c 3T3 cells. Role of phospholipase activation. *J. Biol. Chem.*, **264**, 18128–36.

133 Larrick, J. W. and Wright, S. C. (1990). Cytotoxic mechanism of tumour necrosis factor-α. *FASEB J.*, **4**, 3215–23.

134 Schmid, D. S., Hornung, R., McGrath, K. M., Paul, N., and Ruddle, N. H. (1987). Target cell DNA fragmentation is mediated by lymphotoxin and tumour necrosis factor. *Lymphokine Res.*, **6**, 195–202.

135 Dealtry, G. B., Naylor, M. S., Fiers, W., and Balkwill, F. R. (1987). DNA fragmentation and cytotoxicity caused by tumour necrosis factor is enhanced by interferon-γ. *Eur. J. Immunol.*, **17**, 689–93.

136 Rubin, B. Y., Smith, L. J., Hellermann, G. R., Lunn, R. M., Richardson, N. K., and Anderson, S. L. (1988). Correlation between the anti-cellular and DNA fragmenting activities of tumour necrosis factor. *Cancer Res.*, **48**, 6006–10.

137 Elias, L., Moore, P. B., and Rose, S. M. (1988). Tumour necrosis factor induced DNA fragmentation of HL-60 cells. *Biochem. Biophys. Res. Commun.*, **157**, 963–9.

138 Agarwal, S., Drysdale, B.-E., and Shin, H. S. (1988). Tumour necrosis factor-mediated cytotoxicity involves ADP ribosylation. *J. Immunol.*, **140**, 4187–92.

139 Browning, J. and Ribolini, A. (1989). Studies on the differing effects of tumour necrosis factor and lymphotoxin on the growth of several human tumour lines. *J. Immunol.*, **143**, 1859–67.

140 Brenner, D. A., O' Hara, M., Angel, P., Chojkier, M., and Karin, M. (1989). Prolonged activation of *jun* and collagenase genes by tumour necrosis factor-α. *Nature*, **337**, 661–3.

141 Haliday, E. M., Ramesha, C. S., and Ringold, G. (1991). TNF induces *c-fos* via a novel pathway requiring conversion of arachidonic acid to a lipoxygenase metabolite. *EMBO J.*, **10**, 109–15.

142 Lenardo, M. J. and Baltimore, D. (1989). NFκB: a pleiotropic mediator of inducible and tissue-specific gene control. *Cell*, **58**, 227–9.

143 Urban, M. B., Schreck, R., and Baeuerle, P. A. (1991). NFκB contacts DNA by a heterodimer of the p50 and p65 subunit. *EMBO J.*, **10**, 1817–25.

144 Israël, A., Le Bail, O., Hatat, D., Piette, J., Kieran, M., Logeat, F., Wallach, D., Fellous, M., and Kourilsky, P. (1989). TNF stimulates expression of mouse MHC Class I genes by inducing an NFκB-like enhancer binding activity which displaces constitutive factors. *EMBO J.*, **8**, 3793–800.

145 Libermann, T. A. and Baltimore, D. (1990). Activation of interleukin-6 gene expression through the NFκB transcription factor. *Mol. Cell. Biol.*, **10**, 2327–34.

146 Zhang, Y., Lin, J.-X., and Vilček, J. (1990). Interleukin-6 induction by tumour necrosis factor and interleukin-1 in human fibroblasts involves activation of a nuclear factor binding to a κB-like sequence. *Mol. Cell. Biol.*, **10**, 3818–23.

147 Shimizu, H., Mitomo, K., Watanabe, T., Okamoto, S., and Yamamoto, K. (1990). Involvement of a NFκB-like transcription factor in the activation of the interleukin-6 gene by inflammatory lymphokines. *Mol. Cell. Biol.*, **10**, 561–8.

148 Hohmann, H.-P., Remy, R., Pöschl, B., and Van Loon, A. P. G. M. (1990). Tumour necrosis factors-α and -β bind to the same two types of tumour necrosis factor receptors and maximally activate the transcription factor NFκB at low receptor occupancy and within minutes after receptor binding. *J. Biol. Chem.*, **265**, 15183–8.

149 Hohmann, H.-P., Brockhaus, M., Baeuerle, P. A., Remy, R., Kolbeck, R., and Van Loon, A. P. G. M. (1990). Expression of the types A and B tumour necrosis factor (TNF) receptors is independently regulated, and both receptors mediate activation of the transcription factor NFκB. TNFα is not needed for induction of a biological effect via TNF receptors. *J. Biol. Chem.*, **265**, 22409–17.

150 Hohmann, H.-P., Remy, R., Scheidereit, C., and Van Loon, A. P. G. M. (1991). Maintenance of NFκB activity is dependent on protein synthesis and the continuous presence of external stimuli. *Mol. Cell. Biol.*, **11**, 259–66.

151 Meyer, R., Hatada, E. N., Hohmann, H.-P., Haiker, M., Bartsch, C., Röthlisberger, U., Lahm, H.-W., Schlaeger, E. J., Van Loon, A. P. G. M., and Scheidereit, C. (1991). Cloning of the DNA-binding subunit of human nuclear factor κB: the level of its mRNA is strongly regulated by phorbol ester or tumour necrosis factor-α. *Proc. Natl. Acad. Sci. U.S.A.*, **88**, 966–70.

152 Lowenthal, J. W., Ballard, D. W., Bogerd, H., Böhnlein, E., and Greene, W. C. (1989). Tumour necrosis factor-α activation of the IL-2 receptor-α gene involves the induction of κB-specific DNA binding proteins. *J. Immunol.*, **142**, 3121–8.

153 Hohmann, H.-P., Kolbeck, R., Remy, R., and Van Loon, A. P. G. M. (1991). Cyclic AMP-independent activation of transcription factor NFκB in HL-60 cells by tumour necrosis factors α and β. *Mol. Cell. Biol.*, **11**, 2315–18.

154 Feuillard, J., Gouy, H., Bismuth, G., Lee, L. M., Debré, P., and Körner, M. (1991). NFκB activation by tumour necrosis factor-α in the Jurkat T cell line is

independent of protein kinase A, protein kinase C, and Ca^{2+} regulated kinases. *Cytokine*, **3**, 257–65.

155   Schreck, R., Rieber, P., and Baeuerle, P. A. (1991). Reactive oxygen intermediates as apparently widely used messengers in the activation of the NFκB transcription factor and HIV-1. *EMBO J.*, **10**, 2247–58.

156   Vandevoorde, V., Haegeman, G., and Fiers, W. (1991). Tumour necrosis factor-induced interleukin-6 expression and cytoxicity follow a common signal transduction pathway in L929 cells. *Biochem. Biophys. Res. Commun.*, **178**, 993–1001.

157   Collins, T., Lapierre, L. A., Fiers, W., Strominger, J. L., and Pober, J. S. (1986). Recombinant human tumour necrosis factor increases mRNA levels and surface expression of HLA-A, B antigens in vascular endothelial cells and dermal fibroblasts *in vitro*. *Proc. Natl. Acad. Sci. U.S.A.*, **83**, 446–50.

158   Kurt-Jones, E. A., Fiers, W., and Pober, J. S. (1987). Membrane interleukin-1 induction on human endothelial cells and dermal fibroblasts. *J. Immunol.*, **139**, 2317–24.

159   Pober, J. S. and Cotran, R. S. (1990). The role of endothelial cells in inflammation. *Transplantation*, **50**, 537–44.

160   Bussolino, F., Camussi, G., and Baglioni, C. (1988). Synthesis and release of platelet activating factor by human vascular endothelial cells treated with tumour necrosis factor or interleukin-1α. *J. Biol. Chem.*, **263**, 11856–61.

161   Kilbourn, R. G. and Belloni, P. (1990). Endothelial cell production of nitrogen oxides in response to interferon-γ in combination with tumour necrosis factor, interleukin-1, or endotoxin. *J. Natl. Cancer Inst.*, **82**, 772–6.

162   Robaye, B., Mosselmans, R., Fiers, W., Dumont, J. E., and Galand, P. (1991). Tumour necrosis factor induces apoptosis (programmed cell death) in normal endothelial cells *in vitro*. *Am. J. Pathol.*, **138**, 447–53.

163   Leibovich, S. J., Polverini, P. J., Shepard, H. M., Wiseman, D. M., Shively, V., and Nuseir, N. (1987). Macrophage-induced angiogenesis is mediated by tumour necrosis factor-α. *Nature*, **329**, 630–2.

164   Gamble, J. R., Harlan, J. M., Klebanoff, S. J., and Vadas, M. A. (1985). Stimulation of the adherence of neutrophils to umbilical vein endothelium by human recombinant tumour necrosis factor. *Proc. Natl. Acad. Sci. U.S.A.*, **82**, 8667–71.

165   Bevilacqua, M. P., Wheeler, M. E., Pober, J. S., Fiers, W., Mendrick, D. L., Cotran, R. S., and Gimbrone, M. A. (1987). Endothelial-dependent mechanisms of leucocyte adhesion: regulation by interleukin-1 and tumour necrosis factor. In *Leukocyte emigration and its sequelae* (ed. H. Z. Movat), pp. 79–93. Karger, Basel.

166   Shalaby, M. R., Aggarwal, B. B., Rinderknecht, E., Svedersky, L. P., Finkle, B. S., and Palladino Jr, M. A. (1985). Activation of human polymorphonuclear neutrophil functions by interferon-γ and tumour necrosis factor. *J. Immunol.*, **135**, 2069–73.

167   Larrick, J. W., Graham, D., Toy, K., Lin, L. S., Senyk, G., and Fendly, B. M. (1987). Recombinant tumour necrosis factor causes activation of human granulocytes. *Blood*, **69**, 640–4.

168   Scheurich, P., Thoma, B., Ücer, U., and Pfizenmaier, K. (1987). Immunoregulatory activity of recombinant human tumour necrosis factor (TNF)-α: induction of TNF receptors on human T cells and TNFα-mediated enhancement of T cell responses. *J. Immunol.*, **138**, 1786–90.

169   Yokota, S., Geppert, T. D., and Lipsky, P. E. (1988). Enhancement of antigen and mitogen-induced human T lymphocyte proliferation by tumour necrosis factor-α. *J. Immunol.*, **140**, 531–6.

170   Ehrke, M. J., Ho, R. L. X., and Hori, K. (1988). Species-specific TNF induction of thymocyte proliferation. *Cancer Immunol. Immunother.*, **27**, 103–8.

171   Plaetinck, G., Declercq, W., Tavernier, J., Nabholz, M., and Fiers, W. (1987). Recombinant tumour necrosis factor can induce interleukin-2 receptor expression and cytolytic activity in a rat × mouse T cell hybrid. *Eur. J. Immunol.*, **17**, 1835–8.

172   Ranges, G. E., Bombara, M. P., Aiyer, R. A., Rice, G. G., and Palladino Jr, M. A. (1989). Tumor necrosis factor-α as a proliferative signal for an IL-2-dependent T cell line: strict species specificity of action. *J. Immunol.*, **142**, 1203–8.

173   Jelinek, D. F. and Lipsky, P. E. (1987). Enhancement of human B cell proliferation and differentiation by tumour necrosis factor-α and interleukin-1. *J. Immunol.*, **139**, 2970–6.

174   Kehrl, J. H., Miller, A., and Fauci, A. S. (1987). Effect of tumour necrosis factor-α on mitogen-activated human B cells. *J. Exp. Med.*, **166**, 786–91.

175   Dayer, J. M., Beutler, B., and Cerami, A. (1985). Cachectin/tumour necrosis factor stimulates collagenase and prostaglandin E_2 production by human synovial cells and dermal fibroblasts. *J. Exp. Med.*, **162**, 2163–8.

176   Fiers, W., Beyaert, R., Brouckaert, P., Everaerdt, B., Grooten, J., Haegeman, G., Libert, C., Suffys, P., Takahashi, N., Tavernier, J., Van Bladel, S., Vanhaesebroeck, B., Van Ostade, X., and Van Roy, F. (1989). Tumour necrosis factor and interleukin-6: structure and mechanism of action of the molecular, cellular, and *in vivo* level. In *Vectors as tools for the study of normal and abnormal growth and differentiation* (NATO ASI Series, Vol. H 34). (ed. H. Lother, R. Dernick, and W. Ostertag), pp. 229–40. Springer, Berlin.

177   Sugarman, B. J., Aggarwal, B. B., Hass, P. E., Figari, I. S., Palladino Jr, M. A., and Shepard, H. M. (1985). Recombinant human tumour necrosis factor-α: effects on proliferation of normal and transformed cells *in vitro*. *Science*, **230**, 943–5.

178   Vilček, J., Palombella, V. J., Henriksen-DeStefano, D., Swenson, C., Feinman, R., Hirai, M., and Tsujimoto, M. (1986). Fibroblast growth enhancing activity of tumour necrosis factor and its relationship to other polypeptide growth factors. *J. Exp. Med.*, **163**, 632–43.

179   Kohase, M., Henriksen-DeStefano, D., May, L. T., Vilček, J., and Sehgal, P. B. (1986). Induction of β_2-interferon by tumour necrosis factor: a homeostatic mechanism in the control of cell proliferation. *Cell*, **45**, 659–66.

180   Defilippi, P., Poupart, P., Tavernier, J., Fiers, W., and Content, J. (1987). Induction and regulation of mRNA encoding 26 kDa protein in human cell lines treated with recombinant human tumour necrosis factor. *Proc. Natl. Acad. Sci. U.S.A.*, **84**, 4557–61.

181   Le, J. M., Weinstein, D., Gubler, U., and Vilček, J. (1987). Induction of membrane-associated interleukin-1 by tumour necrosis factor in human fibroblasts. *J. Immunol.*, **138**, 2137–42.

182   Zhang, Y., Lin, J.-X., and Vilček, J. (1988). Synthesis of interleukin-6 (interferonβ_2/B cell stimulatory factor 2) in human fibroblasts is triggered by an increase in intracellular cyclic AMP. *J. Biol. Chem.*, **263**, 6177–82.

183 Piguet, P. F., Collart, M. A., Grau, G. E., Sappino, A.-P., and Vassalli, P. (1990). Requirement of tumour necrosis factor for development of silica-induced pulmonary fibrosis. *Nature*, **344**, 245–7.

184 Beutler, B., Mahoney, J., Le Trang, N., Pekala, P., and Cerami, A. (1985). Purification of cachectin, a lipoprotein lipase-suppressing hormone secreted by endotoxin-induced RAW 264.7 cells. *J. Exp. Med.*, **161**, 984–95.

185 Grunfeld, C. and Feingold, K. R. (1991). The metabolic effects of tumour necrosis factor and other cytokines. *Biotherapy*, **3**, 143–58.

186 Fried, S. K. and Zechner, R. (1989). Cachectin/tumour necrosis factor decreases human adipose tissue lipoprotein lipase mRNA levels, synthesis, and activity. *J. Lipid Res.*, **30**, 1917–23.

187 Sherry, B. and Cerami, A. (1988). Cachectin/tumour necrosis factor exerts endocrine, paracrine, and autocrine control of inflammatory responses. *J. Cell Biol.*, **107**, 1269–77.

188 Beutler, B. and Cerami, A. (1986). Cachectin and tumour necrosis factor as two sides of the same biological coin. *Nature,* **320**, 584–8.

189 Ferraiolo, B. L., Moore, J. A., Crase, D., Gribling, P., Wilking, H., and Baughman, R. A. (1988). Pharmacokinetics and tissue distribution of recombinant human tumour necrosis factor-α in mice. *Drug Metab. Dispos.*, **16**, 270–5.

190 Taguchi, T. and Sohmura, Y. (1991). Clinical studies with TNF. *Biotherapy*, **3**, 177–86.

191 Dinarello, C. A., Cannon, J. G., Wolff, S. M., Bernheim, H. A., Beutler, B., Cerami, A., Figari, I. S., Palladino Jr, M. A., and O'Connor, J. V. (1986). Tumour necrosis factor (cachectin) is an endogenous pyrogen and induces production of interleukin-1. *J. Exp. Med.*, **163**, 1433–50.

192 Rothwell, N. J. (1990). Mechanisms of the pyrogenic actions of cytokines. *Eur. Cytok. Network*, **1**, 211–13.

193 Kettelhut, I. C., Fiers, W., and Goldberg, A. L. (1987). The toxic effects of tumour necrosis factor *in vivo* and their prevention by cyclo-oxygenase inhibitors. *Proc. Natl. Acad. Sci. U.S.A.*, **84**, 4273–77.

194 Grunfeld, C., Wilking, H., Neese, R., Gavin, L. A., Moser, A. H., Gulli, R., Serio, M. K., and Feingold, K. R. (1989). Persistence of the hypertriglyceridaemic effect of tumour necrosis factor despite development of tachyphylaxis to its anorectic/cachectic effects in rats. *Cancer Res.*, **49**, 2554–60.

195 Takahashi, N., Brouckaert, P., and Fiers, W. (1991). Induction of tolerance allows separation of lethal and anti-tumour activities of tumour necrosis factor in mice. *Cancer Res.*, **51**, 2366–72.

196 Weinberg, J. R., Wright, D. J. M., and Guz, A. (1988). Interleukin-1 and tumour necrosis factor cause hypotension in the conscious rabbit. *Clin. Sci.*, **75**, 251–5.

197 Schiller, J. H., Storer, B. E., Witt, P. L., Alberti, D., Tombes, M. B., Arzoomanian, R., Proctor, R. A., McCarthy, D., Brown, R. R., Voss, S. D., Remick, S. C., Grem, J. L., Borden, E. C., and Trump, D. L. (1991). Biological and clinical effects of intravenous tumour necrosis factor-α administered three times weekly. *Cancer Res.*, **51**, 1651–8.

198 Kilbourn, R. G., Gross, S. S., Jubran, A., Adams, J., Griffith, O. W., Levi, R., and Lodato, R. F. (1990). N^G-methyl-L-arginine inhibits tumour necrosis factor-induced hypotension: implications for the involvement of nitric oxide. *Proc. Natl. Acad. Sci. U.S.A.*, **87**, 3629–32.

199 Busse, R. and Mülsch, A. (1990). Induction of nitric oxide synthase by cyto-
     kines in vascular smooth muscle cells. *FEBS Lett.*, **275**, 87–90.
200 Everaerdt, B., Brouckaert, P., Shaw, A., and Fiers, W. (1989). Four different
     interleukin-1 species sensitize to the lethal action of tumour necrosis factor.
     Biochem. Biophys. Res. Commun., **163**, 378–85.
201 Brouckaert, P. G., Everaerdt, B., Libert, C., Takahashi, N., and Fiers, W.
     (1989). Species specificity and involvement of other cytokines in endotoxic shock
     action of recombinant tumour necrosis factor in mice. *Agents Actions*, **26**, 196–8.
202 Brouckaert, P., Libert, C., Everaerdt, B., and Fiers, W. (1992). Selective species
     specificity of tumour necrosis factor for toxicity in the mouse. *Lymphokine
     Cytokine Res.*, **11**, 193–6.
203 Okusawa, S., Gelfand, J. A., Ikejima, T., Connolly, R. J., and Dinarello,
     C. A. (1988). Interleukin-1 induces a shock-like state in rabbits. Synergism with
     tumour necrosis factor and the effect of cyclo-oxygenase inhibition. *J. Clin.
     Invest.*, **81**, 1162–72.
204 Waage, A. and Espevik, T. (1988). Interleukin-1 potentiates the lethal effect of
     tumour necrosis factor α/cachectin in mice. *J. Exp. Med.*, **167**, 1987–92.
205 Wallach, D., Holtmann, H., Engelmann, H., and Nophar, Y. (1988). Sensitiza-
     tion and desensitization to lethal effects of tumour necrosis factor and IL-1.
     J. Immunol., **140**, 2994–9.
206 Libert, C., Van Bladel, S., Brouckaert, P., Shaw, A., and Fiers, W. (1991).
     Involvement of the liver, but not of IL-6, in IL-1-induced desensitization to the
     lethal effects of tumour necrosis factor. *J. Immunol.*, **146**, 2625–32.
207 Lehmann, V., Freudenberg, M. A., and Galanos, C. (1987). Lethal toxicity of
     lipopolysaccharide and tumour necrosis factor in normal and D-galactosamine
     treated mice. *J. Exp. Med.*, **165**, 657–63.
208 Starnes Jr, H. F., Pearce, M. K., Tewari, A., Yim, J. H., Zou, J.-C., and Abrams,
     J. S. (1990). Anti-IL-6 monoclonal antibodies protect against lethal *Escherichia
     coli* infection and lethal tumour necrosis factor-α challenge in mice. *J. Immunol.*,
     145, 4185–91.
209 Hirano, T., Akira, S., Taga, T., and Kishimoto, T. (1990). Biological and clinical
     aspects of interleukin-6. *Immunol. Today*, **11**, 443–9.
210 Matsuda, T. and Hirano, T. (1990). Interleukin-6 (IL-6). *Biotherapy*, **2**, 363–73.
211 Van Snick, J. (1990). Interleukin-6: an overview. *Annu. Rev. Immunol.*, **8**,
     253–78.
212 Wolvekamp, M. C. J., and Marquet, R. L. (1990). Interleukin-6: historical
     background, genetics, and biological significance. *Immunol. Lett.*, **24**, 1–10.
213 Hirano, T. (1991). Interleukin-6. In *The cytokine handbook* (ed. A. W. Thomson),
     pp. 169–90. Academic Press, London.
214 Brouckaert, P., Spriggs, D. R., Demetri, G., Kufe, D. W., and Fiers, W. (1989).
     Circulating interleukin-6 during a continuous infusion of tumour necrosis factor
     and interferon-γ. *J. Exp. Med.*, **169**, 2257–62.
215 Libert, C., Brouckaert, P., Shaw, A., and Fiers, W. (1990). Induction of
     interleukin-6 by human and murine recombinant interleukin-1 in mice. *Eur.
     J. Immunol.*, **20**, 691–4.
216 Brouckaert, P., Everaerdt, B., and Fiers, W. (1992). The glucocorticoid anta-
     gonist RU38486 mimics IL-1 in its sensitization to the lethal and IL-6-inducing
     properties of TNF. *Eur. J. Immunol.*, **22**, 981–6.
217 Playfair, J. H. L., Taverne, J., and Matthews, N. (1984). What is tumour
     necrosis factor really for? *Immunol. Today*, **5**, 165–6.

218 Playfair, J. H. L and Taverne, J. (1987). Anti-parasitic effects of tumour necrosis factor *in vivo* and *in vitro*. In *Tumour necrosis factor and related cytotoxins* (Ciba Foundation Symposium 131) (ed. G. Bock and J. Marsh), pp. 192–205. John Wiley and Sons, Chichester.

219 Rook, G. A. W., Taverne, J., and Playfair, J. H. L. (1991). Evaluation of TNF as anti-viral, anti-bacterial, and anti-parasitic agent. *Biotherapy*, **3**, 167–75.

220 Kongshavn, P. A. and Ghadirian, E. (1988). Effect of tumour necrosis factor on growth of *Trypanosoma musculi in vivo* and *in vitro*. *Adv. Exp. Biol. Med.*, **239**, 257–62.

221 Grau, G. E., Piguet, P. F., Vassalli, P., and Lambert, P. H. (1989). Tumour necrosis factor and other cytokines in cerebral malaria. Experimental and clinical data. *Immunol. Rev.*, **112**, 49–70.

222 Grau, G. E. (1990). Implications of cytokines in immunopathology: experimental and clinical data. *Eur. Cytok. Network*, **1**, 203–10.

223 Fiers, W., Brouckaert, P., Goldberg, A., Kettelhut, I., Suffys, P., Tavernier, J., Vanhaesebroeck, B., and Van Roy, F. (1987). Structure–function relationship of tumour necrosis factor and its mechanism of action. In *Tumour necrosis factor and related cytotoxins* (Ciba Foundation Symposium 131) (ed. G. Bock and J. Marsh), pp. 109–23. John Wiley and Sons, Chichester.

224 Beutler, B., Milsark, I. W., and Cerami, A. C. (1985). Passive immunization against cachectin/tumour necrosis factor protects mice from lethal effect of endotoxin. *Science*, **229**, 869–71.

225 Tracey, K. J., Fong, Y., Hesse, D. G., Manogue, K. R., Lee, A. T., Kuo, G. C., Lowry, S. F., and Cerami, A. (1987). Anti-cachectin/TNF monoclonal antibodies prevent septic shock during lethal bacteraemia. *Nature*, **330**, 662–4.

226 Waage, A., Halstensen, A., and Espevik, T. (1987). Association between tumour necrosis factor in serum and fatal outcome in patients with meningococcal meningitis. *Lancet*, **i**, 355–7.

227 Waage, A., Halstensen, A., Brandtzaeg, P., Shalaby, R., and Espevik, T. (1990). Tumour necrosis factor, interleukin-1, and interleukin-6 in meningococcal disease. In *Tumour necrosis factor: structure, mechanism of action, role in disease and therapy*. (ed. B. Bonavida and G. Granger), pp. 162–7. Karger, Basel.

228 Ohlsson, K., Björk, P., Bergenfeldt, M., Hageman, R., and Thompson, R. C. (1990). Interleukin-1 receptor antagonist reduces mortality from endotoxin shock. *Nature*, **348**, 550–2.

229 Calandra, T., Baumgartner, J. D., Grau, G. E., Wu, M. M., Lambert, P. H., Schellekens, J., Verhoef, J., and Glauser, M. P. (1990). Prognostic values of tumour necrosis factor/cachectin, interleukin-1, interferon-α, and interferon-γ in the serum of patients with septic shock. *J. Infect. Dis.*, **161**, 982–7.

230 Cross, A. S., Sadoff, J. C., Kelly, N., Bernton, E., and Gemski, P. (1989). Pre-treatment with recombinant murine tumour necrosis factor-α/cachectin and murine interleukin-1α protects mice from lethal bacterial infection. *J. Exp. Med.*, **169**, 2021–7.

231 Wong, G. H. W., and Goeddel, D. V. (1986). Tumour necrosis factors α and β inhibit virus replication and synergize with interferons. *Nature*, **323**, 819–22.

232 Mestan, J., Digel, W., Mittnacht, S., Hillen, H., Blohm, D., Möller, A., Jacobson, H., and Kirchner, H. (1986). Anti-viral effects of recombinant tumour necrosis factor *in vitro*. *Nature*, **323**, 816–19.

233   Doherty, P. C., Allan, J. E., and Clark, I. A. (1989). Tumour necrosis factor inhibits the development of viral meningitis or induces rapid death depending on the severity of inflammation at the time of administration. *J. Immunol.*, **142**, 3576–80.

234   Matsuyama, T., Hamamoto, Y., Soma, G., Mizuno, D., Yamamoto, N., and Kobayashi, N. (1989). Cytocidal effect of tumour necrosis factor on cells chronically infected with human immunodeficiency virus (HIV): enhancement of HIV replication. *J. Virol.*, **63**, 2504–9.

235   Aboulafia, D., Miles, S. A., Saks, S. R., and Mitsuyasu, R. T. (1989). Intravenous recombinant tumour necrosis factor in the treatment of AIDS-related Kaposi's sarcoma. *J. Acq. Imm. Defic. Syndr.*, **2**, 54–8.

236   Lahdevirta, J., Maury, C. P., Teppo, A. M., and Repo, H. (1988). Elevated levels of circulating cachectin/tumour necrosis factor in patients with acquired immunodeficiency syndrome. *Am. J. Med.*, **85**, 289–91.

237   Piguet, P. F., Grau, G. E., Allet, B., and Vassalli, P. (1987). Tumour necrosis factor/cachectin is an effector of skin and gut lesions of the acute phase of graft-versus-host disease. *J. Exp. Med.*, **166**, 1280–9.

238   Höller, E., Kolb, H. J., Möller, A., Kempeni, J., Liesenfeld, S., Pechumer, H., Lehmacher, W., Rückdeschel, G., Gleixner, B., and Riedner, C. (1990). Increased serum levels of tumour necrosis factor-α precede major complications of bone marrow transplantation. *Blood*, **75**, 1011–16.

239   Kunkel, S. L., Strieter, R. M., Chensue, S. W., Campbell, D. A., and Remick, D. G. (1991). The role of TNF in diverse pathologic processes. *Biotherapy*, **3**, 135–41.

240   Maury, C. P. and Teppo, A. M. (1987). Raised serum levels of cachectin/tumour necrosis factor-α in renal allograft rejection. *J. Exp. Med.*, **166**, 1132–7.

241   Abramowicz, D., Schandene, L., Goldman, M., Crusiaux, A., Vereerstraeten, P., De Pauw, L., Wybran, J., Kinnaert, P., Du Pont, E., and Toussaint, C. (1989). Release of tumour necrosis factor, interleukin-2, and γ-interferon in serum after injection of OKT3 monoclonal antibody in kidney transplant recipients. *Transplantation*, **47**, 606–8.

242   Saxne, T., Palladino, M. A., Heinegard, D., Tatal, N., and Wollheim, F. A. (1988). Detecting of tumour necrosis factor-α but not tumour necrosis factor-β in rheumatoid arthritis synovial fluid and serum. *Arthr. Rheum.*, **31**, 1041–5.

243   Saklatvala, J. (1986). Tumour necrosis factor-α stimulates resorption and inhibits synthesis of proteoglycan in cartilage. *Nature*, **322**, 547–9.

244   Selmaj, K. W. and Raine, C. S. (1988). Tumour necrosis factor mediates myelin and oligodendrocyte damage *in vitro*. *Ann. Neurol.*, **23**, 339–46.

245   Pujol-Borrell, R., Todd, I., Doshi, M., Franco Bottazzo, G., Sutton, R., Gray, D., Adolf, G. R., and Feldmann, M. (1987). HLA Class II induction in human islet cells by interferon-γ plus tumour necrosis factor or lymphotoxin. *Nature*, **326**, 304–6.

246   Jacob, C. O., Aiso, S., Michie, S. A., McDevitt, H. O., and Acha-Orbea, H. (1990). Inhibition of adoptive transfer and development of spontaneous diabetes mellitus in non-obese diabetic mice by TNFα. In *Tumour necrosis factor: structure, mechanism of action, role in disease and therapy*. (ed. B. Bonavida and G. Granger), pp. 222–7. Karger, Basel.

247   Grossman, R. H., Krueger, J., Yourish, D., Granelli-Piperno, A., Murphy, D. P., May, L. T., Kupper, T. S., Seghal, P. B., and Gottlieb, A. B. (1989). Interleukin-6 is expressed in high levels in psoriatic skin and stimulates proli-

feration of cultured human keratinocytes. *Proc. Natl. Acad. Sci. U.S.A.*, **86**, 6367–71.

248   Prens, E. P., Benne, K., Van Damme, J., Bakkus, M., Brakel, K., Benner, R., and Van Joost, T. (1990). Interleukin-1 and interleukin-6 in psoriasis. *J. Invest. Dermatol.*, **95**, 121S-4S.

249   Skoven, I. and Thormann, J. (1979). Lithium compound treatment and psoriasis. *Arch. Dermatol.*, **115**, 1185–7.

250. Sasaki, T., Saito, S., Aihara, M., Ohsawa, J., and Ikezawa, Z. (1989). Exacerbation of psoriasis during lithium treatment. *J. Dermatol.* Tokyo, **16**, 59–63.

251   Beyaert, R., Schulze-Osthoff, K., Van Roy, F., and Fiers, W. (1992). Synergistic induction of IL-6 by TNF and LiCl: possible role in the triggering and exacerbation of psoriasis by lithium treatment. *Eur. J. Immunol.*, **22**, 2181–4.

252   Langstein, H. N. and Norton, J. A. (1991). Mechanisms of cancer cachexia. *Hematol./Oncol. Clin. North America*, **5**, 103–23.

253   Patton, J. S., Peters, P. M., McCabe, J., Crase, D., Hansen, S., Chen, A. B., and Liggitt, D. (1987). Development of partial tolerance to the gastrointestinal effects of high doses of recombinant tumour necrosis factor-α in rodents. *J. Clin. Invest.*, **80**, 1587–96.

254   Norton, J. A., Moley, J. F., and Green, M. V. (1985). Parabiotic transfer of cancer anorexia/cachexia in male rats. *Cancer Res.*, **45**, 5547–53.

255   Socher, S. H., Friedman, A., and Martinez, D. (1988). Recombinant human tumour necrosis factor induces acute reductions in food intake and body weight in mice. *J. Exp. Med.*, **167**, 1957–62.

256   Tracey, K. J., Wei, H., Manogue, K. R., Fong, Y., Hesse, D. G., Nguyen, H. T., Kuo, G. C., Beutler, B., Cotran, R. S., Cerami, A., and Lowry, S. F. (1988). Cachectin/tumour necrosis factor induces cachexia, anaemia, and inflammation. *J. Exp. Med.*, **167**, 1211–27.

257   Oliff, A., Defeo-Jones, D., Boyer, M., Martinez, D., Kiefer, D., Vuocolo, G., Wolfe, A., and Socher, S. H. (1987). Tumours secreting human TNF/cachectin induce cachexia in mice. *Cell*, **50**, 555–63.

258   Vanhaesebroeck, B., Mareel, M., Van Roy, F., Grooten, J., and Fiers, W. (1991). Expression of the tumour necrosis factor gene in tumour cells correlates with reduced tumourigenicity and reduced invasiveness *in vivo*. *Cancer Res.*, **51**, 2229–38.

259   Tracey, K. J., Morgello, S., Koplin, B., Fahey, T. J., Fox, J., Aledo, A., Manogue, K. R., and Cerami, A. (1990). Metabolic effects of cachectin/tumour necrosis factor are modified by site of production. Cachectin/tumour necrosis factor-secreting tumour in skeletal muscle induces chronic cachexia, while implantation in brain induces predominately acute anorexia. *J. Clin. Invest.*, **86**, 2014–24.

260   Shimomura, K., Manda, T., Mukumoto, S., Kobayashi, K., Nakano, K., and Mori, J. (1988). Recombinant human tumour necrosis factor alpha: thrombus formation is a cause of anti-tumour activity. *Int. J. Cancer*, **41**, 243–7.

261   Asami, T., Imai, M., Tanaka, Y., Hosaka, Y., Kato, K., Nakamura, N., Horisawa, Y., Ashida, Y., Kanamori, T., Nobuhara, M., and Kurimoto, M. (1989). *In vivo* anti-tumour mechanism of natural human tumour necrosis factor involving a T cell-mediated immunological route. *Jpn. J. Cancer Res.*, **80**, 1161–4.

262   Palladino Jr, M. A., Shalaby, M. R., Kramer, S. M., Ferraiolo, B. L., Baughman, R. A., Deleo, A. B., Crase, D., Marafino, B., Aggarwal, B. B.,

Figari, I. S., Liggitt, D., and Patton, J. S. (1987). Characterization of the anti-tumour activities of human tumour necrosis factor-α and the comparison with other cytokines: induction of tumour-specific immunity. *J. Immunol.*, **138**, 4023–32.

263 Mareel, M., Dragonetti, C., Tavernier, J., and Fiers, W. (1988). Tumour-selective cytotoxic effects of murine tumour necrosis factor (TNF) and interferon gamma (IFN-gamma) in organ culture of B16 melanoma cells and heart tissue. *Int. J. Cancer*, **42**, 470–3.

264 Brouckaert, P. G. G., Leroux-Roels, G. G., Guisez, Y., Tavernier, J., and Fiers, W. (1986). *In vivo* anti-tumour activity of recombinant human and murine TNF, alone and in combination with murine IFN-gamma, on a syngeneic murine melanoma. *Int. J. Cancer*, **38**, 763–9.

265 Marquet, R. L., IJzermans, J. N. M., De Bruin, R. W. F., Fiers, W., and Jeekel, J. (1987). Anti-tumour activity of recombinant mouse tumour necrosis factor (TNF) on colon cancer in rats is promoted by recombinant rat interferon gamma; toxicity is reduced by indomethacin. *Int. J. Cancer*, **40**, 550–3.

266 Gresser, I., Belardelli, F., Tavernier, J., Fiers, W., Podo, F., Federico, M., Carpinelli, G., Duvillard, P., Prade, M., Maury, C., Bandu, M. T., and Maunoury, M. T. (1986). Anti-tumour effects of interferon in mice injected with interferon-sensitive and interferon-resistant Friend leukaemia cells. V. Comparisons with the action of tumour necrosis factor. *Int. J. Cancer*, **38**, 771–8.

267 Mahony, S. M. and Tisdale, M. J. (1989). Role of prostaglandins in tumour necrosis factor induced weight loss. *Br. J. Cancer*, **60**, 51–5.

268 Fraker, D. L., Stovroff, M. C., Merino, M. J., and Norton, J. A. (1988). Tolerance to tumour necrosis factor in rats and the relationship to endotoxin tolerance and toxicity. *J. Exp. Med.*, **168**, 95–105.

269 Balkwill, F. R., Lee, A., Aldam, G., Moodie, E., Thomas, J. A., Tavernier, J., and Fiers, W. (1986). Human tumour xenografts treated with recombinant human tumour necrosis factor alone or in combination with interferons. *Cancer Res.*, **46**, 3990–3.

270 Balkwill, F. R., Ward, B. G., Moodie, E., and Fiers, W. (1987). Therapeutic potential of tumour necrosis factor-α and γ-interferon in experimental human ovarian cancer. *Cancer Res.*, **47**, 4755–8.

271 Malik, S. T. A., Griffin, D. B., Fiers, W., and Balkwill, F. R. (1989). Paradoxical effects of tumour necrosis factor in experimental ovarian cancer. *Int. J. Cancer*, **44**, 918–25.

272 Malik, S. T. A., Naylor, M. S., East, N., Oliff, A., and Balkwill, F. R. (1990). Cells secreting tumour necrosis factor show enhanced metastasis in nude mice. *Eur. J. Cancer*, **26**, 1031–4.

273 Demetri, G. D., Spriggs, D. R., Sherman, M. L., Arthur, K. A., Imamura, K., and Kufe, D. W. (1989). A phase I trial of recombinant human tumour necrosis factor and interferon-γ: effects of combination cytokine administration *in vivo*. *J. Clin. Oncol.*, **7**, 1545–53.

274 Räth, U., Kaufmann, M., Schmid, H., Hofmann, J., Wiedenmann, B., Kist, A., Kempeni, J., Schlick, E., Bastert, G., Kommerell, B., and Männel, D. (1991). Effect of intraperitoneal recombinant human tumour necrosis factor-α on malignant ascites. *Eur. J. Cancer*, **27**, 121–5.

275 Pauli, U., Beutler, B., and Peterhans, E. (1989). Porcine tumour necrosis factor alpha: cloning with the polymerase chain reaction and determination of the nucleotide sequence. *Gene*, **81**, 185–91.

276 Drews, R. T., Coffee, B. W., Prestwood, A. K., and McGraw, R. A. (1990). Gene sequence of porcine tumour necrosis factor alpha. *Nucleic Acids Res.*, **18**, 5564.

277 Goeddel, D. V., Aggarwal, B. B., Gray, P. W., Leung, D. W., Nedwin, G. E., Palladino, M. A., Patton, J. S., Pennica, D., Shepard, H. M., Sugarman, B. J., and Wong, G. H. W. (1986). Tumour necrosis factors: gene structure and biological activities. In *Molecular biology of Homo sapiens* (Cold Spring Harbor Symposia on Quantitative Biology, Vol. 51), pp. 597–609. Cold Spring Harbor Laboratory, Cold Spring Harbor.

278 Young, A. J., Hay, J. B., and Chan, J. Y. C. (1990). Primary structure of ovine tumour necrosis factor alpha cDNA. *Nucleic Acids Res.*, **18**, 6723.

279 McGraw, R. A., Coffee, B. W., Otto, C. M., Drews, R. T., and Rawlings, C. A. (1990). Gene sequence of feline tumour necrosis factor alpha. *Nucleic Acids Res.*, **18**, 5563.

280 Ito, H., Shirai, T., Yamamoto, S., Akira, M., Kawahara, S., Todd, C. W., and Wallace, R. B. (1986). Molecular cloning of the gene encoding rabbit tumour necrosis factor. *DNA*, **5**, 157–65.

281 Shirai, T., Shimizu, N., Horiguchi, S., and Ito, H. (1989). Cloning and expression in *Escherichia coli* of the gene for rat tumour necrosis factor. *Agric. Biol. Chem.*, **53**, 1733–6.

282 Pennica, D., Hayflick, J. S., Bringman, T. S., Palladino, M. A., and Goeddel, D. V. (1985). Cloning and expression in *Escherichia coli* of the cDNA for murine tumour necrosis factor. *Proc. Natl. Acad. Sci. U.S.A.*, **82**, 6060–4.

283 Vilček, J. and Lee, T. H. (1991). Tumour necrosis factor. New insights into the molecular mechanisms of its multiple actions. *J. Biol. Chem.*, **266**, 7313–6.

5 The complement system

K. WHALEY AND C. LEMERCIER

1 Introduction

The complement system comprises a series of plasma (Table 5.1) and cell membrane (Table 5.2), proteins which are involved in host defence against microbial infections and in the pathogenesis of immunologically mediated diseases. The initial description of complement as a heat-sensitive constituent of a heat-sensitive bactericidal activity of serum was later shown to depend on heat-stable antibody as well as a heat-labile factor which was initially labelled alexin and later complement (1). It is well known that antibody activates the complement system through the classical pathway. In addition to antibody-dependent activation of complement there are a number of antibody-independent mechanisms by which complement is activated, the best known being the alternative pathway. Antibody-independent activation of the classical pathway is also beginning to be understood (Figure 6.5). The primary humoral immune response requires several days to occur and therefore in the early stages of host defence, antibody-independent mechanisms of complement activation are extremely important. This is clear from the effects of deficiencies of complement components, particularly the alternative pathway components. Lack of these proteins increases susceptibility to infection. During complement activation pro-inflammatory peptides, anaphylatoxins, are released from the activated complement components, complement components bind to the surface of micro-organisms to prepare them for phagocytosis and intracellular killing, and a multimeric cytolytic membrane attack complex is assembled and inserted into the membranes of micro-organisms to destroy them directly. The advantage of antibody-mediated activation of complement is that the antibody molecule directs complement activation to the target of the immune response whereas antibody-independent activation tends to be more widespread and more likely to attack the cells and tissues of the host. Protection of host cells against complement-mediated attack is conferred by a series of membrane-bound proteins which regulate both the early stages of complement activation and the insertion of the cytolytic membrane attack complex into host cell membranes.

2 Nomenclature

The constituent proteins of the classical pathway and the terminal sequence are termed components and each is given a number pre-fixed by the symbol

Table 5.1 Components of the human plasma complement system

Classical pathway	Serum conc. ($\mu g/ml$)	Molecular weight	Number of polypeptide chains	Number of genetic loci	Chromosomal assignment
C1q	75	410 kDa	3(A--B.C) × 6	3(A,B,C)	1p34.1-36.3
C1r	30	170 kDa	Homodimer	1	12p13
C1s	30	85 kDa	Single but forming Ca^{2+}-dependent dimer	1	12p13
C4	450	204 kDa	3(β--α--γ)	2(C4A,C4B)	6p21.3 (MHC Class III)
C2	20	95 kDa	1	1	6p21.3 (MHC Class III)
Alternative pathway					
Factor B	200	95 kDa	1	1	6p21.3 (MHC Class III)
Factor D	2	25 kDa	1	1	ND
Factor P	30	220 kDa	cyclic polymers	1	Xp 11.23-21.1
Terminal sequence					
C3	1000	190 kDa	2(β--α)	2(β--α)	19q
C5	75	196 kDa	2(β--α)	2(β--α)	9q 32-24
C6	60	128 kDa	1	1	5
C7	60	110 kDa	4	1	5
C8	80	150 kDa	3(α--γ,β)	3($\alpha\beta\gamma$)	α, β 1p32
C9	60	71 kDa	1	1	-9q

Table 5.1 (*continued*)

Control proteins	Serum conc. ($\mu g/ml$)	Molecular weight	Number of polypeptide chains	Number of genetic loci	Chromosomal assignment
C1 inhibitor	200	105 kDa	1	1	11q11–13.1
C4bp	250	550 kDa	$8(7\alpha - 1\beta)$	$2(\alpha,\beta)$	1q32 (RCA cluster)
Factor I	50	90 kDa	1	1	4q25
Factor H	300	150 kDa + 2 minor species	1	1 (probably a second locus for one of minor bands)	1q28 (RCA cluster)
S protein (vitronectin)	150	80 kDa	1	1	?
SP40-40 (clusterin)	65	80 kDa	$2(\alpha - \beta)$	1	8
Carboxypeptidase N (anaphylatoxin inactivator)	35	280 kDa	$4(H,L \times 2)$	?	?

ND, not determined.

Table 5.2 Complement receptors and membrane control proteins

Protein	Ligand	Molecular weight (kDa)	Cell distribution	Biological activitiy	Chromosomal assignment
C1qR	C1q Collagen-like region	65	B lymphocytes, neutrophils, monocytes	Triggers respiratory burst, phagocytosis, degradation of immune complexes	?
C3a/C4aR	C3a/C4a	?	Mast cells, granulocytes, some T lymphocytes	Increased vascular permeability, granulocyte degranulation and aggregation, immunomodulation	?
C5aR	C5a	50	Mast cells, granulocytes, monocytes/macrophages,	Increased vascular permeability, chemotaxis, granulocyte secretion and aggregation, platelet aggregation and secretion	?
C3b/C4bR (CR1)	C3b, C4b, iC3b	Four allotypes 190, 220, 160, 250	Erythrocytes, monocytes/ macrophages, neutrophils, eosinophils, B cells, some T cells, kidney podocytes, follicular dendritic cells	Clearance of immune complexes, phagocytosis, and killing of bacteria. Accelerates decay of classical and alternative pathway. Cofactor for factor I in C3b/C4b, C3, and C5	1q32
C3dR (CR2)	iC3b, C3dg, C3d	140	B lymphocytes, follicular dendritic cells	Modulates lymphocyte production and antibody production	1q32
iC3bR (CR3)	iC3b, C3dg, C3d	α 165 β 95	Monocytes/macrophages, neutrophils, NK cells, some T lymphocytes	Phagocytosis and killing of bacteria	α 16p11–13.1 β 21q22.1–qter

Table 5.2 (*continued*)

Protein	Ligand	Molecular weight (kDa)	Cell distribution	Biological actitivity	Chromosomal assignment
p150/95 (CR4)	iC3b, C3dg, C3d	α 150 β 95	Granulocytes, mast cells, T cells, B cells	? phagocytosis	α 16p11–13.1 β 21q22.1–qter
DAF	Classical and alternative pathway, C3 and C5 convertases	75	Widespread	Accelerates decay of classical and alternative pathway C3 and C5 convertases	1q32
MCP	C3b/C4b	45–70	Widespread	Cofactor for factor I cleavage of C3b/C4b	1q32
CD59/MIRL/HRF20	C5b–8	18	Widespread	Prevents polymerization of C9	?
HRF/C8BP	C5b–8	65	Widespread	Prevents polymerization of C9	?

C, e.g. C1, C2, C3, C4, C5, C6, C7, C8, and C9. The proteins of the alternative pathway are called factors and they are represented by a letter, e.g. factor B, factor D, properdin (factor P). These are usually abbreviated to B, D, and P respectively. The control proteins are referred to by the abbreviated forms of their trivial names, e.g. C1 inhibitor (C1inh), C4 binding protein (C4bp). However because of the crucial roles of factors I and H in the regulation of the alternative pathway they are referred to by their full names or alternatively by their abbreviated forms I and H respectively.

Activated C1 and its subcomponents C1r and C1s have horizontal bars over the number and cleavage fragments are indicated by suffixed lower case letters, e.g. C4a, C4b, C4c, C4d. The polypeptide subunit chains of components are suffixed with the greek letters starting with α for the largest, then β and γ, e.g. C4α, C4β, and C4γ.

3   Chemistry and reaction mechanisms

3.1   The classical pathway (Figure 5.1)

The components of the classical pathway are C1, C4, C2, and C3, which are responsible for the formation of the classical pathway C3 activating enzyme (C3 convertase; C4b2a) and C5 activating enzyme (C5 convertase; C4b2a3b). Activation of the classical pathway occurs mainly following the binding of antibody to antigen although non-antibody activation may occur (see Chapter 6). Activation of C1 by antibody–antigen complexes will be considered

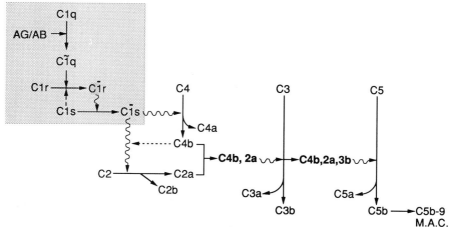

Fig. 5.1   Classical pathway activation by antigen–antibody complexes. The *shaded area* represents the processes involved in activation of CL. The *dashed arrow* indicates the facilitation of C1s-mediated activation of C2 by C4b. (From Whaley, K. (1987). Introduction to complement. In *Complement in health and disease*. (ed. K. Whaley), MTP Press — by permission of the publishers.)

as it provides a basis for comparison of C1 activation in the absence of specific antibody. C1 is activated by antibodies of the IgM or IgG classes (subclasses IgG_1, IgG_2, and IgG_3 only). C1 is a macromolecule comprising the three subcomponents C1q, C1r, and C1s in a molar ratio of 1:2:2 held together in a calcium-dependent complex (2). The C1q subcomponent consists of six identical collagen-like stalks radiating from a central core, each terminating in a globular protein head. Each strand is composed of three polypeptide chains (A, B, C) (3), encoded by a separated gene (4). The globular protein heads interact with the Fc pieces of immunoglobulin. The C1r and C1s molecules which are zymogens of serine proteases are joined end-to-end as an elongated tetramer which is arranged around the collagen-like stalks. Although the precise arrangement has not been ascertained, the most probable is a figure of eight in which the catalytic domains of C1r and C1s are in contact within the cage formed by the C1q stalks (2).

Each of the globular protein heads of C1q can bind to the Fc region of immunoglobulin, the CH2 domain of IgG, or the CH3 domain of IgM, but multivalent attachment of C1q is required for C1 activation (5). In solution IgM exists as a pentameric, planar molecule to which C1q binds weakly. Once IgM antibody binds to a multivalent antigen it assumes a 'staple' conformation which allows at least two C1q heads to bind to separate Fc pieces. Thus a single pentameric IgM molecule is sufficient to activate C1. Natural antibodies are of the IgM class and are therefore extremely efficient complement activators. As IgG is monomeric at least two molecules are required to cross-link the globular heads of C1q and activate C1. On particulate antigens several thousand IgG molecules may have to bind to ensure that two are within 40 nm of each other to form a stable binding site for C1q. Therefore, on particulate antigens IgG antibody is a far less efficient complement activator than IgM (6). When IgG antibody binds to soluble antigens, complexes formed at equivalence or in the zone of slight antibody excess are better activators of C1 than those formed in antigen excess or marked antibody excess (7, 8), again because at this ratio the IgG molecules are closest together.

Following binding to antibody C1q undergoes a conformational change, which results in activation of C1r (2). It is thought that one molecule of C1r in the tetramer activates the other C1r by proteolysis. $\overline{C1r}$ has one natural substrate, C1s, which is converted to its proteolytically active form as a result of a single proteolytic cleavage. $\overline{C1s}$, the active 'extrovert' enzyme of C1, has two natural substrates, C4 and C2. $\overline{C1s}$ cleaves a 6 kDa fragment, C4a, from the amino-terminus of the α chain of C4, and an internal thiolester bond in the α' chain of the major product C4b is exposed (Figure 5.2). This thiolester links the sulfydryl group of the cysteine in position 991 to the carbonyl group of a glutamine residue in position 994 (9). Nucleophilic attack of the thiolester bond by exposed hydroxyl groups or amino groups on nearby surfaces results in the formation of ester or amide bonds respectively (10). Thus for a few microseconds, nascent C4b with an exposed thiolester is able

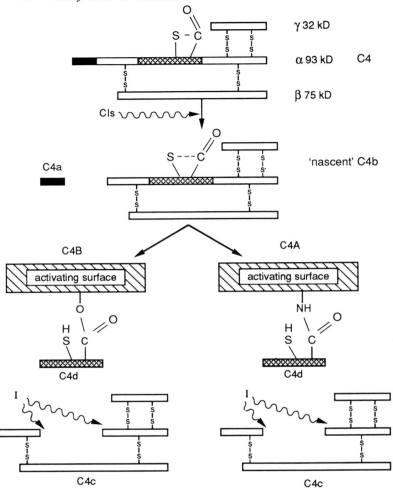

Fig. 5.2 Activation of C4 by C̄1s involves cleavage of the N-terminus of the α chain to release C4a (6 kDa). A thiolester bond in the α chain of C4b reacts with OH groups to form ester bonds or amino groups to form amide bonds. Although both C4A and C4B can form either type of bond, C4A has a greater propensity to form amide bonds than C4B. Thus C4A is shown as forming amide bonds and C4B as forming ester bonds.

Inactivation of C4b occurs by enzymatic attack of factor I and a cofactor (C4bp or membrane cofactor protein) to release C4c and leave C4d bound to the target.

Disulfide bridges are shown schematically.

to bind covalently to targets. C4b which does not form ester or amide bonds within this period loses its binding site as the thiolester reacts with water to become inactive fluid-phase C4b in which the thiolester becomes hydrolysed and the residue corresponding to 994 becomes glutamate.

C2 binds to C4b in a Mg^{2+}-dependent reaction to form a pro-convertase (11) before being cleaved by C̄1s into C2b, which bears the original C4b binding site, and C2a which develops a binding site for C4b and also expresses serine protease activity (12). The C4b2a complex is the classical pathway C3 convertase which cleaves the α chain of C3 to release a 9 kDa fragment, C3a, from the amino-terminus and exposes an internal thiolester bond in the α chain of C3b (13). As with C4b the thiolester becomes the subject of nucleophilic attack and forms covalent ester or amide bonds with surface hydroxyl or amino groups; usually ester bonds are formed (Figure 5.3). Only a small proportion (up to ten per cent) of C3 binds covalently to a complement-activating surface. The thiolester of the majority of the activated C3 reacts with water so that inactive fluid-phase C3b is formed.

Some C3b binds to C4b in C4b2a and acts as a receptor for C5. This complex, C4b2a3b, is the classical pathway C5 convertase. A 12 kDa peptide (C5a) is released from the amino-terminus of C5 and the major cleavage product, C5b is available for the assembly of the cytolytic membrane attack complex.

Humans, and some other species produce two types of C4 molecules, C4A and C4B, each being the product of a distinct gene. The importance of this distinction is that C4A has a greater propensity to form amide bonds than C4B (14–16), probably because its thiolester is more stable than that of C4B (17) (Figure 5.2). Only minor structural differences exist between C4A and C4B, and are located within the C4d region of the α chain which contains the thiolester (18). Different experiments, including site-directed mutagenesis have shown that the important difference is related to the presence of aspartic acid at position 1106 in C4A while histidine is present in C4B (19).

3.2 Regulation of the classical pathway

Classical pathway activation is localized by the binding of antibody to the target antigen and the extreme lability of the thiolester bonds of C4b and C3b which focuses subsequent activation of the cascade to the site of initial interaction with C1. The short half-lives (approximately 90 seconds at 37 °C) of the C3 and C5 convertases also limits complement activation.

In addition to these regulatory mechanisms there are a series of plasma and membrane proteins which regulate complement activation.

C1 inhibitor is a member of the SERPIN (serine protease inhibitor) family of proteins. It binds to the active sites of $\overline{C1r}$ and $\overline{C1s}$ and so prevents further activation of C4 and C2 (20). It acts as a 'false' substrate, becomes cleaved by the enzyme but forms an acyl intermediate. This covalently linked C1r:C1s:C1 inhibitor complex (molar ratio 1:1:2) dissociates from C1 leaving C1q bound to the original activation site (21, 22).

C1 inhibitor interacts locally with the C1r zymogen the C1 molecule to prevent spontaneous C1 activation (23). C1 inhibitor also acts as an inhibitor in the Hageman factor-dependent pathways of blood coagulation where it inhibits activated Hageman factor, its fragments, kallikrein and plasmin.

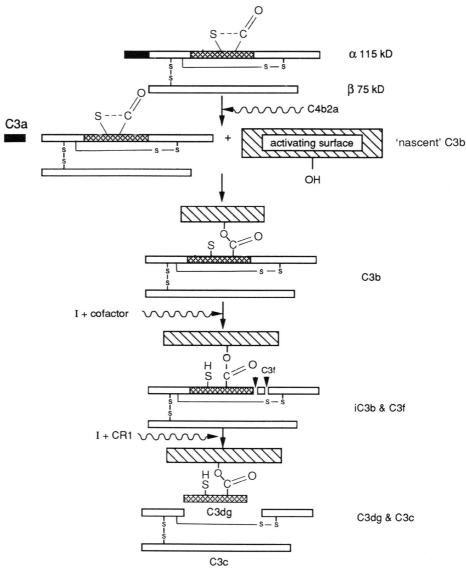

Fig. 5.3 Activation of C3 by C3 convertases (C4b2a or C3bBbP) results in the release of C3a (9 kDa) from the N-terminus of the α chain. The thiolester bond in the α chain of C3b forms covalent (ester or amide, but usually the former) bonds with the complement-activating surface. Inactivation of C3b occurs in two stages, both of which are catalysed by factor I. In the first step, involving factor H or membrane cofactor protein as co-factor, two closely adjacent cleavages occur in the α chain to release a small-fragment (C3f; 3 kDa) and iC3b is formed which cannot bind C5 or factor R. A further cleavage, possibly involving CR1 as a cofactor, releases C3c and leaves C3dg bound to the target. The cross-hatched region is C3dg.

C4bp binds to C4b and acts as a cofactor for factor I-mediated degradation of C4b (Figure 5.2). The α' chain of C4b is cleaved twice to release C4c into the fluid-phase, leaving C4d covalently attached to the surface (24). Thus assembly of C4b2a is restricted. C4bp also binds to C4b which is part of C4b2a and increases the rate of decay of this already very unstable enzyme (25).

Two membrane proteins, decay acceleration factor (DAF) and membrane cofactor protein (MCP) are the principle regulators of the expression of C3 and C5 convertases on host cells. Both are encoded by genes in the regulation of complement activation (RCA) gene cluster on chromosome 1q in man, along with complement receptor types 1 (CR1) and 2 (CR2), C4bp, and factor H (26–28). Both proteins MCP and DAF are widely distributed on mammalian cells. MCP is a transmembrane protein which acts as a cofactor for factor I in the degradation of C4b and C3b on the cell surface (29), while DAF has a glycolipid anchor and accelerates the decay of the C3 and C5 convertases of the classical and alternative pathways (30). In contrast to MCP and DAF, CR2 has a more limited cell distribution being formed principally of circulating cells in the blood, tissue macrophages, follicular dendritic cells, and kidney podocytes. CR1 possesses both cofactor and decay accelerating activity. Although it is less potent than either MCP or DAF (31) *in vitro*, *in vivo* experiments in which a soluble form of CR1 has been used suggest CR1 is a most potent regulator in minimising complement-mediated tissue damage following myocardial infarction, for example (32).

3.3   Non-immune activation of the classical pathway

Heterozygous deficiency of C1 inhibitor gives rise to spontaneous fluid-phase activation of C1, C4, and C2 and the clinical syndrome of hereditary angiooedema (33). An acquired form of the disease also exists, most cases being due to the presence of a circulating auto-antibody to C1 inhibitor (34).

C-reactive protein (CRP), an acute phase reactant binds to bacterial capsular polysaccharides to form a C1 activating particle (35). Serum CRP levels increase dramatically during the early phase of infection due to cytokine stimulated hepatic synthesis. This mechanism plays an important role in host defence during the early stages of the humoral immune response. Certain viruses (36) and Gram-negative bacteria (37) can bind and activate C1 directly, while Gram-positive bacteria will only activate the classical pathway when anti-bacterial antibody is present (37).

Mitochondria will bind C1 and activate the classical pathway (38).

It has been suggested that such complement activation is important in the pathogenesis of tissue injury following myocardial infarction (39). Reduction in complement activation with recombinant CR1 reduces the size of experimentally induced myocardial infarctions (32).

Mannan-binding protein (MBP) is structurally similar to C1q and can bind the C1r:C1s tetramer. Following binding to mannan, MBP undergoes a conformational change with activation of C1r and C1s (40). Thus MBP may substitute for C1q and activate the classical pathway in the absence of antibody. MBP and other related molecules are discussed further in Chapter 6.

4   The alternative pathway

The alternative pathway is thought to be phylogenetically more primitive than the classical pathway. Alternative pathway activators tend to be molecules with repeating chemical structures such as polysaccharides, lipopolysaccharides, and teichoic acid, all of which are present on the surfaces of bacteria. Activation can occur in the absence of immunoglobulin, C4, or C2 but requires C3. Activation of the alternative pathway involves three processes: initiation, amplification, and recognition (Figure 5.4).

4.1   Inititation

The alternative pathway is undergoing continuous low-grade fluid-phase turnover because the thiolester of C3 undergoes slow spontaneous hydrolysis to form $C3(H_2O)$ (41) which, for less than one second, can bind factor B to form the $C3(H_2O)B$ complex in which factor B is susceptible to cleavage and activation by factor D to form $C3(H_2O)Bb$, a fluid-phase C3 convertase. This stage is regulated by degradation of a proportion of $C3(H_2O)$

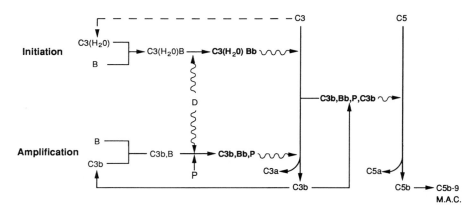

Fig. 5.4   Activation of the alternative pathway. Initiation is thought to occur as the result of spontaneous hydrolysis of the thiolester in C3 to form a molecule $C3(H_2O)$ which has C3b-like properties. Amplification occurs by the positive feedback loop which is regulated by factors H and I. (From Whaley, K. (1987). Introduction to complement. In *Complement in health and disease*. (ed. K. Whaley), MTP Press — by permission of the publishers.)

molecules by factor I in the presence of its cofactor, factor H, and by factor H binding to C3(H$_2$O) in the C3(H$_2$O)Bb complex and accelerating the rate of decay of this already unstable enzyme.

4.2 Amplification

C3(H$_2$O)Bb cleaves C3 into C3a and C3b at exactly the same site as the classical pathway C3 convertase, C4b2a. The C3b formed can bind to surfaces by means of its thiolester bond. Surface-bound C3b can bind factor B which is then cleaved by factor D to form C3bBb, the unstable alternative pathway C3 amplification convertase, which has a half-life of approximately 90 seconds at 37 °C. The convertase is stabilized by the non-covalent binding of properdin to form the complex C3bBbP (42). As this convertase also cleaves C3 into C3a and C3b, a positive feedback amplification loop is established as one of the products (C3b) of the action of the enzyme on its substrate is a constituent of the enzyme. Turnover of this amplification loop is regulated by factors H and I. Factor H binds to cell bound C3b and promotes inactivation of C3b by the enzyme factor I (43). The inactivated product, iC3b (Figure 5.3) is unable to bind factor B so that convertase formation is prevented. In addition to its cofactor activity factor H will also bind to C3b in the C3bBb and C3bBbP complexes to displace Bb from them (43, 44). Thus factor H accelerates the decay of these two enzymes.

4.3 Recognition

C3b formed as a result of alternative pathway activation binds to any surface and recognition occurs only after C3b binding.

On host cell membranes factor H will bind to C3b with approximately 100 times the affinity of factor B for C3b (45), thus the balance favours C3b degradation. However, on the surface of alternative pathway activators the affinity of factor H for C3b is decreased to a level which is similar to that of factor B for C3b so that the balance is shifted away from regulation to amplification. In this way amplification is confined to the surface of the activating agent. The surface structures which determine whether it is an alternative pathway activator or a non-activator must be diverse. Some activators have little surface sialic acid and some non-activators such as sheep erythrocytes, can be converted to activators by removal of surface sialic acid (46).

Although antibody is not required for alternative pathway activity, IgG antibody promotes activation (47–52). Carbohydrate groups on the Fab regions of some IgG subclasses may be involved (53) and C3b bound to IgG may be relatively resistant to the actions of factors H and I (54, 55).

4.4   C5 convertase formation

Although C3b is an integral part of the alternative pathway C3 convertase, C5 cleavage can only occur when a second C3b molecule has bound to the original C3b molecule to act as a receptor for C5 prior to C5 cleavage by Bb (56). Thus the alternative pathway C5 convertase is C3bBbPC3b and is directly comparable to the classical pathway C5 convertase.

4.5   Regulation of the alternative pathway

In addition to factors H and I, the membrane proteins DAF, MCP, and CR1 are able to regulate alternative pathway activity. MCP and CR1 act as cofactors for factor I in the inactivation of C3b, and DAF and CR1 are both able to accelerate the decay of the C3 and C5 convertases.

4.6   C3 degradation (Figure 5.3)

Although membrane-bound C3b can be inactivated slowly by factor I (43), for rapid inactivation of the bound C3b and inactivation of fluid-phase C3b the presence of its plasma cofactor, factor H, or the membrane cofactors CR1 or MCP is required.

In the presence of any one of these three cofactors, factor I produces two closely adjacent cleavages in the α chain of C3b, releasing a fragment of 3 kDa (57). The residual fragment iC3b is functionally different from C3b. The iC3b fragment cannot interact with factor B to form the alternative pathway C3 convertase nor can it recognise C5 so that both classical and alternative pathway C5 convertase activity is lost. Binding to CR1 is also greatly reduced when C3b is converted to iC3b. iC3b consists of two α chain fragments (68 kDa and 43 kDa) and the intact β chain. A further cleavage of the α chain is produced possibly by factor I using CR1 as its cofactor (58). This cleavage results in the release of C3c and leaves a fragment C3dg, which because it contains the thiolester, remains covalently attached to the complement-activating surface.

5   The membrane attack complex

Once C5 has been cleaved by C5 convertase the membrane attack complex (MAC) is assembled from C5, C6, C7, C8, and C9. C6, C7, C8, and C9 are structurally homologous amphipathic molecules. They are relatively hydrophobic with amino and carboxyl-termini which contain repetitive hydrophilic sequences.

Cleavage of C5 by either the classical or alternative pathway C5 convertases results in the formation of C5a and the larger fragment, C5b. Although C5 is structurally similar to C4 and C3 it lacks an internal thiolester bond (59). C5b remains bound to the C3b subunit of the C5 convertase and acts as a receptor for C6. The C5b binding site for C6 decays rapidly, having a half-life of approximately two minutes at 37 °C. The C5b6 complex may remain bound to C3b and serve as an acceptor for C7 or if C7 does not bind, it is released into the fluid-phase where it can complex with C7 and be inserted into other cell membranes for subsequent binding of C8 and C9. This process is called reactive lysis (60).

The binding of C7 to C5b6 produces an irreversible transition from hydrophilic precursor to the amphiphilic C5b67 complex. This transition is achieved by conformational changes which expose internal hydrophobic domains in C6 an C7 (61). As a result of this change the C5b67 complex becomes inserted into the cell membrane and its ability to bind C8 and C9 remains for long periods. If the complement activating agent does not possess a lipid bilayer, (e.g. immune complexes or zymosan particles) the C5b67 complex is incapable of binding and is released into the fluid-phase where it can bind to host cells and target them for destruction. 'Innocent bystander' lysis is prevented by a number of plasma proteins (see below and Chapters 9 and 11). C8 binds the C5b67 by its β chain while the C8α-γ subunit becomes inserted into the cell membrane. Formation of the C5b–8 complex in the membrane creates small pores of approximately 10 Å diameter which probably result from the aggregation of two or more C5b–8 complexes (61). The formation of C5b–8 pores in certain *in vitro* systems, (e.g. complement activation on the surface of sheep erythrocytes) results in 'low grade' lysis (62). For rapid lysis C9 must be incorporated into the C5b–8 complex. C9 binds to C8α-γ and undergoes a conformational change which exposes a second C9 binding site to which a second molecule of C9 binds and under-goes the same changes. Thus a tubular polymer consisting of 10–16 C9 molecules (63) forms having an internal diameter of 9–12 nm, and an everted lysis on the outer aspect of the cell membrane, with an external diameter of 22 nm (64). The C9 polymer penetrates the cell membrane and produces lysis. The mechanism of lysis is still unclear. The formation of transmem-brane channels in anucleate cells may result in osmotic lysis. When large numbers of MACs are inserted into a cell membrane a dramatic increase in surface area occurs in the absence of osmotic swelling. This swelling may disrupt the integrity of the cell membrane and cause cell death independently of ion fluxes through transmembrane channels (65).

Membrane C5b–9 pores allow entry of Na$^+$ and Ca^{2+} and efflux of K$^+$. Increased intracellular Ca^{2+} is associated with random triggering of a number of intracellular pathways and rapid depletion of ATP and high energy phos-phates. All these factors may contribute to cell death. Damage to the cell membrane by the MAC does not always result in cell death: there is good evidence that cells may recover. Recovery is associated with 'capping' and vesiculation of the MAC and associated cell membrane (66). Non-lethal complement attack of neutrophils and macrophages results in secretion of inflammatory mediators such as arachidonic acid metabolites (Chapters 12 and 13) and toxic oxygen species.

The potent effects of the MAC require that its activity is regulated to prevent damage to host cells. 'Innocent bystander lysis' by fluid-phase C5b67 is restricted by C8, S protein (vitronectin) (Chapter 11), lipoproteins, and clusterin (SP40–40). C8 binding to fluid-phase C5b67 prevents the complex from being inserted into cell membranes, possibly because the membrane binding site has become too bulky, while lipoproteins allow C5b67 to bind to their lipid core by means of the membrane binding site (67). Two or three molecules of S protein bind to fluid-phase C5b67 and convert it to a hydrophilic complex, rendering it water soluble and blocking its membrane binding site (68). The resultant SC5b–7 complex can still bind C8 and C9 to form a fluid-phase complex but C9 polymerization is restricted and only two to three molecules of C9 are bound. The action of clusterin may be similar to S protein.

Host cells are protected from MAC insertion by two proteins, homologous restriction factor (69) (HRF, also called membrane inhibitory protein and C8 binding protein) and CD59 (70) (also called HRF-20; membrane inhibitor of reactive lysis and protectin), both of which are widely distributed on different cells and are attached by glycolipid anchors. CD59 binds to C8 in the inserted C5b–8 complex and although the molecule of C9 binds to the complex, polymerization is prevented so that the biologically active mature MAC is not formed. It is probable that HRF acts in the same way (see Chapter 9 for further discussion).

6   Complement receptors (Table 5.2)

In addition to the plasma proteins and the membrane regulatory proteins described above there are a number of cell membrane proteins which are receptors which have complement components as their ligands (71, 72). These include the C1q receptor, the C3b/C4b receptor (CR1), the iC3b receptor (CR3), the C3dg receptors (CR2 and CR4), and the anaphylatoxin receptors (the C3a/C4a receptor and the C5a receptor). The C1q receptor has only recently been isolated and little is known about its biological role, although C1q binding to neutrophils probably facilitates phagocytosis and stimulates the respiratory burst. Although CR1, CR2, CR3, and CR4 are receptors for cleavage peptides of C3 and C4, they are structurally distinct and each has a unique tissue distribution (71–73) The C5a receptor has been cloned and sequenced and shown to be present in neutrophils and monocytes (74). In contrast the C3a receptor is less well characterized but is thought to be present on mast cells, vascular endothelium, and guinea pig ileum (75).

7 Biological activities of complement activation

As a result of complement activation a number of different biological activities are generated which can be divided into pro-inflammatory, opsonic, and cytolytic.

The pro-inflammatory activities are mainly the result of the generation of the anaphylatoxins C4a, C3a, and C5a. All three anaphylatoxins cause mast cells to degranulate and thereby increase vascular permeability (76). C4a is the least potent and C5a the most potent. C5a is also a potent chemotactic agent for monocytes and neutrophils (77–79) and is also a powerful neutrophil activator increasing adhesiveness, stimulating the respiratory burst, and degranulation (77, 80). Anaphylatoxin activity is regulated by the active enzyme carboxypeptidase N which rapidly removes the carboxy-terminal arginine, and inactivates the anaphylatoxic activities (81). The desArg form of C5a however retains its chemotactic activities probably through interaction with vitamin D binding protein and serum cochemotaxin (82–84). An α chain fragment of C3, C3e, promotes the mobilization of neutrophils from the bone marrow (85–87), although C5a also produces neutrophilia (88). In addition to these peptides, non-lethal membrane attack by complement stimulates phagocytic cells to release arachidonic acid metabolites and toxic oxygen metabolites.

Opsonization is mediated by the covalent binding of C3b and C4b to antibody molecules or to cell surfaces. The binding of C3b to immune complexes containing soluble antigens during their formation prevents them from becoming insoluble and so prevents tissue injury (89). This process, prevention of immune precipitation, depends upon the classical pathway (90) which deposits C3b on the antigen and antibody moieties of the complex, which reduces the possibility of excessive cross-linking (91). If the complex remains relatively insoluble after complement activation, the immune complex will bind via C3b to CR1 on the surface of erythrocytes on which they will be transported to the Kupffer cells of the liver (92). The mechanism of transfer of complexes from erythrocyte CR1 to Kupffer cell CR3 or Fcγ receptors is not understood. In contrast to the formation of immune complexes in the presence of complement, exposure of insoluble pre-formed complexes to serum results in their solubilization. This process depends upon the alternative pathway (93) and is mediated by the binding of C3b to both antigen and antibody with disruption of Fc–Fc interactions and the primary antigen–antibody bonds (91).

Opsonization of bacteria with C4b and/or C3b allows them to bind to CR1, while iC3b can bind to CR3, which if on the surface of phagocytic cells and particularly if co-opsonized with IgG antibody, allows the bacteria to be phagocytosed and killed (94). There is also evidence which suggests that terminal components may be required for the intracellular killing of some organisms. For example, *E coli* ingested by neutrophils may not be killed unless at least some of the terminal components are present on the organisms (95–97).

The assembly of the membrane attack complex on the bacterial cell wall may also lead to bacteriolysis and death, which are independent events. These events only occur with Gram-negative organisms and probably an active bacterial metabolic response in response to MAC insertion is required for the lethal effect (98). The early classical pathway components exert anti-viral activity particularly neutralization (C4) while activation of the classical pathway in the absence of antibody and assembly of the MAC destroys RNA tumour viruses (99). Activation of the alternative pathway by IgG antibody coated virus (RNA or DNA virus) infected cells leads to their lysis (99).

There is now good evidence that complement plays a role in the modulation of immune responses (100). Most of the evidence implicates a central role for C3. C3 fragments (C3a and the kallikrein derived fragment of C3dg) enhance or inhibit T and B cell responses *in vivo* depending on the concentration of the fragment (101, 102), trapping of immune complexes in germinal centres requires C3 (103), and ligation of CR2 on B cell membranes enhances antibody production (104). Guinea pigs and some humans who are deficient in C4, C2, or C3 produce poor primary immune responses to the T-dependent antigen, bacteriophage ϕX174 (105, 106), and C3 deficient animals produce poor secondary immune responses and fail to undergo isotype switching (105, 107). Recently it has been suggested that the human C4A isotype is more effective than the C4B isotype in overcoming the reduced immune response in C4 deficient guinea pigs (108).

8   Complement deficiency

With the exception of C1 inhibitor deficiency (autosomal dominant) and properdin deficiency (X-linked recessive) deficiencies of all complement components are autosomal recessive (Table 3). C1 inhibitor deficiency may result from either failure to secrete C1 inhibitor protein from the transcript of the abnormal gene (85 per cent of cases) or because the transcript of the abnormal gene encodes a functionally inactive protein (15 per cent of cases). The clinical picture of episodes of subcutaneous and submucous oedema are characteristic. Prior to the advent of modern therapy the disease had a mortality of 30–40 per cent due to asphyxia occurring secondary to laryngeal-oedema (33).

Deficiencies of the classical pathway components (C1q, C1r/C1s, C4, C2, and C3) are associated with a high incidence of immune complex and chronic rheumatic disease, possibly because of the importance of the classical pathway components in the prevention of immune precipitation (see above) (109). There is also an increased incidence of recurrent pyogenic infections including meningitis and septicaemia (110, 111).

Complete deficiencies of either factor H or factor I result in uncontrolled turnover of the alternative pathway with secondary deficiencies of C3 and factor B due to depletion. These patients also have a high incidence of immune complex disease and severe systemic bacterial infections (meningitis, septicaemia, septic arthritis).

Deficiencies of the alternative pathway components factor D and factor P have been documented but there are no reported cases of primary factor B deficiency. Factor D deficiency is associated with recurrent meningitis, septicaemia, and respiratory infections while a large proportion of patients with factor P deficiency develop fatal meningococcal disease (75 per cent mortality). Some patients with factor P deficiency are asymptomatic and others may develop less severe bacterial infections of the lower respiratory tract.

Deficiencies of C5, C6, C7, C8β, C8α, and C9 have been reported and all are associated with increased risk of systemic *Neisserial* infection, usually meningococcal meningitis. In contrast to the high mortality seen in patients with factor P deficiency, meningitis in these patients has a lower mortality and tends to be recurrent.

Deficiency of C4bp has been reported in one kindred in association with Behçet's syndrome and angio-oedema (112).

CR3 is a member of the integrin family of cell membrane proteins (113). Deficiency occurs as part of the leucocyte adhesion deficiency syndrome in which patients are unable to synthesize normal amounts of the functionally active β chain of the heterodimer (114). These individuals are unable to express CR3, LFA-1, and p150–95, all of which share a common β chain (114). They have defects in leucocyte adhesion and their leucocytes cannot adhere to endothelial cells. Leucocyte migration is impaired and bacterial phagocytosis and killing is severely impaired (115, 116). Delayed umbilical cord separation, recurrent bacterial infections of soft tissues, mucosal surfaces, and intestinal tract occur, often progressing to necrosis.

Deficiency of DAF, HRF, and CD59 occur in patients with paroxysmal nocturnal haemoglobinuria (117–121). In this acquired clonal disorder of bone marrow cells, GPI-anchored proteins cannot be inserted in the cell membrane so that they are unduly susceptible to complement lysis (122–24). Thus any complement activation will generate C5b–9 complexes which may be formed on erythrocytes or other blood cells and result in their lysis as GPI-anchored membrane complement control proteins are not expressed.

9   Complement biosynthesis

Most plasma complement components are synthesized by hepatocytes (125–127), although many components are synthesized by other cells, particularly mononuclear phagocytes, endothelial cells, fibroblasts, and the epithelial cells of the genitourinary and gastrointestinal tracts (126, 127) (Table 5.4). The importance of extrahepatic complement synthesis is unknown but may be important in local host defence (opsonization) (128) or contribute to local complement activation at sites of inflammation where complement activation

Table 5.3 Complement deficiency syndromes

Missing complement	No. of cases reported	Mode of inheritance	Functional defect	Associated disease
Classical pathway				
C1 (C1q, C1r/C1s)	31	Autosomal recessive	Impaired immune complex handling and loss of classical pathway	IC/ICTD (48%). Infection with encapsulated bacteria (22%). Both 18%. Healthy 12%.
C4	21	Autosomal recessive		
C2	109	Autosomal recessive		
Alternative pathway				
D	3	X-linked	Impaired complement activation in the absence of specific antibody	Infection (usually meningococcal) 74%. Healthy 26%.
P	70	Autosomal recessive		
C3	19	Autosomal recessive	Absent classical and alternative pathway activity. Impaired immune complex handling. Absent serum bactericidal activity. Impaired opsonization/phagocytosis. Impaired chemotaxis,	IC/ICTD 79%. Infections with encapsulated bacteria 71%.
Terminal sequence				
C5	27	Autosomal recessive	Impaired chemotaxis. Absent serum bactericidal activity	Infection (Neisseria spp especially meningococcal 59%).
C6	77	Autosomal recessive	Absent serum bactericidal activity	IC/ICTD 4%. Both 1%. Healthy 25%.
C7	73	Autosomal recessive		
C8	73	Autosomal recessive		
C9	18	Autosomal recessive	Reduced serum bactericidal activity	Healthy 92%. Infection 8%.

Table 5.3 (Continued)

Missing complement	No. of cases reported	Mode of inheritance	Functional defect	Associated disease
Plasma proteins				
C1 inhibitor	Many	Autosomal, dominant or acquired	Lack of regulation of C1 activation and of enzymes in Hageman factor-dependent results in generation of inflammatory mediator	Hereditary angio-oedema. ICD/ICTD 2–5%.
C4bp	3	Autosomal recessive	Impaired regulation of C4b2a	Angio-oedema + Behcet's-like syndrome in one patient.
Factor H	13	Autosomal recessive	Uncontrolled alternative pathway turnover → secondary deficiencies of C3 and factor B	ICD/ICTD 40%. ICD/ICTD + infections with encapsulated organisms 40%. Healthy 20%.
Factor I	14	Autosomal recessive	Uncontrolled alternative pathway turnover → secondary deficiencies of C3 and factor B	Infections with encapsulated organisms 100%.
Membrane proteins				
DAF/CD59/HRF	Many	Acquired	Impaired regulation of C3 and C5 convertases of both pathways and impaired regulation of MAC assembly → lysis of blood cells	Paroxysmal nocturnal haemoglobinuria.
CR3	>20	Autosomal recessive	Impaired neutrophil adhesive functions, e.g. margination, chemotaxis, iC3b mediated opsonization, and phagocytosis	Infections (*S. aureus*, *Pseudomonas Sp*) 100%.

ICD: immune complex disease; ICTD: immune complex type disease.

Table 5.4   Sites of synthesis of complement proteins

	Classical pathway	Alternative pathway	Terminal sequence	Regulatory proteins
Hepatocyte	C1r, C1s, C4, C2	C3, factor B	C3, C5, C6, C7, C8, C9	C1 inh, C4bp, factors H, I
Mononuclear phagocytes	C1q, C1r, C1s, C4, C2	C3, factors B, D, P	C3, C5, C8	C1 inh, factors H, I, C4bp
Fibroblasts	C1q, C1r, C1s, C4, C2	C3, factor B	–	C1 inh, factor H
Endothelial cells	C2	C3, factor B	C3	C1 inh, factors H, I
Epithelial cells	C1q, C1r, C1s	C3 factor B	C3	–

leads to severe depletion. It is important to note that complement component synthesis by these cells responds rapidly to cytokines and synthesis rates may increase by many orders of magnitude (126, 127). In one *in vivo* study of C3 metabolism, local synthesis of C3 within an inflamed joint accounted for up to 50 per cent of the C3 present in the joint fluid (129).

10   Summary

The complement system is of major importance as an initial defence mechanism in the absence of antibody. It precedes the acute phase response, although the acute phase can potentiate complement-mediated reactions. Complement activation also leads to recruitment of other inflammatory cells and mediators to the site of infection. The structure of the complement components and biochemistry of complement activation are now reasonably well understood. The major challenges remaining are the understanding of the biological activities of complement, defining the genetic mutations which give rise to complement deficiencies, understanding how the expression of complement genes is regulated, and determining the role of extrahepatic complement synthesis.

Acknowledgements

The authors' work is supported by grants from the Arthritis and Rheumatism Council, the Wellcome Trust, the Scottish Home and Health Department, and the European Community.

References

1   Ross, G. D. (1986). Introduction and history of complement research. In *Immunobiology of the complement system* (ed. G. D. Ross), pp. 1–19. Academic Press Inc., Orlando.

2   Colomb, R. G., Arland, G. J., and Villiers, C. L. (1984). Activation of C1. *Philos. Trans. R. Soc. London B*, **306**, 283–92.

3   Porter, R. R. and Reid, K. B. M. (1978). The biochemistry of complement. *Nature*, **275**, 699–704.

4   Sellar, G. C., Blake, D. J., and Reid, K. B. M. (1990). Characterization of the genes encoding the A-B- and C-chains of human complement component C1q. The complete derived amino acid sequence of C1q. *Biochem. J.*, **274**, 481–90.

5   Hughes-Jones, N. C. (1986). The classical pathway. In *Immunobiology of the complement system* (ed. G. D. Ross), pp. 20–44. Academic Press Inc., Orlando.

6   Borsos, T and Rapp, H. J. (1965). Complement fixation on cell surfaces by 19S and 7S antibodies. *Science*, **150**, 505–7.

7   Auda G. R. (1991). PhD Thesis. University of Glasgow.

8   Fust, G., Medgyesi, G. A., Rajnavelgyi, E., Csecsi-Nagy, M., Czikora, K., and Gergely, J. (1978). Possible mechanism of the first step of the classical complement activation pathway: binding and activation of C1. *Immunology*, **35**, 873–84.

9   Belt, K. T., Carroll, M. C., and Porter, R. R. (1984). The structural basis of the multiple forms of human complement component C4. *Cell*, **36**, 907–14.

10 Campbell, R. D., Gagnon, J., and Porter, R. R. (1981). Amino acid sequence around the thiol and reactive acyl groups of human complement component C4. *Biochem. J.*, **199**, 359–70.

11 Villiers, M-B., Thielens, N. M., and Colomb, M. G. (1985). Soluble C3 proconvertase and convertase of the classical pathway of human complement: conditions for stabilization *in vitro*. *Biochem. J.*, **226**, 429–36.

12 Kerr, M. A. (1980). The human complement system: assembly of the classical pathway C3 convertase. *Biochem. J.*, **189**, 173–81.

13 Tack, B. F., Harrison, R. A., Janatova, J., Thomas, M. L., and Prahl, J. W. (1980). Evidence for the presence of an internal thiolester bond in the third component of human complement. *Proc. Natl. Acad. Sci. U.S.A.*, **77**, 5764–8.

14 Dodds, A. W., Law, S. K., and Porter, R. R. (1985). The origin of the very viable haemolytic activities of the common human complement component C4 allotypes including C4-A6. *EMBO J.*, **4**, 2239–44.

15 Law, S. K., Dodds, A. W., and Porter, R. R. (1984). A comparison of the properties of two classes C4A and C4B of the human complement component C4. *EMBO J.*, **3**, 1819–23.

16 Isenman, D. E. and Young, J. R. (1984). The molecular basis for the difference in immune haemolysis activity of the Chido and Rodgers isotypes of human complement component C4. *J. Immunol.*, **132**, 3019–27.

17 Law, S. K. A., Sepp, A., and Dodds, A. W. (1991). Specificity of the thiolester-mediated binding reaction. *Complement and inflammation*, **3**, 181 (abstract).

18 Sim, E. and Dodds, A. W. (1987). The fourth component of human complement —towards understanding an enigma of variations. In *Complement in health and disease* (ed. K. Whaley), pp. 99–124. MTP Press.

19 Carroll, M., Fathallah, D., Bergamaschini, L., Alicot, E., and Isenman, D. (1990). Substitution of a single amino acid (aspartic acid for histidine) converts the functional activity of human complement C4B to C4A. *Proc. Natl. Acad. Sci. U.S.A.*, **87**, 6868–72.

20 Harpel, P. C. and Cooper, NR (1975). Studies on human plasma C1 inactivator–enzyme interactions. I. Mechanisms of interaction with C1s, plasmin, and trypsin. *J. Clin. Invest.*, **55**, 593–604.

21 Sim, R. B., Arlaud, G. J., and Colomb, M. G. (1979). C1 inhibitor-dependent dissociation of human complement component C1 bound to immune complexes. *Biochem. J.*, **179**, 449–57.

22 Ziccardi, R. J., and Cooper, N. R. (1979). Active disassembly of the first complement component C1 by C1 inactivator. *J. Immunol.*, **123**, 788–92.

23 Cooper, N. R. (1985). The classical complement pathway: activation and regulation of the first complement component. *Adv. Immunol.*, **37**, 151–216.

24 Fujita, T. and Nussenzweig, V. (1979). The role of C4 binding protein and β1H in proteolysis of C4b and C3b. *J. Exp. Med.*, **150**, 267–76.

25 Gigli, I., Fujita, T., and Nussenzweig, V. (1980). Modulation of the classical pathway C3 convertase by the plasma protein C4bp and C3bIna. *J. Immunol.*, **124**, 1521 (abstract).

26 Kristensen, T., D'Eustachio, P., Ogata, R. T., Chung, L. P., Reid, K. B., and Tack, B. F. (1987). The superfamily of C3b/C4b-binding proteins. *Fed. Proc.*, **46**, 2463–9.

27 Reid, K. B. M., Bentley, D. R., Campbell, R. D., Chung, L. P., Sim, R. B., Kristensen, T., and Tack, B F. (1986). Complement system proteins which interact with C3b or C4b. A superfamily of structurally related proteins. *Immuno. Today*, **7**, 230–4.

28 Atkinson, J. P. and Farries, T. (1987). Separation of self from non-self in the complement system. *Immunol. Today*, **8**, 212–15.

29 Seya, T., Turner, J. R., and Atkinson, J. P. (1986). Purification and characterization of a membrane protein (gp45–70) that is a cofactor for cleavage of C3b and C4b. *J. Exp. Med.*, **163**, 837–55.

30 Nicholsen-Weller, A., Burge, J., Fearon, D. T., Weller, P. F., and Austen, K. F. (1982). Isolation of a human erythrocyte membrane glycoprotein with decay accelerating activity for C3 convertases of the complement system. *J. Immunol.*, **129**, 184–9.

31 Holers, V. M., Cole, J., Lublin, D. M., Seya, T., and Atkinson, J. P. (1985). Human C3b- and C4b-regulator proteins: a new multigene family. *Immunol, Today*, **6**, 188–92.

32 Weisman, H. F., Bartow, T., Leppo, M. K., Marsh, H. C., Carson, G. R., Concino, M. F., Boyle, M. P., Roux, K. H., Weisfeldt, M. L., and Fearon, D. T. (1990). Soluble human complement receptor type *in vivo* inhibitor of complement suppressed post-ischaemic myocardial inflammation and necrosis. *Science*, **249**, 146–51.

33 Kerr, M. A. and Yeung-Laiwah, A. C. (1987). C1 inhibitor deficiency and angiooedema. In *Complement in health and disease* (ed. K. Whaley), pp. 53–78. MTP Press.

34 Jackson, J., Sim, R. B., Whelan, A., and Feighery, C. (1986). An IgG autoantibody which activates C1 inhibitor. *Nature*, **323**, 722–4.

35 Claus, D. R., SiegeL, J., Petras, K., Skor, D., Osmond, P., and Gewurz, H. (1977). Complement activation by interaction of multiple polyanions and polycations in he presence of C-reactive protein. *J. Immunol.*, **118**, 83–7.

36 Cooper, N. R., Jensen, F. C., Welsh, R. M., and Oldstone, M. B. A. (1976). Lysis of RNA tumour viruses by human serum: direct antibody-independent triggering of the classical complement pathway. *J. Exp. Med.*, **144**, 970–84.

37 Cias, F. and Loos, M. (1987). Complement and bacteria. In *Complement in health and disease* (ed. K. Whaley), pp. 201–231. MTP Press.

38 Giclas, P. C., Pinkard, R. N., and Olson, M. S. (1979). *In vivo* activation of complement by isolated human heart subcellular membranes. *J. Immunol.*, **122**, 146–51.

39 Yasuda, M., Takeuchi, K., Hiruma, M., Iida, H., Tahara, A., Itagane, H., Akioka, K., Teragaki, M., Oku, H., Kanayama, Y., Takeda, T., Kolb, W. P., and Tamerius, J. D. (1990). The complement system in ischaemic heart disease. *Circulation*, **81**, 156–63.

40 Lu, J., Thiel, S., Wiedemann, H., Timpl, R., and Reid, K. B. M. (1990). Binding of the pentamer/hexamer forms of mannan-binding protein to zymosan activates the pro-enzyme $C1r_2C1s_2$ complex, of the classical pathway of complement, without development of C1q. *J. Immunol.*, **144**, 2287–94.

41 Isenman, D., Kells, D. I. C., Cooper, N. R., Müller-Eberhard, H. J., and Pangburn, M. K. (1981). Nucleophilic modification of human complement protein C3: correlation of conformational changes with acquisition of C3b-like functional properties. *Biochemistry*, **19**, 4458–7.

42 Fearon, D. T. and Austen, K. F. (1975). Properdin: binding to C3b and stabilization of the C3b-dependent C3 convertase. *J. Exp. Med.*, **142**, 856–63.

43 Whaley, K. and Ruddy, S. (1976). Modulation of the alternative complement pathway by β1H globulin. *J. Exp. Med.*, **144**, 1147–63.

44 Weiler, J. M., Daha, M. R., Austen, K., and Fearon, D. T. (1976). Control of the amplification convertase of complement by the plasma protein β1H. *Proc. Natl. Acad. Sci. U.S.A.*, **73**, 3268–72.

45 Kazatchkine, M. D., Fearon, D. T., and Austen, K. F. (1979). Human alternative complement pathway: membrane associated sialic acid regulates the competition between B and β1H for cell-bound C3b. *J. Immunol.*, **122**, 75–81.

46 Fearon, D. T. (1978). Regulation by membrane sialic acid of β1H-dependent decay-dissociation of the amplification C3 convertase of the alternative pathway. *Proc. Natl. Acad. Sci. U.S.A.*, **75**, 1971–5.

47 Nelson, B. and Ruddy, S. (1979). Enhancing role of IgG in lysis of rabbit erythrocytes by the alternative pathway of human complement. *J. Immunol.*, **122**, 1994–9.

48 Nicholson-Weller, A., Daha, M. R., and Austen, K. F. (1981). Different functions for specific guinea pig IgG1 and IgG2 in the lysis of sheep erythrocytes by C4 deficient guinea pig serum. *J. Immunol.*, **126**, 1800–4.

49 Ratnoff, W. D., Fearon, D. T., and Austen, K. F. (1983). The role of antibody in the activation of the alternative complement. *Springer Semin. Immunopathol.*, **6**, 361–71.

50 Schenkein, H. A. and Ruddy, S. (1981). The role of immunoglobulins in alternative complement pathway activation by zymosan. I. Human IgG with specificity for zymosan enhances alternative pathway activation by zymosan. *J. Immunol.*, **126**, 7–10.

51 Schenkein, H. A. and Ruddy, S. (1981). The role of immunoglobulins in alternative pathway activation by zymosan. II. The effect of IgG on the kinetics of the alternative pathway. *J. Immunol.*, **126**, 11–5.

52 Winkelstein, J. A. and Shin, H. S. (1974). The role of immunoglobulin in the interaction of pneumococci and the properdin pathway: evidence for its specificity and lack of requirement for the Fc portion of the molecule. *J. Immunol.*, **112**, 1635–42.

53 Capel, P. J., Groeneboer, O., Grosveld, G., and Pondman, K. W. (1978). The binding of activated C3 to polysaccharides and immunoglobulins. *J. Immunol.*, **121**, 2566–72.

54 Fries, L. F., Gaither, T. A., Hammer, C. H., and Frank, M. M. (1984). C3b covalently bound to IgG demonstrates a reduced rate of inactivation by factors H and I. *J. Exp. Med.*, **160**, 1640–55.

55 Joiner, K. A., Fries, L. F., Schmetz, M. A., and Frank, M. M. (1985). IgG bearing covalently bound C3b has enhanced bactericidal activity for *Escherichia coli* 0111. *J. Exp. Med.*, **162**, 877–89.

56 Kinoshita, T., Takata, Y., Kozono, H., Takeda, J., Hong, K., and Inoue, K. (1988). C5 convertase of the alternative pathway: covalent linkage between two C3b molecules within the trimolecular complex enzyme. *J. Immunol.*, **141**, 3895–901.

57 Harrison, R. A. and Lachmann, P. J. (1980). The physiological breakdown of the third component of complement. *Mol. Immunol.*, **17**, 9–20.

58 Medof, M. E., Iida, K., Mold, C., and Nussenzweig, V. (1982). Unique role for the complement receptor CR1 in the degradation of C3b associated with immune complexes. *J. Exp. Med.*, **156**, 1739–54.

59 Lundwall, A. B., Wetsel, R. A., Kristensen, T., Whitehead, A. S., Woods, D. E., Ogden, R. C., Colten, H. R., and Tack, B. F. (1985). Isolation and sequence analysis of a cDNA clone encoding the fifth complement component. *J. Biol. Chem.*, **260**, 2108–12.

60 Lachmann, P. J., and Thompson, R. A. (1970). Reactive lysis: the complement-mediated lysis of unsensitized cells. II. The characterization of activated reactor as C5b and the participation of C8 and C9. *J. Exp. Med.*, **131**, 643–57.

61 Podack, E. R. (1986). Assembly and functions of the terminal components. In *Immunology of the complement system* (ed. G. D. Ross), pp. 115–37. Academic Press Inc., Orlando.

62 Stolfi, R. L. (1968). Immune lytic transformation: a state of irreversible damage generated as a result of the reaction of the eighth component of the guinea pig complement system. *J. Immunol.* **100**, 46–54.

63 Tschopp, J., Engel, A., and Podack, E. R. (1984). Molecular weight of poly (C9): 12–18 molecules form the transmembrane channel of complement. *J. Biol. Chem.*, **259**, 1922–8.

64 Tschopp, J. (1984). Ultrastructure of the membrane attack complex of complement. Heterogeneity of the complex caused by different degrees of C3 polymerization. *J. Biol. Chem.*, **259**, 7857–63.

65 Esser, A. F., Kolb, W. P., Podack E. R., and Müller-Eberhard, H. J. (1979). Molecular reorganization of lipid bilayers by complement: a possible mechanism for membranolysis. *Proc. Natl. Acad. Sci. U.S.A.*, **76**, 1410–4.

66 Morgan, B. P., Dankert, J. P., and Esser, A. F. (1985). Recovery of human neutrophils from complement attack: production of membrane vesicles bearing the membrane attack complex. *Complement*, **2**, 56 (abstract).

67 Lint, T. F., Behrends, C. L., and Gewurz, H. (1977). Serum lipoproteins and C567-Inh activity. *J. Immunol.*, **119**, 883–8.

68 Dahlbach, B. and Podack, E. R. (1985). Characterization of human S protein, an inhibitor of the membrane attack complex of complement. Demonstration of a free reactive thiol group. *Biochemistry*, **24**, 2368–74.

69 Zahlman, L. S., Wood, L. M., and Müller-Eberhard, H. J. (1986). Isolation of a human erythrocyte membrane protein capable of inhibiting expression of homologous complement transmembrane channels. *Proc. Natl. Acad. Sci. U.S.A.*, **83**, 6975–9.

70 Davies, A., Simmons, D. L., Hale, G., Harrison, R. A., Tighe, H., Lachmann, P. J., and Weldman, H. (1989). CD59 an LY-6-like protein expressed in human lymphoid cells regulates the action of the complement membrane attack complex on homologous cells. *J. Exp. Med.*, **170**, 637–50.

71 Fearon, D. T. and Wong, W. W. (1983). Complement ligand–receptor interactions that mediate biological responses. *Annu. Rev. Immunol.*, **1**, 243–71.

72 Ross. G. D. and Medof, M. E. (1985). Membrane complement receptors specific for bound fragments of C3. *Adv. Immunol.*, **37**, 217–67.

73 Wilson, J. G., Andriopoulos, N. A., and Fearon, D. T. (1987). CR1 and the cell membrane proteins that bind C3 and C4. A basic and clinical review. *Immunol. Res.*, **6**, 192–209.

74 Gerard, N. P. and Gerard, C. (1991). The chemotactic receptor for human C5a anaphylatoxin. *Nature*, **349**, 614–7.

75 Hugli, T. E. (1983). Biological activities of fragments derived from human complement components. *Prog. Immunol.*, **5**, 419–26.

76 Johnson, A. R., Hugli, T. E., and Müller-Eberhard, H. J. (1975). Release of histamine from rat mast cells by the complement peptides C3a and C5a. *Immunology*, **28**, 1067–80.

77 Damerau, B., Zimmermann, B., Grunefeld, E., Czorniak, K., and Vogt, W. (1980). Biological activities of C5a and C5a desArg from hog serum. *Int. Arch. Allergy Appl. Immunol.*, **63**, 408–14.

78 Damerau, B., Grunefeld, E., and Vogt, W. (1978). Chemotactic effects of the complement-derived peptides C3a, C5ai, and C5a (classical anaphylatoxin) on rabbit and guinea pig polymorphonuclear leucocytes. *Arch. Pharmacol.*, **305**, 181–4.

79 Fernandez, H. N., Henson, P. M., Otani, A., and Hugli, T. E. (1978). Chemotactic response to human C3a and C5a anaphylatoxins. I. Evaluation of C3a and C5a leucotaxis *in vitro* and under simulated *in vivo* conditions. *J. Immunol.*, **120**, 109–14.

80 Tonnensen, M. G., Smedly, L. A., and Henson, P. M. (1984). Neutrophil–endothelial cell interactions. Modulation of neutrophil adhesiveness induced by complement fragments C5a and C5a desArg and formyl-methionyl-leucyl-phenylalanine *in vitro*. *J. Clin. Invest.*, **74**, 1581–2.

81 Bokisch, V. A. and Müller-Eberhard, H. J. (1970). Anaphylatoxin inactivator of human plasma: its isolation and characterization as a carboxypeptidase. *J. Clin. Invest.*, **49**, 2427–36.

82 Kew, R. R. and Webster, R. O. (1988). Gc-globulin (vitamin D binding protein) enhances the neutrophil chemotactic activity of C5a and C5a desArg. *J. Clin. Invest.*, **82**, 364–9.

83 Perez, H. D., Goldstein, I. M., Chernoff, D., Webster, R. O., and Henson, P. M. (1980). Chemotactic activity of C5a desArg. Evidence of a requirement for an anionic polypeptide ('Helper Factor') in normal serum. *J. Immunol.*, **124**, 1535 (abstract).

84   Perez, H. D., Hooper, C., Volanakis, J., and Ueda, A. (1987). Specific inhibitor of complement (C5)-derived chemotactic activity in systemic lupus erythematosus related antigenically to the Bb fragment of human factor B. *J. Immunol.*, **139**, 484–9.

85   McCall, C. E., de Chatelet, L. R., Brown, D., and Lachmann, P. J. (1974). New biological activity following intravascular activation of the complement cascade. *Nature*, **249**, 841–3.

86   Ghebrehiwet, s. and Müller-Eberhard, H. J. (1979). C3e: an acidic fragment of human C3 with leucocytosis inducing activity. *J. Immunol.*, **123**, 616–21.

87   Ghebrehiwet, B. (1984). The release of lysosomal enzymes from human polymorphonuclear leucocytes by human C3e. *Clin. Immunol. Immunopathol.*, **30**, 321–9.

88   Kajita, T. and Hugli, T. E. (1990). C5a-induced neutrophilia. A primary humoral mechanism for recruitment of neutrophils. *Am. J. Pathol.*, **137**, 467–77.

89   Schifferli, J., Bartolotti, S. R., and Peters, D. K. (1980). Inhibition of immune precipitation by complement. *Clin. Exp., Immunol.*, **42**, 387–92.

90   Naama, J. K., Hamilton, A. O., Yeung-Laiwah, A., and Whaley, K. (1984). Prevention of immune precipitation in rheumatic disease: a clinical and laboratory study: *Scand. J. Rheumatol.*, **58**, 486–92.

91   Johnson, A., Auda, G. A., Kerr, M. A., Steward, M. A., and Whaley, K. (1991). Dissociation of primary antigen–antibody bonds is essential for complement mediated solubilization of immune complex. *Mol. Immunol.*, **29**, 659–65.

92   Cornacoff, J. B., Hebert, L. A., Smead, W. L., Van Aman, M. E., Birmingham, D. J., and Waxman, F. J. (1983). Primate erythrocyte immune complex-clearing mechanism. *J. Clin. Invest.*, **71**, 236–47.

93   Czop, J. and Nussenzweig, V. (1976). Studies on the mechanism of solubilization of immune precipitates by serum. *J. Exp. Med.*, **143**, 615–30.

94   Densen, P. and Mandell, G. L. (1990). Granulocytic phagocytes. In *Principles and practice of infectious diseases* (ed. G. L. Mandell, R. G. Douglas Jr, and J. E. Bennett), pp. 81–101. Churchill Llvingstone, New York.

95   Mannion, B. A., Weiss, J., and Elsbach, P. (1990). Separation of sublethal and lethal effects of polymorphonuclear leucocytes on *Escherichia coli*. *J. Clin. Invest.*, **86**, 631–41.

96   Tedesco, F., Rottini, G., and Patriarca, P. (1981). Modulating effect of the late-acting components of the complement system on the bactericidal activity of human polymorphonuclear leucocytes on *E. coli* 0111:B4. *J. Immunol.*, **127**, 1910–5.

97   Tedesco, F., Rottini, G., Roncelli, L., Basaglia, M., Menegazzi, R., and Patriarca, P. (1986). Bactericidal activities of human polymorphonuclear leucocyte proteins against *Escherichia coli* 0111:B4 coated with C5 or C8. *Infect. Immun.*, **54**, 250–4.

98   Taylor, P. W. (1983). Bactericidal and bacteriolytic activity of serum against Gram-negative bacteria. *Microbiol. Rev.*. **47**, 46–83.

99   Cooper, N. R. and Nemerow, G. R. (1986). Complement-dependent mechanisms of virus neutralization. In *Immunobiology of the complement system* (ed. G. D. Ross), pp. 139–62. Academic Press Inc., Orlando, Fla.

100   Weiler, J. M. (1987). Complement and the immune response. In *Complement in health and disease* (ed. K. Whaley), pp. 289–315. MTP Press.

101   Laham, M. N., Caldwell, J. R., and Panush, R. S. (1982). Modulation of lymphocyte proliferative responses in mitogens and antigens by complement components C1, C4, and C2. *J. Clin. Lab. Immunol.*, **9**, 39–47.

102 Weiler, J., Ballas, Z., Needleman, B., Hobbs, M. V., and Feldbush, T. L. (1982). Complement fragments suppress lymphocyte immune responses. *Immunol. Today*, **3**, 236–47.

103 Papamichail, M., Gutierrez, C., Embling, P., Johnson, P., Holborow, E. J., and Pepys, M. B. (1975). Complement dependence of localization of aggregated IgG in germinal centre. *Scand. J. Immunol.*, **43**, 343–7.

104 Cooper, N. R., Moore, M. D., and Nemerow, G. R. (1988). Immunobiology of CR2 and B lymphocyte receptor for Epstein–Barr virus and the C3d complement fragment. *Annu. Rev. Immunol.*, **6**, 85–113.

105 Bottger, E. C. and Bitter-Suermann, D. (1987). Complement and the regulation of humoral immune responses. *Immunol. Today*, **8**, 261–4.

106 Ochs, H. D., Wedgwood, R. J., Heller, S. R., and Beatty, P. G. (1986). Complement, membrane glycoproteins, and complement receptors: their role in regulation of the immune response. *Clin. Immunol. Immunopathol.*, **40**, 94–104.

107 O'Neil, K. M. H., Ochs, D., Heller, S. R., Cork, L. C., Morrris, J. M., and Winkelstein, J. A. (1988). Role of C3 in humoral immunity. Defective antibody production in C3 deficient dogs. *J. Immunol.*, **140**, 1939–45.

108 Finco, O., Li, S., Cuccia, M., Rosen, F. S., and Carroll, M. C. (1992). Structural differences between the two human complement C4 isotypes affect the humoral immune response. *J. Exp. Med.*, **175**, 537–43.

109 Atkinson, J. P. (1989). Complement deficiency: predisposing factor to auto-immune syndromes. *Clin. Exp. Rheumatol.*, **7**, 95–101.

110 Ross, S. C. and Densen, P. (1984). Complement deficiency states and infection: epidemiology, pathogenesis, and consequences of *Neisseria* and other infections in an immune deficiency. *Medicine* (Baltimore), **63**, 243–73.

111 Figueroa, J. E. and Densen, P. (1991). Infectious diseases associated with complement deficiencies. *Clin. Microbiol. Rev.*, **4**, 359–95.

112 Trapp, R. G., Fletcher, M., Forristal, J., and West, C. D. (1987). C4 binding protein deficiency in a patient with atypical Behcet's disease. *J. Rheumatol.*, **14**, 135–8.

113 Hynes, R. O. (1987). Integrins: a family of cell surface receptors. *Cell*, **48**, 549–54.

114 Springer, T. A., Thompson, W. S., Miller, L. J., Schmalstieg, F. C., and Anderson, D. C. (1984). Inherited deficiency of the Mac-1, LFA-1, p150,95 glycoprotein family and its molecular basis. *J. Exp. Med.*, **160**, 1901–18.

115 Anderson, D. C., Schmalsteig, F. C., Finegold, M. J., Hughes, B. J., Rothlein, R., Miller, L. J., Kohl, S., Tosi, M. F., Jacobs, R. L., and. Waldrop, T. C. (1985). The severe and moderate phenotyes of heritable Mac-1, LFA-1 deficiency: their quantitative definition and relation to leucocyte dysfunction and clinical features. *J. Infect. Dis.*, **152**, 668–89.

116 Anderson, D. C. and Springer, T. A. (1987). Leucocyte adhesion deficiency: an inherited defect in the Mac-1, LFA-1, and p169,95 glycoproteins. *Annu. Rev. Med.*, **38**, 1975–94.

117 Hansch, G. M., Schonermark, S., and Roelcke, D. (1987). Paroxysmal nocturnal haemoglobinuria type III. Lack of an erythrocyte membrane protein restricting the lysis by C5b–9. *J. Clin. Invest.*, **80**, 7–12.

118 Holguin, M. H., Fredrick, L. R., Bernshaw, N. J., Wilcox, L. A., and Parker, C. J. (1989). Isolation and characterization of a membrane protein from normal human erythrocytes that inhibits reactive lysis of the erythrocytes of paroxysmal nocturnal haemoglobinuria. *J. Clin. Invest.*, **84**, 7–17.

119 Nicholson-Weller, A., March, J. P., Rosenfeld, S. I., and Austen, K. F. (1983). Affected erythrocytes of patients with paroxysmal nocturnal haemoglobinuria are deficient in the complement regulatory protein, decay accelerating factors. *Proc. Natl. Acad. Sci. U.S.A.*, **80**, 5066–70.

120 Pangburn, M. K., Schreiber, R. D., and Müller-Eberhard, H. J. (1983). Deficiency of an erythrocyte membrane protein with complement regulatory activity in paroxysmal nocturnal haemoglobinuria. *Proc. Natl. Acad. Sci. U.S.A.*, **80**, 5430–4.

121 Hansch, G., Hammer, C., and Vanguri, P. (1981). Homologous species restriction in lysis of erythrocytes by terminal complement proteins. *Proc. Natl. Acad. Sci. U.S.A.*, **78**, 5118–21.

122 Rosse, W. F. (1972). Paroxysmal nocturnal haemoglobinuria. In *Haematology* (ed. W. J. Williams, E. Beutler, A, J. Erslev, and R. W. Rundles), pp. 460–74. McGraw-Hill Book Co., New York.

123 Rosse, W. F. (1990). Phosphatidylinositol-linked proteins and paroxysmal nocturnal haemoglobinuria. *Blood*, **75**, 1595–601.

124 Rosse, W. F. and Parker, C. J. (1985). Paroxysmal nocturnal haemoglobinuria. *Clin. Haematol.* **14**, 105–25.

125 Alper, C. A., Raum, A. D., Awdeh, Z. L., Petersen, B. H., Taylor, P. D., and Starzl, T. E. (1980). Studies of hepatic synthesis *in vivo* of plasma proteins, including orosomucoid, transferrin, alpha-1-antitrypsin,, C8, and factor B. *Clin. Immunol. Immunopathol.*, **16**, 84–9.

126 Lappin, D. F. and Whaley, K. (1992). Synthesis of complement by macrophages. *Blood Reviews*, (In press).

127 Colten, H. R. and Strunk, R. C. (1992). Extrahepatic complement synthesis. In *Complement in health and disease* 2nd ed (ed. K. Whaley, M. Loos, and J. Weiler). Kluwer Publication, Amsterdam (In press).

128 Ezekowitz, R. A. R., Sim, R. B., Hill, M., and Gordon, S. (1984). Local opsonization by secreted macrophage complement components. Role of receptors for complement in uptake of zymosan. *J. Exp. Med.*, **159**, 244–60.

129 Ruddy, S. and Colten, H. R. (1974). Rheumatoid arthritis. Biosynthesis of complement proteins by synovial tissues. *N. Engl. J. Med.*, **290**, 1284–5.

6 C1q and related molecules in defence

K. B. M. REID AND S. THIEL

1 Introduction

Activation of the classical and alternative pathways of complement leads to the utilization of a number of effector mechanisms in the blood which are of importance in defence by the generation of inflammation and through lysis and clearance of pathogens. Either pathway can be activated by both antibody-dependent and antibody-independent mechanisms although it is usually considered that the classical pathway is triggered primarily via antibody while the alternative pathway mainly provides antibody-independent activation. Immune aggregates containing antibody IgM, or certain subclasses of antibody IgG, are very efficient activators of the C1 complex of the classical pathway (via the Fc regions in the antibodies) while antibody IgG is not a pre-requisite for efficient alternative pathway activation (although it can have an enhancing effect, via the F(ab')$_2$ region, on this pathway). Apart from alternative pathway activation, the non-antibody-dependent mechanisms which appear to be of some importance in terms of defence, via complement activation and the generation of inflammation, involve acute phase proteins such as C-reactive protein (CRP), and mannan-binding protein (MBP), which can efficiently activate the classical pathway after direct interaction with ligands such as Pneumoccal C-polysaccharide (for CRP) or with terminal N-acetyl gluclosamine and/or mannose residues (for MBP) on glycoproteins. However, CRP still utilizes C1q to bring about classical pathway activation while MBP can replace C1q by mimicking its action. The observation that the binding of MBP to carbohydrate ligands can activate complement is quite recent (1–3) and there is already good evidence indicating that the serum level of MBP may be important in dealing with pathogenic organisms in the very young (4, 5) or in immunodeficient individuals. The MBP molecule contains distinct globular and collagen-like domains and therefore in view of its overall structural similarity to C1q it is perhaps not too surprising that it can mimic C1q's role in terms of classical pathway activation. Several other lectins, which include serum conglutinin and the lung surfactant molecules SP-A and SP-D, also contain collagen-like domains and it appears that they can all bind to the C1q receptor (C1qR) (6)—although this remains to be shown in the case of SP-D. Interaction of these lectins, presumably via their collagen-like regions, with C1qR could be of considerable physiological importance since the C1qR is found on a wide range of cells (such as fibroblasts, platelets, endothelial cells, and most leucocytes) and it has been reported that binding to the receptor triggers a wide range of biological effects (7).

A complete understanding of the possible roles that C1q and related molecules may play in antibody-independent defence requires some knowledge of their structures as detailed in the first part of this review. In general, the globular 'head' regions of these structurally related molecules play a recognition role. The collagen-like regions in the molecules are involved in the triggering of the complement cascade (C1q and MBP) or in interaction with cell surface receptors (C1q, MBP, SP-A, conglutinin, and possibly SP-D). The effects mediated by these molecules are described in the second half of the review.

2   Structural aspects

2.1   C1q

The C1q molecule contains 18 polypeptide chains (six A-, six B-, and six C-chains), each being approximately 225 amino acid residues long and containing a collagen-like region of approximately 81 residues near the N-terminus, and a C-terminal globular region of approximately 136 residues (Figure 6.1; (8)). The chains of human C1q have been cloned at the cDNA and genomic levels (9), and the genes encoding the chains have been shown to be aligned $\overrightarrow{5'/3'}$, in the same orientation, in the order A-C-B, on a 24 kb stretch of DNA within the region 1p34.1–1p36.3 on chromosome 1 (9).

The 18 chains of C1q are linked by interchain disulfide-bonds, located near the N-terminal end of each chain, to yield 6A-B dimer subunits and 3C-C dimer subunits which associate, via strong non-covalent bonds, to yield the intact hexameric C1q molecule of 46 kd (8). This model is consistent with electron microscopy studies which show C1q to be composed of six globular 'heads' linked via six collagen-like stalks to a fibril-like central region (Figure 6.2; (10)). The collagen-like regions of C1q interact with the Ca^{2+}-dependent, $C1r_2C1s_2$ pro-enzyme complex (360 kDa) to yield C1, the first component of complement. The globular 'heads' of C1q can interact with the Fc regions of IgG and IgM antibodies, once these antibodies have bound to antigens and this brings about activation of the C1 pro-enzyme complex. The activated $C1r_2C1s_2$ enzyme complex comes under the control of the C1 inhibitor molecule which binds covalently to the activated C1r and C1s enzymes thus causing their inactivation and rapid dissociation from the C1 complex. This leaves the collagen-like regions of the C1q molecule free to interact with the C1q receptor (6) found on a wide range of lymphoid cells thus allowing presentation of the C1q–antibody–antigen complex to these cells.

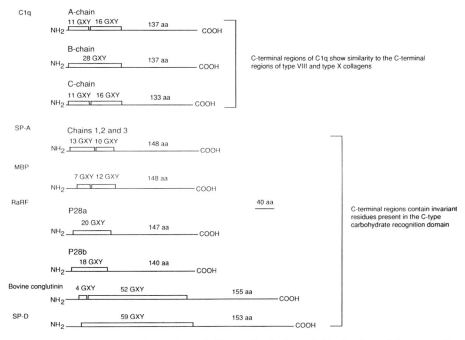

Fig. 6.1 The polypeptide chains of C1q and of the soluble lectins which contain collagen-like sequences: G-X-Y and the *open box* indicate the presence of Gly-Xaa-Yaa triplet repeats. The regions between open boxes are points of disruption in the Gly-Xaa-Yaa repeating structure. The C-terminal regions of the chains of C1q show a strong similarity to the non-collagen-like C-terminal regions of the type VIII and type X collagens. The C-terminal regions of all the other chains shown in this figure contain the conserved residues seen in the C-type lectin domains (see Figure 6.3).

An unusual structural feature in C1q is the presence of a 'bend' approximately half-way along each triple helix (Figure 6.2) which is known to be a result of interruptions to the Gly-Xaa-Yaa triplet sequences in the A- and C-chains. This structural feature correlates with the intron/exon boundaries seen in the A- and C-chain genes. It is possible that this type of structural feature, also seen in MBP and SP-A, may be of importance in interaction with $C1r_2C1s_2$ or with the C1q receptor.

2.2 Mannan-binding protein (MBP)

MBP is a member of the family of C-type lectins (as defined in the legend for Figure 6.3) and has been given a variety of names such as, mannan-binding protein, mannose-binding protein, and core-specific lectin. Mannan-binding protein was the first name used for the molecule (11) therefore it

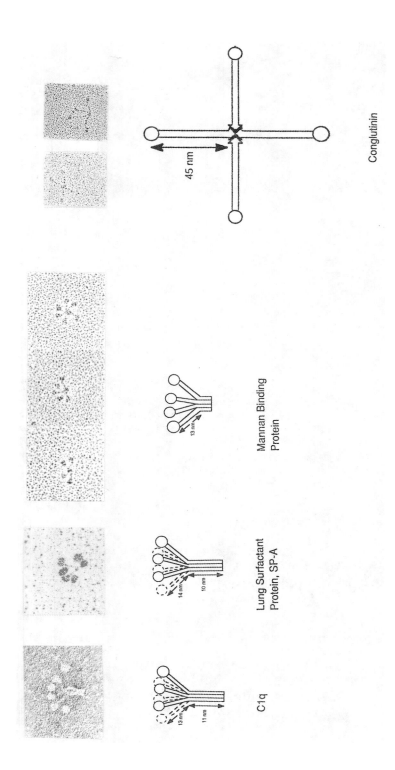

Fig. 6.2 Electron microscopy pictures of (from *left* to *right*): human C1q, human SP-A, human MBP, and bovine conglutinin. *Underneath* each picture is a schematic drawing of each protein showing the dimensions obtained by electron microscopy measurements. The SP-A and C1q electron micrographs were kindly provided by Dr J. Engel and Dr H. Isliker respectively and the MBP and conglutinin electron micrographs were provided by Dr R. Timpl.

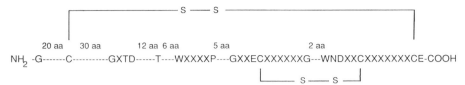

Fig. 6.3   The conserved residues found in the COOH-terminal carbohydrate re-cognizing domains (CRDs) of C-type lectins. The number of amino acids found between conserved residues is variable and in each case is indicated by a *broken line* plus the average number of amino acids as calculated from a variety of C-type lectins (18).

seems appropriate to use this nomenclature, especially since this distinguishes it from proteins such as the macrophage mannose-specific lectin.

The cDNAs and genes coding for MBP in rat and man have been cloned and sequenced (12–15). In man the mature MBP consists of three regions: (a) an NH_2-terminal segment of 21 amino acids with three cysteines probably involved in the formation of interchain disulfide-bonds which stabilize multi-meric forms of the protein, (b) a collagen-like domain consisting of 19 repeats of the sequence Gly-Xaa-Yaa (but with one disruption), and (c) a COOH-terminal C-type carbohydrate recognition domain of 148 amino acids (see Figure 6.1 and Figure 6.3).

When serum MBP is analysed by SDS-PAGE, in non-reducing conditions, it migrates as a large (>200 kDa) molecule and reduced it behaves as a 31 kDa polypeptide chain (3). MBP is synthesized in hepatocytes (14, 16). In man the MBP gene is located on chromosome 10 and is split in four exons (15, 17). The first exon encodes the NH_2-terminal part of the protein; the next two exons encode the collagen region. The second exon codes up to the disruption seen in the collagen sequence (see Figure 6.1), the third exon encodes the remaining part of the collagen region. The last exon codes for the COOH-terminal carbohydrate recognizing region. Due to the non-separated exon coding for the carbohydrate recognition domain, MBP is also termed a C-type lectin (18).

The 5'-flanking region of the gene for the human MBP contains a region similar to the Drosophila heat-shock promoter consensus sequence and three further regions are similar to consensus sequences for glucocorticoid respon-sive elements (15, 17). Consistent with these findings, it has been found that the level of MBP mRNA is probably increased following an acute phase response (14). Studies of the serum concentrations of MBP before and after major surgery confirms that MBP is an acute phase reactant (S. Thiel unpublished). It is noteworthy that the heat-shock consensus sequences also are present in the 5'-flanking region of the human CRP gene (19). CRP is a classical acute phase reactant, increasing dramatically (up to 1000-fold) during inflammation (20) (see Chapter 1).

Electron microscopy studies show that purified human serum MBP is composed of a mixture of trimers, tetramers, pentamers, and hexamers of an approximate 90 kDa structural unit (3, 21). The hexameric form of MBP is similar in overall structure to C1q as both molecules are composed of six globular heads each joined by connecting strands to a central structure (Figure 6.2). As discussed later, only fractions of purified MBP containing pentamer/hexamer forms of the molecule appear capable of efficiently activating the complement system.

2.3   Conglutinin

Bovine conglutinin is a serum protein which is able to mediate the agglutination (conglutination) of serum reacted erythrocytes (22–25). Initial studies on the structure of conglutinin indicated that it contained collagen-like features (26–28) and this was confirmed when the complete amino acid sequence was determined, at the protein level (29). Conglutinin contains one type of polypeptide chain which has an NH_2-terminal 25 amino acid globular segment followed by a 171 residue long collagenous domain, with a 155 amino acid long globular, C-terminal, domain (see Figure 6.1). A C-type carbohydrate recognition domain is present in the COOH C-terminal domain. The collagen-like stretch contains 56 Gly-Xaa-Yaa repeats with one interruption (Cys 38 instead of Gly 38) which could introduce flexibility into the collagenous arms of conglutinin.

When analysed by SDS-PAGE the bovine conglutinin appears as a 300 kDa molecule in the unreduced state, and upon reduction protein bands at 48 and 42 kDa are seen (27, 30, 31). These two bands are due to limited proteolysis producing a truncated form of the conglutinin polypeptide chain which lacks the N-terminal 54 residues (J. Lu, S. Thiel and A. C. Willis, unpublished observations).

In the electron microscope, bovine conglutinin appears as a tetramer of four 'lollipop' structures emanating from a central hub (32) (see Figure 6.2). The 45nm long 'arms' seem very flexible, probably as a result of the interruption of the triplet Gly-Xaa-Yaa sequence (see Figure 6.1). Strang *et al.* (32) have proposed a model for bovine conglutinin in which four disulfide-linked trimers are associated, via their N-terminal regions, to form the intact macromolecule as viewed in the electron microscope (see Figure 6.2). This would predict that the macromolecule has a molecular weight of approximately 576 kDa (12 times approximately 48 kDa).

2.4   Ra reactive factor

Ra reactive factor (RaRF) is a complement-dependent bactericidal factor present in sera of a wide variety of vertebrates (33, 34). It binds specifically to rough Ra chemotype strains of *Salmonella* and to rough R2 strains of

E. coli (35, 36). RaRF is a 300 kDa, Ca^{2+}-dependent, complex of proteins which dissociates into two fractions on treatment with EDTA. One is composed of multimers of two 28 kDa polypeptides (P28a and P28b) and the other is composed of 70 kDa (P70) and 29 kDa (P29) disulfide-linked polypeptides. The P28a and P28b form an RaLPS recognizing structure whereas the P70 and P29 are involved in the activation of C4 (Figure 6.4) (35, 37). P28a and P28b each have a short NH_2-terminal segment followed by a collagenous domain and a COOH-terminus comprising a C-type CRD (Figure 6.1) (38). It is therefore possible that the P28a and P28b will also form a 'tulip-like' structure. Identity in sequence, over the lectin domains, of mouse P28a and P28b with the recently published cDNA derived sequences of mouse MBP-C, and mouse MBP-A, respectively (39) strongly suggests that the P28a and P28b components of mouse RA reactive factor are MBP-C and MBP-A.

2.5   SP-A and SP-D

Two lung glycoproteins, SP-A and SP-D, have been found to show a structural similarity to the serum proteins discussed above (40, 41).

2.5.1   SP-A

SP-A, formerly referred to as apolipoprotein A, glycoprotein A, SP 28–36 and SAP-35 (nomenclature reviewed in Possmayer, (42)), is the most abundant lung-specific surfactant protein. The protein has been identified in all mammalian species examined so far, including rodents, ruminants, and primates as well as in chicken, frog, and fish (43–47). In man the cell type

Classical Pathway Activation

	Antibody-dependent	Antibody-independent			
	C1	C1/C1q LPS	CRP-C1q	MBP	RaRF
Ligand	Fc portion of immunoglobulin	Lipopolysaccharides on Gram-negative bacteria Sub cellular components	C-Polysaccharide on Streptococci pneumonia	Mannose or N-acetylglucosamine at oligosaccharide termini	Rough core RaLPS
Recognition molecule	C1q	C1q	CRP	MBP	P28a/b
Activating enzyme complex	$C1r_2 C1s_2$	$C1r_2 C1s_2$	$C1r_2 C1s_2$	$C1r_2 C1s_2$	P70/P29

Fig. 6.4   Outline of C4 activation by antibody-dependent and antibody-independent routes involving C1q, CRP, MBP, and RaRF. It appears that C1q, CRF–C1q, and MBP all activate C4 via an activation of C1r in the $C1r_2C1s_2$ complex, whereas RaRF activates C4 after binding to RaLPS by activation of P70/P29. See text for details.

responsible for the synthesis of SP-A, as determined by *in situ* hybridization, is the alveolar type II cell (48).

The polypeptide chain in the fully mature protein has a short seven amino acid long N-terminal segment (containing a cysteine residue) followed by 73 residues of a collagen-like, -Gly-Xaa-Yaa-, sequence. This sequence is interrupted at the 13th Gly-Xaa-Yaa triplet due to an insertion of an extra proline residue and the substitution of a glycine by cysteine. This is followed by a 148 residue long C-terminal globular region (see Figure 6.1 and Figure 6.2) (49). The COOH-terminal part contains a C-type CRD with four cysteines which may be connected as shown in Figure 6.3. When analysed by SDS-PAGE under reducing conditions the SP-A migrates as two major bands at 28 and 35 kDa (50). These represent an unglycosylated and a glycosylated form of the polypeptide chain, respectively. Native SP-A is considered to contain 18 polypeptide chains, each approximately 35 kDa, yielding an intact molecule of approximately 630 kDa.

One genomic sequence of human SP-A (situated on chromosome 10) has been described and at least two cDNA's have been characterized (49, 51). The slightly different translation products from these cDNA's may be required to form triple helices consisting of heterodimers (see later). Recombinant SP-A, obtained by transfection of Chinese hamster ovary (CHO) cells with a single genomic construct, is not well assembled into the oligomeric form although the protein is functionally active in some instances (40, 52). The overall appearance of the protein, when examined by electron microscopy (Figure 6.2), is indistinguishable from that of C1q (40). The interruption of the Gly-Xaa-Yaa sequence in each chain in the molecule correlates with the presence of a 'kink' in the stalk region of SP-A (Figure 6.2).

2.5.2   SP-D

SP-D, formerly referred to as collagenous protein 4 (CP-4), has been isolated from the culture medium of isolated type II pneumocytes (rat), from bronchoalveolar lavage (rat and man) (53, 54), and human amniotic fluid (55). The protein has a molecular weight of approximately 630 kDa in non-dissociating conditions, and on SDS-PAGE, in reducing conditions, it migrates as a 43 kDa polypeptide. The derived amino acid sequence of human SP-D has been obtained by analysis of cDNA clones (55) and the protein is highly homologous (66 per cent identity) to bovine conglutinin and has an N-terminal, collagen-like domain and a C-terminal, C-type lectin, carbohydrate-binding domain. Despite this high degree of homology, human SP-D shows quite a different sugar binding specificity to that of conglutinin. SP-D shows strong binding to maltose (and the related isomaltose and maltotriose) which is calcium-dependent with lesser binding to glucose and mannose and essentially no binding is observed to *N*-acetylglucosamine and *N*-acetylgalactosamine (41). Furthermore, the protein can be eluted from crude lung surfactant with maltose, indicating that the association of SP-D with surfactant is mediated by carbohydrate-dependent interactions with specificity for, α-glucosyl residues (41).

3 Functional aspects

3.1 The role of C-reactive protein (CRP) in C1q mediated, non-antibody-dependent activation of the classical pathway of complement

The roles of antibody IgG, or IgM, in the binding and activation of the C1 complex are well documented (see Chapter 5) (56). The C1q-binding site, in the C_H2 domain of the Fc region of IgG, appears to reside in the charged motif $Glu_{(318)}$-X-$Lys_{(320)}$-Y-$Lys_{(322)}$ (57). A motif in the C_H3 domain of IgM, perhaps involving only two charged amino acids, may be the site of IgM–C1q interaction (58). By interaction of the acute phase C-reactive protein (CRP) with C1q, the antibody requirement, for bringing about activation of the $C1r_2C1s_2$ pro-enzyme complex, is bypassed. CRP is composed of five identical, non-covalently linked, subunits, each of 24 kDa. It has a Ca^{2+}-dependent binding specificity for phosphocholine present in the cell walls and membranes of *Streptococci pneumoniae*. It is well known, from *in vitro* studies, that CRP can activate the classical pathway after interaction with pneumococcal C-polysaccharide (59) or certain polycations (60). Recently, by utilizing CRP-trimers prepared by cross-linking, Jiang *et al.* (61), have proposed that the site of CRP-C1q interaction lies at the junction where the collagen-like regions of C1q merge into the globular heads and they demonstrated that this site was distinct from the IgG-C1q interaction site located in the globular heads of C1q. In addition, CRP has been shown to be involved in the promotion of phagocytosis by polymorphonuclear leucocytes and thus appears to play a general role in host defence against certain bacterial infections. This view is supported by the observation that human CRP can be used to provide passive protection of mice from a lethal infection of *Streptococci pneumoniae*, in the absence of antibody and by use of a complement-dependent mechanism (62).

C1q can also directly interact with lipopolysaccharides and porins from Gram-negative bacteria (63, 64), and with a wide variety of the products of tissue damage, such as mitochondrial cardiolipin, mitochondrial proteins, and nucleic acids. The antibody-independent interaction of C1q with these highly charged polymers can result in activation of the classical pathway resulting in the complement-mediated enhanced clearance of these substances from the blood. It may be of significance that in disorders with defective immune complex clearance, the antibody specificities are directed against subcellular components which will lead to activation of the classical complement pathway. As described in Chapter 5, complement deficiencies, particularly of the classical pathway components are associated with immune complex deposition.

3.2   C1q-C1q receptor interaction and involvement of molecules related to C1q

In the blood the majority of the C1q protein is associated, via its collagen-like region, with the pro-enzyme $C1r_2\text{-}Ca^{2+}\text{-}C1s_2$ complex (65, 66). When the activation of the pro-enzymes C1r and C1s has been triggered by the ionic interaction between the 'heads' of C1q and the Fc regions of IgG, or IgM, the activated C1 complex comes under control of the C1 inhibitor and are rapidly removed from the C1 activator complex, thus leaving the collagen-like regions free to interact with the C1q receptor (C1qR). The C1qR is found at levels of $10^5\text{--}10^6$ molecules/cell on the surface of endothelial cells, fibroblasts, B and T lymphocytes, monocytes/macrophages, and a variety of cultured cells such as Raji, Daudi, U937, Wil$_2$WT with lower levels, of approximately 4×10^3 molecules/cell, as well as being found on platelets (7). The C1qR, as isolated from human tonsils or U937 cells has been shown to be an acidic glycoprotein of 56 kDa on SDS-PAGE in both reducing and non-reducing conditions (67). The C1qR contains 15–20 per cent carbohydrate and the detergent solubilized protein behaves as a dimer of 115 kDa and remains soluble in the absence of detergent. Preparations of C1qR from other cells such as Raji appear to show a higher molecular weight of 65–80 kDa on SDS-PAGE (7) and there is another report of C1qR preparations from U937 cells, monocytes, and neutrophils which all have a molecular weight of 123 kDa on SDS-PAGE, in both reducing and non-reducing conditions (68). It is therefore possible that there is more than one type of C1qR or that C1qR is composed of more then one chain. It is clear that when the collagen-like regions of C1q, in the C1q–antibody–antigen complex, are presented to C1qR then a wide range of phenomena can be triggered such as cell-mediated cytotoxicity, increased oxidative metabolism, enhanced phagocytosis, modulation of cytokine and immunoglobulin secretion, and polymorph–endothelium interaction (biological properties reviewed by Ghebrehiwet (7)).

3.3   Mannan-binding protein

3.3.1   Binding specificities of MBP

The most potent sugar inhibitors of the Ca^{2+}-dependent binding between mannan and MBP are N-acetyl-D-glucosamine and mannose. Other monosaccharides are poor inhibitors (11, 69, 70). It is perhaps of more importance to evaluate the binding of MBP to oligosaccharides as these probably will represent physiologically more relevant binding structures. Oligosaccharide recognition by MBP has been investigated by using as probes a series of structurally characterized glycolipids separated by thin layer chromatography (71). When the binding to N-linked biantennary complex-type oligosaccharides was investigated MBP showed preferential reactivities with those containing two peripheral N-acetylglucosamine residues. Substitution with galactose masked reactivity. Similarly, mannose residues have to be exposed i.e. non-reducing, to be effective in binding. Fucose when bound in the $\alpha 1-4$, or $\alpha 1-3$ configuration to GlcNAc at the ends of complex-type oligosaccharides is also a ligand for MBP. Clearly, MBP has the potential to react with several glycoconjugates, but a major determining factor is likely to be the accessibility of the oligosaccharides which may be influenced by the structure of the protein chain to which they are covalently attached (28, 72).

3.3.2 Interaction with the complement system—functional, as well as structural, similarity of MBP to C1q

Purified MBP from man, rabbit, and rat in the presence of serum can mediate classical pathway-dependent lysis of sheep erythrocytes coated with mannan (1). Further studies, indicate that C1s, but only when C1r is also present, binds to MBP, when the MBP is bound to mannan-coated erythrocytes (2). In another functional study, the ligand for MBP was zymosan and activation of the complement system was followed by measurement of the activation of pro-enzyme C1s in the $C1s_2C1r_2$ complex (3). Importantly, it was shown that only the hexamer/pentamer forms of MBP (supported by electron microscopy studies of the relevant fractions), and not smaller forms of the molecule, could activate C1s. This is in agreement with Ikeda *et al.* (1) who observed that only MBP purified from serum, but not MBP purified from liver (which has a considerably lower apparent molecular weight compared to the serum MBP), mediated activation of the complement system.

In another approach, sera were analysed for their ability to deposit complement factors, via classical pathway activation, onto mannan-coated microtitre wells (73). Analysis of 176 healthy blood donors revealed that the levels of complement factors, bound to the mannan-coated surface, correlated with the amount of MBP in the sera. In contrast to these studies, Schweinle *et al.* (74) have reported activation of the alternative pathway of complement by Gram-negative bacteria coated with MBP.

3.3.3 Anti-microbial and anti-viral activity

Since it is known that high mannose oligosaccharides are present on several viruses (75, 76) these could be potential ligands for MBP (and conglutinin and SP-A). For example, the membrane proteins, the outer membrane gp120, and the transmembrane gp41, of human immunodeficiency virus type 1 have been shown to be heavily glycosylated. About 50 per cent of the gp120 molecule is comprised of N-linked oligosaccharides of the high mannose type as well as of hybrid and complex types (77, 78). It may also contain some O-linked carbohydrates (79). CD4 antigen on the surface of target cells provides recognition structures for the attachment of the virion (80, 81). gp120 is the molecule on the virus which mediates the binding to CD4 (82, 83). It appears that glycosylation of gp120 may influence the infection of the target cells with HIV-1, but somewhat conflicting results have been reported (84–88). Molecules interacting with gp120 or CD4 could possibly prevent infection of target cells.

In accordance with this it has been reported that certain plant lectins, with the potential to bind to carbohydrates on gp120, inhibit viral replication when added to cultures of HIV-1 and target cells (89). As plant lectins are generally highly toxic and immunogenic these proteins are not of direct therapeutic interest. Investigation of the potential of mammalian lectins to inhibit viral infection of cells has therefore been started.

One study has investigated the interaction between HIV-1 and MBP (90). Purified human serum MBP was found to bind to HIV-1 infected CD4$^+$H9 cells and to HIV-1 infected cells of the monocytic cell line U937. Also a direct, divalent cation-dependent, binding of MBP to a recombinant form of the membrane protein gp120 was observed. Further it was found that pre-incubation of HIV-1 with MBP inhibits subsequent infection of H9 lymphoblast with HIV-1.

Another approach to the study of mannose-binding proteins and their ability to interact with virus is presented in a study on the β-inhibitors of influenza virus A (91). These inhibitors are identified as heat-labile components of normal sera that have virus neutralizing as well as haemagglutination inhibiting activity. Investigation into the nature of the interaction of β-inhibitors with influenza virus revealed that these are mannose-binding lectins, (i.e. the haemagglutination inhibiting activity is inhibited by mannose) (91). These inhibitors may be identical to one of the known mannose-binding proteins, MBP or conglutinin.

MBP is also able to mediate bactericidal activity dependent on the classical pathway of complement (92). When a rough strain of *Escherichia coli* (strain K-12 and B) has been sensitized with MBP and complement is added, then classical pathway-dependent killing of the bacteria is seen. When *Salmonella montevideo* (strain SH5770) is sensitized with MBP, a serum-mediated killing of the bacteria can be observed (74). A direct opsonizing effect and increased killing was demonstrated when human MBP was bound to *Salmonella montevideo* (strain SH5770 expressing a mannose rich O-polysaccharide within its LPS), the bacteria washed, and then mixed with polymorphonuclear leucocytes (PMN) or monocytes.

As discussed above, it has been found that MBP is able to interact with the C1qR (6). The interaction with C1qR suggests that there are two ways MBP can opsonize micro-organisms; (a) a direct opsonizing function by binding to the micro-organism, mediating phagocytosis via C1qR and (b) an indirect opsonizing effect by binding to a micro-organism and then activating the complement system where the deposited complement factors (especially C3b and iC3b) will have an opsonic effect. The last function is probably the most important one due to the amplification factor gained by activating the complement system.

3.3.4 Clinical observations

The failure of serum to opsonize bakers yeast (*Saccharomyces cerevisiae*) for phagocytosis by normal polymorphonuclear leucocytes has been reported in a series of children with frequent unexplained infections (93), in association with chronic diarrhoea of infancy (94), and in association with otitis media in infants (95). The defect is surprisingly common (5–7 per cent) in the general population (93, 96, 97). An association between this defect to opsonize yeast and a lowered ability to deposit C3b/iC3b fragments on the yeast surface has been established (97). An association of low levels of MBP in the serum with the defect in opsonization has been established (4). Furthermore purified MBP corrected the opsonizing defect in the sera in a dose-dependent manner. Previous observations have shown that people with the opsonic defect deposit lower levels of C3b not only on *Candida albicans*, but also on *Staphylococcus aureus* and *Escherichia coli* (98) which suggests that low levels of MBP may result in suboptimal responses to a wide range of common bacterial infections. It is clear that disease is not inevitably associated with low levels of MBP as low levels of MBP are found in about ten per cent of normal healthy children. A deficiency of the lectin may become pathologically important in individuals where the other immunological responses toward polysaccharides (either humoral or cellular) are weakened. This is most likely to occur in infants aged 6–18 months as they will have no residual maternal antibodies and their own immune system will still not have reached a fully mature state (99). With the maturation of the antibody repertoire and the cellular immune response the host will depend less on antigen non-specific immune mechanisms such as MBP, and the clinical relevance of low levels of the lectin in these circumstances is less clear.

Recently, MBP deficiency has been shown to be the result of a point mutation at base 230 of exon 1 in the MBP gene—which results in the replacement of a glycine by aspartic acid thus disrupting the fifth Gly-Xaa-Yaa repeating triplet within the collagen-like region of the MBP chain (5). This mutation appears to prevent triple helix formation and results in low, or zero, levels of functionally active MBP. Analysis of families, in which one or more members have low MBP levels, showed autosomal dominant co-inheritance of the mutation.

3.4   Conglutinin

3.4.1   Carbohydrate specificity

The ligand for conglutinin in the agglutination of serum reacted erythrocytes has been determined to be iC3b derived from C3b deposited on the cells (100–102). It has been found that conglutinin binds to the carbohydrates on the α chain of iC3b (103). Certain carbohydrates are able to inhibit the agglutination better than others (104, 105). Thus a 'scale of inhibiting capacity' can be made: GlcNAc, chitobiose > L-fucose and Man ≫ GalNAc, ManNAc, D-fucose, and galactose. The lack of reactivity of conglutinin with native C3, and its reaction with enzymatically degraded fragments of C3b, indicates that the folding of the protein chain hinders accessibility of the oligosaccharides for reaction with conglutinin. Enhanced oligosaccharide accessibility is therefore likely to be the biochemical basis for the binding of conglutinin to the proteolytically generated, and cell-bound, iC3b fragment. Oligosaccharides that in theory should mediate conglutinin binding are also present in, for example IgG, IgM, thyroglobulin, and ovalbumin. However, no binding is seen to IgG and IgM in their non-denatured states, again indicating that the polypeptide chain of the protein is able to cover, or maybe restrict the possible forms of the carbohydrate structures which are the putative ligands for conglutinin.

Another approach to the study of carbohydrate specificity of lectins is, as described for MBP, the use of glycolipids separated on thin layer chromatography as solid-phase oligosaccharide probes. Overlaying a spectrum of glycolipids (constructed using complex-type and high mannose-type oligosaccharides from N-glycosylated proteins) with [^{125}I]bovine conglutinin indicate that complex-type chains with unsubstituted terminal *N*-acetylglucosamine residues on their outer branches and unsubstituted mannose residues in their core regions are recognized by conglutinin, as well as the terminal mannose residues of high mannose-type chains (106). Based on these and other data (72) it is predicted that bovine conglutinin has the potential to bind an array of glycoconjugates other than C3, if the oligosaccharides are accessible.

3.4.2 Anti-microbial activity

Several observations strongly indicate that bovine conglutinin is consumed during infection of cattle with organisms, such as *Mycobacterium tuberculosis* (107), *Cowdria rumination* (108), and the parasite *Anaplasma marginale* (109), and that it therefore may in some way participate in anti-microbial defence mechanisms (110). In general, the lowest levels of conglutinin are seen at the peak of infection and they return to normal levels after infection

3.4.3 Interaction with micro-organisms

As discussed above the membrane-bound glycoproteins of several micro-organisms have high mannose oligosaccharides attached to their polypeptide chains. *In vivo* studies of a possible anti-bacterial effect of bovine conglutinin have shown that mice injected with a conglutinin containing euglobulin fraction of ox serum had higher survival rates following subsequent challenge with Gram-negative bacteria (111, 112). It was also reported that the rate of clearance of *Salmonella typhimurium* from blood circulation was markedly enhanced in mice which had been injected one day previously with the conglutinin containing euglobulin fraction from ox serum (112). These results have been confirmed and the supposition of an anti-bacterial activity of bovine conglutinin has been substantiated using highly purified bovine conglutinin in *in vitro* experiments (31). These experiments indicated that the effect of conglutinin required complement activation which resulted in the calcium-dependent binding of conglutinin to iC3b (a major product of complement activation). The presence of peritoneal exudate, or spleen cells was also essential for the anti-bacterial effect mediated by conglutinin (31). These results indicate that bovine conglutinin is able to enhance opsonization and phagocytosis by promoting contact between iC3b-coated bacteria and effector cell. The C1q receptor has been found to bind conglutinin (6) and it may be that the opsonizing effect of conglutinin is mediated through a binding to C1qR on phagocytic cells. As discussed, MBP was the first of the animal lectins found to be able to interact with HIV-1 and the macrophage mannose-specific receptor has been found to bind to gp120, the major glycoprotein of HIV-1 (87). It appears that bovine conglutinin may also interact with HIV-1 glycoproteins since it has been shown that a recombinant form of the viral protein gp160 (the precursor molecule that is cleaved to yield gp120 and gp41), is a possible ligand for conglutinin (113).

3.5   Ra reactive factor

The strains of bacteria which are susceptible to Ra reactive factor have in common a rough core LPS, and the determinant to which RaRF binds probably consists of GlcNAc, glucose, and L-glycero-D-mannoheptosyl residues present in the non-reducing termini of the polysaccharide chains of all these strains (114). The binding of Ra reactive factor to the Ra LPS is Ca^{2+}-dependent and it is inhibited in the presence of GlcNAc and glucose (34). After binding to bacteria, RaRF is able to activate the classical pathway of the complement system and thereby kill the bacteria (35, 115).

3.6   SP-A

It has been demonstrated, by means of affinity chromatography, that SP-A binds to immobilized carbohydrate in a calcium-dependent manner, the preferred ligands being mannose, fucose, galactose, or glucose (116). No binding was seen to immobilized *N*-acetylglucosamine or *N*-acetylgalactosamine. Several structural and metabolic roles have been attributed to SP-A, e.g. in the regulation of surfactant homeostasis and in the regulation of the formation of tubular myelin (reviewed by Weaver and Whitsett (117)). Although these functions are of major importance this review will only be dealing with the possible role of SP-A in host defence.

Several reports indicate that SP-A is able to interact with macrophages. Following binding of SP-A to alveolar macrophages various biological responses have been demonstrated. SP-A thus has been shown to enhance phagocytosis of bacteria opsonized by serum and of immunoglobulin and complement-coated erythrocytes (68, 118). Further, SP-A is shown to increase phagocytosis of herpes simplex virus by alveolar macrophages (119). Also, binding of SP-A to cells is shown to induce production of oxygen radicals by the cells (118). Enhanced phagocytosis described for different experimental systems may be due to a stimulation of the cell by SP-A which causes a signal to increase the phagocytic pathways; however, a direct opsonizing effect of SP-A cannot be excluded. The binding site of SP-A on alveolar macrophages is unknown, but a likely candidate would be the C1qR. Binding of SP-A to this receptor has been confirmed and the cell response to this binding is being explored (6, 120). Increased phagocytosis of micro-organisms due to an opsonizing effect of SP-A would therefore provide an alternative mechanism for clearing certain pathogens from the lung, in addition to antibody and complement-mediated phagocytosis.

It is surprising that, despite its marked overall similarity to C1q, SP-A (bound to carbohydrate) does not appear to activate complement (J. Haurum, unpublished observation). The reason for this functional difference is unclear since the overall molecular structure of SP-A is very similar to that of C1q, while MBP, which can activate complement, is a smaller molecule than C1q. One reason could be the more hydrophobic and amphiphatic nature of the SP-A as compared to C1q and MBP.

3.7   Macrophage scavenger cell receptor

The macrophage scavenger cell receptor contains an extracellular collagen-like region (an unbroken stretch of 24 Gly-Xaa-Yaa, triplets). The chains of this receptor are considered to form homotrimers containing a triple-helical structure which is utilized in a defence mechanism which allows scavenger cells to ingest and degrade oxidized and chemically altered proteins (121). The receptor therefore could be regarded as being related in certain respects to C1q and the lectins containing collagen-like sequences. However, the triple-helical region of the receptor appears to be used for direct recognition of the target to be eliminated, e.g. by interaction with low density lipoprotein after it has been modified by acetylation of lysine groups, or has been oxidized by smoking or aging. This implies that the receptor acts as a filter to remove oxidized proteins from the bloodstream but that it behaves differently from C1q, and the lectins containing collagen-like sequences, which utilize their collagen-like regions to trigger the $C1r_2C1s_2$ pro-enzyme complex or to interact with the C1qR.

4   Summary

C1q and the lectins containing collagen-like structure (termed 'collectins', by Sim and colleagues (120)) can clearly participate in a variety of antibody-independent, recognition and clearance mechanisms resulting in the neutralization and elimination of pathogenic organisms (Figure 6.5). It is clear that the C-type lectin domains in the globular heads of the 'collectins' carry the specificity for binding to specific carbohydrate structures on the target.

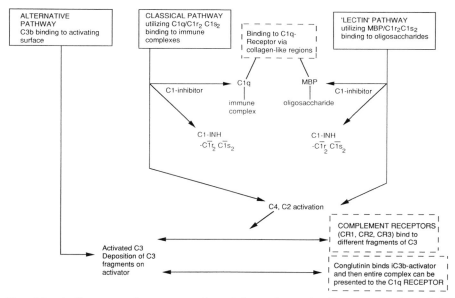

Fig. 6.5 A diagrammatic representation of the pathways leading to activation of the serum complement system.

However, the manner by which the collagen-like 'stalks' of these molecules interact, and trigger, cell surface receptors is not entirely clear and is likely to be the focus of much future research.

References

1 Ikeda, K., Sannoh, T., Kawasaki, N., Kawasaki, T., and Yamashina, I. (1987). Serum lectin with known structure activates complement through the classical pathway. *J. Biol. Chem.*, **262**, 7451–44.

2 Ohta, M., Okada, M., Yamashina, I., and Kawasaki, T. (1990). The mechanism of carbohydrate mediated-complement activation by the serum mannan-binding protein. *J. Biol. Chem.*, **265**, 1980–4.

3 Lu, J., Thiel, S., Wiedemann, H., Timpl, R., and Reid, K. B. M. (1990). Binding of the pentamer/hexamer forms of mannan-binding protein to zymosan activates the pro-enzyme C1r₂C1s₂ complex, of the classical pathway of complement, without involvement of C1q. *J. Immunol.*, **144**, 2287–4.

4 Super, M., Thiel, S., Lu, J., Levinsky, R. J., and Turner, M. W. (1989). Association of low levels of mannan-binding protein with a common defect of opsonization. *Lancet*, **2**, 1236–9.

5 Sumiya, M., Super, M., Tabona, P., Levinsky, R. J., Arai, T., Turner, M. W, and Summerfield, J. A. (1991). Molecular basis of opsonic defect in immunodeficient children. *Lancet*, **337**, 1569–70.

6   Malhotra, R., Thiel, S., Reid, K. B. M., and Sim, R. B. (1990). Human leucocyte C1q receptor binds other soluble proteins with collagen domains. *J. Exp. Med.*, **172**, 955–9.

7   Ghebrehiwet, B. (1989). Functions associated with the C1q receptor. *Behring. Inst. Mitt.*, **84**, 204–15.

8   Reid, K. B. M. (1983). Proteins involved in the activation and control of the two pathways of human complement. *Biochem. Soc. Trans*, **11**, 1–12.

9   Sellar, G. C., Blake, D. J., and Reid, K. B. M. (1991). Characterization and organization of the genes encoding the A-, B-, and C-chains of human complement subcomponent C1q. The complete derived amino acid sequence of human C1q. *Biochem. J.*, **274**, 481–90.

10 Knobel, H. R., Villiger, W., and Isliker, H. (1975). Chemical analysis and electron microscopy studies of human C1q prepared by different methods. *Eur. J. Immunol.*, **5**, 78–82.

11 Kawasaki, T., Etoh, R., and Yamashina, I. (1978). Isolation and characterization of mannan-binding protein from rabbit liver. *Biochem. Biophys. Res. Commun.*, **81**. 1018–24.

12 Drickamer, K., Dordal, M. S., and Reynolds, L. (1986). Mannose-binding proteins isolated from rat liver contain carbohydrate recognition domains linked to collagenous tails. *J. Biol. Chem.*, **261**, 6878–87.

13 Drickamer, K. and McCreary, V. (1987). Exon structure of a mannose-binding protein gene reflects its evolutionary relationship to the asialoglycoprotein receptor and non-fibrillar collagens. *J. Biol. Chem.*, **262**, 2582–9.

14 Ezekowitz, R. A. B., Day, L. E., and Herman, G. A. (1988). A human mannose-binding protein is an acute phase reactant that shares sequence homology with other vertebrate lectins. *J. Exp. Med.*, **167**, 1034–46.

15 Sastry, K., Herman, G. A., Day, L., Deignan, E., Bruns, G., Morton, C. C., and Ezekowitz, R. A. (1989). The human mannose-binding protein gene. Exon structure reveals its evolutionary relationship to a human pulmonary surfactant gene and localization to chromosome 10. *J. Exp. Med.*, **170**, 1175–89.

16 Brownell, M. D., Colley, K. J., and Baenziger, J. U. (1984). Synthesis, processing, and secretion of the core-specific lectin by rat hepatocytes and hepatoma cells. *J. Biol Chem.*, **259**, 3925–32.

17 Taylor, M. E., Brickell, P. M., Craig, R. K., and Summerfield, J. A. (1989). Structure and evolutionary origin of the gene encoding a human serum mannose-binding protein. *Biochem. J.*, **262**, 763–71.

18 Drickamer, K. (1989). Multiple subfamilies of carbohydrate recognition domains in animal lectins. *Ciba Found. Symp.*, **145**, 45–58.

19 Woo, P., Korenberg, J. R., and Whitehead, A. S. (1985). Characterization of genomic and complementary DNA sequence of human C-reactive protein, and comparison with the complementary DNA sequence of serum amyloid P component. *J. Biol. Chem.*, **260**, 13384–8.

20 Macintyre, S. S., Schultz, D., and Kushner, I. (1982). Biosynthesis of C-reactive protein. *Ann. N. Y. Acad. Sci.*, **389**, 76–87.

21 Thiel, S. and Reid, K. B. M. (1989). Structures and functions associated with the group of mammalian lectins containing collagen-like sequences. *FEBS Lett.*, **250**, 78–84.

22 Bordet, J. and Gay, F. P. (1906). Sur les relations des sensibilisatrices avec l'alexine. *Annal. Inst. Pasteur*, **20**, 467–98.

23 Muir, R. and Browning, C. H. (1906). On the action of complement as agglutinin. *J. Hygiene*, **6**, 20–2.

24 Bordet, J. and Streng, O. (1909). Les phenomänes d'adsoption et la conglutinine du serum de boeuf. *Zbl. Bakt.*, **49**, 260–76.

25 Coombs, R. R. A., Coombs, A. M., and Ingram, D. G. (1961). *The serology of conglutination and its relation to disease.* Blackwell Scientific Publications, Oxford.

26 Lachmann, P. J., and Coombs, R. R. A. (1965). In *Complement, conglutinin and immunoconglutinins, Ciba Foundation Symposium* (ed. G. E. W. Walstenholme and J. Knights), pp. 242–61. Little, Brown and Co., Boston, MA.

27 Davis, A. E. and Lachmann, P. J. (1984). Bovine conglutinin is a collagen-like protein. *Biochemistry*, **23**, 2139–44.

28 Kawasaki, N., Kawasaki, T., and Yamashina, I. (1985). Mannan-binding protein and conglutinin in bovine serum. *J. Biochem.*, Tokyo, **98**, 1309–20.

29 Lee, Y. M., Leiby, K. R., Allar, J., Paris, K., Lerch, B., and Okarma, T. B. (1991). Primary structure of bovine conglutinin, a member of the C-type animal lectin family. *J. Biol. Chem.*, **266**, 2715–23.

30 Jensenius, J. C., Thiel, S., Baatrup, G., and Holmskov-Nielsen, U. (1985). Human conglutinin-like protein. *Biosci. Reports*, **5**, 901–5.

31 Friis-Christiansen, P., Thiel, S., Svehag, S. E., Dessau, R., Svendsen, P., Andersen, O., Laursen, S. B., and Jensenius, J. C. (1990). *In vivo* and *in vitro* anti-bacterial activity of conglutinin, a mammalian plasma lectin. *Scand. J. Immunol.*, **31**, 453–60.

32 Strang, C. J., Slayter, H. S., Lachmann, P. J., and Davis, A. E.. (1986). Ultrastructure and composition of bovine conglutinin. *Biochem. J.*, **234**, 381–9.

33 Kawakami, M., Ihara, I., Ihara, S., Suzuki, A., and Fukui, K. (1984). A group of bactericidal factors conserved by vertebrates for more than 300 million years. *J. Immunol.*, **132**, 2578–81.

34 Ihara, S., Takahashi, A., Hatsuse, H., Sumitomo, K., Doi, K., and Kawakami, M. (1991). Major component of Ra reactive factor, a complement-activating bactericidal protein, in mouse serum. *J. Immunol.*, **146**, 1874–9.

35 Ihara, I., Ihara, S., Nagashima, A., Ji, Y. H., and Kawakami, M. (1988). The 28 k and 70 k dalton polypeptide components of mouse Ra reactive factor are responsible for bactericidal activity. *Biochem. Biophys. Res. Commun.*, **152**, 636–41.

36 Kawakami, M., Ihara, I., Suzuki, A., and Harada, Y. (1982). Properties of a new complement-dependent bactericidal factor specific for Ra chemotype salmonella in sera of conventional and germ-free mice. *J. Immunol.*, **129**, 2198–201.

37 Takahashi, A., Kuge, S., Ji, Y. H., Fujita, T., Hatsuse, H., and Kawakami, M. (1989). Functional and structural similarity of Ra reactive factor to C1 component of complement. *Complement and Inflammation*, **6**, 404 (abstract).

38 Kawakami, M. (1989). A family of lectins resemble the C1 component of complement. *Seikagaku*, **61**, 482–6.

39 Sastry, K., Zahedi, K., Lelias, J. M., Whitehead, A. S., and Ezekowitz, R. A. B. (1991). Molecular characterization of the mouse mannan-binding proteins. The mannose-binding protein A but not C is an acute phase reactant. *J. Immunol.*, **147**, 692–7.

40 Voss, T., Eistetter, H., Schafer, K. P., and Engel, J. (1988). Macromolecular organization of natural and recombinant lung surfactant protein SP 28–36.

Structural homology with the complement factor C1q. *J. Mol. Biol.*, **201**, 219–27.

41 Persson, A., Chang, D., and Crouch, E. (1990). Surfactant protein D is divalent cation-dependent carbohydrate-binding protein. *J. Biol. Chem.*, **265**, 5755–60.

42 Possmayer, F. (1988). A proposed nomenclature for pulmonary surfactant associated proteins. *Am. Rev. Respir. Dis.*, **138**, 990–8.

43 Sueishi, K. (1981). Isolation of a major apolipoprotein of canine and murine pulmonary surfactant. Biochemical and immunochemical characteristics. *Biochim. Biophys. Acta*, **665**, 442–53.

44 Phelps, D. S. and Taeusch, H. W. J. (1985). A comparison of the major surfactant associated proteins in different species. *Comp. Biochem. Physiol. B.*, **82**, 441–6.

45 King, R. J. (1989). Isolation of apoproteins from canine surface active material. *Am. J. Physiol.*, **224**, 788–95.

46 Bhattacharyya, S. N. (1976). Isolation and characterization of a unique glycoprotein from lavage of chicken lungs and lamellar organelles. *Am. Rev. Respir. Dis.*, **114**, 843–50.

47 Weaver, T. E. (1988). Pulmonary surfactant associated proteins. *Gen. Pharmacol.*, **19**, 361–8.

48 Phelps, D. S. and Floros, J. (1988). Localization of surfactant protein synthesis in human lung by *in situ* hybridization. *Am. Rev. Respir. Dis.*, **137**, 939–42.

49 White, R. T., Damm, D., Miller, J., Spratt, K., Schilling, J., Hawgood, S., Benson, B., and Cordell, B. (1985). Isolation and characterization of the human pulmonary surfactant apoprotein gene. *Nature,* **317**, 361–3.

50 Whitsett, J. A., Hull, W., Ross, G., and Weaver, T. (1985). Characteristics of human surfactant associated glycoproteins A. *Pediatr. Res.*, **19**, 501–8.

51 Floros, J., Steinbrink, R., Jacobs, K., Phelps, D., Kriz, R., Recny, M., Sultzman, L., Jones, S., Taeusch, H. W., Frank, H. A., and *et al.* (1986). Isolation and characterization of cDNA clones for the 35 kDa pulmonary surfactant associated protein. *J. Biol. Chem.*, **261**, 9029–33.

52 Haagsman, H. P., White, R. T., Schilling, J., Lau, K., Benson, B. J., Golden, J., Hawgood, S., and Clements, J. A. (1989). Studies of the structure of lung surfactant protein SP-A. *Am. J. Physiol.*, **257**, L421–9.

53 Persson, A., Rust, K., Chang, D., Moxley, M., Longmore, W., and Crouch, E. (1988). CP4: a pneumocyte-derived collagenous surfactant associated protein. Evidence for heterogeneity of collagenous surfactant proteins. *Biochemistry*, **27**, 8576–84.

54 Persson, A., Chang, D., Rust, K., Moxley, M., Longmore, W., and Crouch, E. (1989). Purification and biochemical characterization of CP4 (SP-D), a collagenous surfactant associated protein. *Biochemistry*, **28**, 6361–7.

55 Lu, J. (1992). Purification, characterisation, and cDNA cloning of human lung suffactant protein D. D. Phil. Thesis, University of Oxford.

56 Schumaker, V. N., Zavodszky, P., and Poon, P. H. (1987). Activation of the first component of complement. *Annu. Rev. Immunol.*, **5**, 21–42.

57 Duncan, A. R. and Winter, G. (1988). The binding site for C1q on IgG. *Nature*, **332**, 738–40.

58 Perkins, S. J., Nealis, A. S., Sutton, B. J., and Feinstein, A. (1991). The solution structure of human and mouse immunoglobulin M by synchrotron X-ray scattering and molecular graphics modelling: a possible mechanism for complement activation. *J. Mol. Biol.*, **221**, 1345–66.

59   Kaplan, M. H. and Volanakis, J. E. (1974). Interaction of C-reactive protein complexes with the complement system. Consumption of human complement associated with the reaction of C-reactive protein with pneumococcal C-polysaccharide and with the choline phosphatides, lecithin, and spingomyelin. *J. Immunol.*, **112**, 2135–41.

60   Siegel, J., Osmand, A. P., Wilson, M. F., and Gewurz, H. (1978). Interactions of C-reactive protein with the complement system II. C-reactive protein-mediated consumption of complement by polylysine polymers and other polycations. *J. Exp. Med.*, **142**, 709–14.

61   Jiang, H., Siegel, J. N., and Gewurz, H. (1991). Binding and complement activation by C-reactive protein via the collagen-like region of Clq and inhibition of these reactions by monoclonal antibodies to C-reactive protein and Clq. *J. Immunol.*, **146**, 2324–30.

62   Horowitz, J., Volanakis, J. E., and Briles, D. E. (1987). Blood clearance of *Streptococcus pneumoniae* by C-reactive protein. *J. Immunol.*, **138**, 2598–603.

63   Clas, F., Euteneuer, B., Stemmer, F., and Loos, M. (1989). Interaction of fluid-phase C1/Clq and macrophage membrane associated Clq with Gram-negative bacteria. *Behring. Inst. Mitt.*, **84**, 236–54.

64   Zohair, A., Chesne, S., Wade, R. H., and Colomb, M. G. (1989). Interaction between complement subcomponent Clq and bacterial lipopolysaccharides. *Biochem. J.*, **257**, 865–73.

65   Reid, K. B. M., Sim, R. B., and Faiers, A. P. (1977). Inhibition of the reconstitution of the haemolytic activity of the first component of human complement by a pepsin-derived fragment of subcomponent Clq. *Biochem. J.*, **161**, 239–45.

66   Siegel, R. C. and Schumaker, V. N. (1983). Measurement of the association constants of the complexes formed between intact Clq or pepsin treated Clq stalks and the unactivated or activated $C1r_2C1s_2$ tetramers. *Mol. Immunol.*, **20**, 53–66.

67   Malhotra, R. and Sim R. B. (1989). Chemical and hydrodynamic characterization of the human leucocyte receptor for complement subcomponent Clq. *Biochem. J.*, **262**, 625–31.

68   Tenner, A. J., Robinson, S. L., Borchelt, J., and Wright, J. R. (1989). Human pulmonary surfactant protein (SP-A), a protein structurally homologous to Clq, can enhance FcR- and CR1-mediated phagocytosis. *J. Biol. Chem.*, **264**, 13923–8.

69   Townsend, R. and Stahl, P. (1981). Isolation and characterization of a mannose/N-acetylglucosamine/fucose-binding protein from rat liver. *Biochem. J.*, **194**, 209–14.

70   Mizuno, Y., Kozutsumi, Y., Kawasaki, T., and Yamashina, I. (1981). Isolation and characterization of a mannan-binding protein from rat liver. *J. Biol. Chem.*, **256**, 4247–52.

71   Childs, R. A., Drickamer, K., Kawasaki, T., Thiel, S., Mizuochi, T., and Feizi, T. (1989). Neoglycolipids as probes of oligosaccharide recognition by recombinant and natural mannose-binding proteins of the rat and man. *Biochem. J.*, **262**, 131–8.

72   Loveless, R. W., Feizi, T., Childs, R. A., Mizuochi, T., Stoll, M. S., Oldroyd, R. G., and Lachmann, P. J. (1989). Bovine serum conglutinin is a lectin which binds non-reducing terminal N-acetylglucosamine, mannose, and fucose residues. *Biochem. J.*, **258**, 109–13.

73 Super, M., Levinsky, R. J., and Turner, M. W. (1990). The level of mannan-binding protein regulates the binding of complement-derived opsonins to mannan and zymosan at low serum concentrations. *Clin. Exp. Immunol.*, **79**, 144–50.

74 Schweinle, J. E., Ezekowitz, R. A., Tenner, A. J., Kuhlman, M., and Joiner, K. A. (1989). Human mannose-binding protein activates the alternative complement pathway and enhances serum bactericidal activity on a mannose-rich isolate of *Salmonella*. *J. Clin. Invest.*, **84**, 1821–9.

75 Hakomori, S. (1981). Glycosphingolipids in cellular interaction, differentiation, and oncogenesis. *Annu. Rev. Biochem.*, **50**, 733–64.

76 Olden, K., Bernard, B. A., and Humphries, M. J. (1985). Function of glycoprotein glycans. *Trends Biochem. Sci.*, **2**, 78–??.

77 Geyer, H., Holschbach, C., Hunsmann, G., and Schneider, J. (1988). Carbohydrates of human immunodeficiency virus. Structures of oligosaccharides linked to the envelope glycoprotein 120. *J. Biol. Chem.*, 263, 11760–7.

78 Mizuochi, T., Matthews, T. J., Kato, M., Hamako, J., Titani, K., Solomon, J., and Feizi, T. (1990). Diversity of oligosaccharide structures on the envelope glycoprotein gp120 of human immunodeficiency virus 1 from the lymphoblastoid cell line H9. Presence of complex-type oligosaccharides with bisecting N-acetylglucosamine residues. *J. Biol. Chem.*, **265**, 8519–24.

79 Hansen, J. E., Clausen, H., Nielsen, C., Teglbjaerg, L. S., Hansen, L. L., Nielsen, C. M., Dabelsteen, E., Mathiesen, L., Hakomori, S. l., and Nielsen, J. O. (1990). Inhibition of human immunodeficiency virus (HIV) infection *in vitro* by anti-carbohydrate monoclonal antibodies: peripheral glycosylation of HIV envelope glycoprotein gp120 may be a target for virus neutralization. *J. Virol.*, **64**, 2833–40.

80 Weiss, R. A., Clapham, P. R., McClure, M., and Marsh, M. (1989). The CD4 receptor for the AIDS virus. *Biochem. Soc. Trans.*, **17**, 644–7.

81 Sattentau, Q. J. and Weiss, R. A. (1988). The CD4 antigen: physiological ligand and HIV receptor. *Cell*, **52**, 631–3.

82 McDougal, J. S., Maddon, P. J., Dalgleish, A. G., Clapham, P. R., Littman, D. R., Godfrey, M., Maddon, D. E., Chess, L., Weiss, R. A., and Axel, R. (1986). The T4 glycoprotein is a cell surface receptor for the AIDS virus. *Cold. Spring. Harb. Symp. Quant. Biol.*, **51 Pt 2**, 703–11.

83 Maddon, P. J., Dalgleish, A. G., McDougal, J. S., Clapham, P. R., Weiss, R. A., and Axel, R. (1986). The T4 gene encodes the AIDS virus receptor and is expressed in the immune system and the brain. *Cell*, **47**, 333–48.

84 Matthews, T. J., Weinhold, K. J., Lyerly, H. K., Langlois, A. J., Wigzell, H., and Bolognesi, D. P. (1987). Interaction between the human T cell lymphotropic virus type IIIB envelope glycoprotein gp120 and the surface antigen CD4: role of carbohydrate in binding and cell fusion. *Proc. Natl. Acad. Sci. U.S.A.*, **84**, 5424–8.

85 Robinson, W. E. J., Montefiori, D. C., and Mitchell, W. M. (1987). Evidence that mannosyl residues are involved in human immunodeficiency virus type 1 (HIV-1) pathogenesis. *AIDS Res. Hum. Retroviruses*, **3**, 265–82.

86 Gruters, R. A., Neefjes, J. J., Tersmette, M., de-Goede, R. E., Tulp, A., Huisman, H. G., Miedema, F., and Ploegh, H. L. (1987). Interference with HIV-induced syncytium formation and viral infectivity by inhibitors of trimming glucosidase. *Nature*, **330**, 74–7.

87 Larkin, M., Childs, R. A., Matthews, T. J., Thiel, S., Mizuochi, T., Lawson, A. M., Savill, J. S., Haslett, C., Diaz, R., and Feizi, T. (1989). Oligosaccharide-

mediated interactions of the envelope glycoprotein gp120 of HIV-1 that are independent of CD4 recognition. *AIDS*, **3**, 793–8.

88 Fenouillet, E., Gluckman, J. C., and Bahraoui, E. (1990). Role of N-linked glycans of envelope glycoproteins in infectivity of human immunodeficiency virus type 1. *J. Virol.*, **64**, 2841–8.

89 Lifson, J., Coutre, S., Huang, E., and Engleman, E. (1986). Role of envelope glycoprotein carbohydrate in human immunodeficiency virus (HIV) infectivity and virus-induced cell fusion. *J. Exp. Med.*, **164**, 2101–6.

90 Ezekowitz, R. A. B., Kuhlman, M., Groopman, J. E., and Byrn, R. A. (1989). A human serum mannose-binding protein inhibits *in vitro* infection by the human immunodeficiency virus. *J. Exp. Med.*, **169**, 185–96.

91 Anders, E. M., Hartley, C. A., and Jackson, D. C. (1990). Bovine and mouse serum beta inhibitors of influenza A viruses are mannose-binding lectins. *Proc. Natl. Acad. Sci. U.S.A.*, **87**, 4485–9.

92 Kawasaki, N., Kawasaki, T., and Yamashina, I. (1989). A serum lectin (mannan-binding protein) has complement-dependent bactericidal activity. *J. Biochem*, Tokyo, **106**, 483–9.

93 Soothill, J. F. and Harvey, B. A. (1976). Defective opsonsization. A common immunity deficiency. *Arch. Dis. Child.*, **51**, 91–9.

94 Candy, D. C., Larcher, V. F., Tripp, J. H., Harries, J. T., Harvey, B. A., and Soothill, J. F. (1980). Yeast opsonization in children with chronic diarrhoeal states. *Arch. Dis. Child.* **55**, 189–93.

95 Richardson, V. F., Larcher, V. F., and Price, J. F. (1983). A common congenital immunodeficiency predisposing to infection and atopy in infancy. *Arch. Dis. Child.*, **58**, 799–802.

96 Levinsky, R. J., Harvey, B. A., and Paleja, S. (1978). A rapid objective method for measuring the yeast opsonization activity of serum. *J. Immunol. Methods*, **24**, 251–6.

97 Turner, M. W., Mowbray, J. F., and Roberton, D. R. (1981). A study of C3b deposition on yeast surfaces by sera of known opsonic potential. *Clin Exp. Immunol.*, **46**, 412–9.

98 Turner, M. W., Grant, C., Seymour, N. D., Harvey, B., and Levinsky, R. J. (1986). Evaluation of C3b/C3bi opsonization and chemiluminescence with selected yeasts and bacteria using sera of different opsonic potential. *Immunology.*, **58**, 111–5.

99 Turner, M. W., Super, M., Singh, S., and Levinsky, R. J. (1991). Molecular basis of a common opsonic defect. *Clin. Exp. Allergy*, **21**, 182–8.

100 Lachmann, P. J. and Müller-Eberhard, H. J. (1968). The demonstration in human serum of 'conglutinogen-activating factor' and its effect on the third component of complement. *J. Immunol.*, **100**, 691–8.

101 Linscott, W. D., Ranken, R., and Triglia, R. P. (1978). Evidence that bovine conglutinin reacts with an early product of C3b degradation, and an improved conglutination assay. *J. Immunol.*, **121**, 658–64.

102 Brown, E. J., Gaither, T. A., Hammer, C. H., Hosea, S. W., and Frank, M. M. (1982). The use of conglutinin in a quantitative assay for the presence of cell-bound C3bi and evidence that a single molecule of C3bi is capable of binding conglutinin. *J. Immunol.*, **128**, 860–5.

103 Hirani, S., Lambris, J. D., and Müller-Eberhard, H. J. (1985). Localization of the conglutinin binding site on the third component of human complement. *J. Immunol.*, **134**, 1105–9.

104   Leon, M. A. and Yokohari, R. (1964). Conglutination: specific inhibition by carbohydrates. *Science*, **43**, 1327–8.

105   Young, N. M. and Leon, M. A. (1987). The carbohydrate specificity of conglutinin and its homology to proteins in the hepatic lectin family. *Biochem. Biophys. Res. Commun.*, **143**, 645–51.

106   Mizuochi, T., Loveless, R. W., Lawson, A. M., Chai, W., Lachmann, P. J., Childs, R. A., Thiel, S., and Feizi, T. (1989). A library of oligosaccharide probes (neoglycolipids) from N-glycosylated proteins reveals that conglutinin binds to certain complex-type as well as high mannose-type oligosaccharide chains. *J. Biol. Chem.*, **264**, 13834–9.

107   Jettmar, H. M. (1922). Studien Åber die konglutination und Åber das schwaken des konglutingehaltes im serum gesunder und kranker rinder. *Z. Immun. Forsh.*, **36**, 148–99.

108   Du-Plessis, J. L. (1985). The natural resistance of cattle to artificial infection with *Cowdria ruminantium*: the role played by conglutinin. *Onderstepoort. J. Vet. Res.*, **52**, 273–7.

109   Rose, J. E., Amerault, T. E., Roby, T. O., and Martin, W. H. (1978). Serum levels of conglutinin, complement, and immunoconglutinin in cattle infected with *Anaplasma marginale*. *Am. J. Vet. Res.*, **39**, 791–3.

110   Ingram, D. G. (1972). Biological aspects of conglutinin and immunoconglutinins. (ed. U. Rother), pp. 215–29. In *Biological activities of complement*. Karger, Basel.

111   Ingram, D. G. (1959). The conglutination phenomenon. XIII. *In vivo* interactions of conglutinin and experimental bacterial infection. *Immunology*, **2**, 322–45.

112   Ingram, D. G. (1959). The conglutination phenomenon. XIV. The resistance enhancing effect of conglutinin and immunoconglutinin in experimental bacterial infections. *Immunology*, **4**, 334–45.

113   Andersen, O., Sõrensen, A. M., Svehag, S. E., and Fenouillet, E (1991). Conglutinin binds the HIV-1 envelope glycoprotein gp160 and inhibits its interaction with cell membrane CD4. *Scand. J. Immunol.*, **33**, 81–8.

114   Ihara, I., Harada, Y., Ihara, S., and Kawakami, M. (1982). A new complement-dependent bactericidal factor found in non-immune mouse sera: specific binding to polysaccharide of Ra chemotype *Salmonella*. *J. Immunol.*, **128**, 1256–60.

115   Ji, Y. H, Matsushita, M., Okada, H., Fujita, T., and Kawakami, M. (1988). The C4 and C2 but not C1 components of complement are responsible for the complement activation triggered by the Ra reactive factor. *J. Immunol.*, **141**, 4271–5.

116   Haagsman, H. P, Hawgood, S., Sargeant, T., Buckley, D, White, R. T., Drickamer, K., and Benson, B. J. (1987). The major lung surfactant protein, SP 28–36, is a calcium-dependent, carbohydrate-binding protein. *J. Biol. Chem.*, **262**, 13877–80.

117   Weaver, T. E. and Whitsett, J. A. (1991). Function and regulation of expression of pulmonary surfactant associated proteins. *Biochem. J.*, **273**, 249–64.

118   van Iwaarden, F., Welmers, B., Verhoef, J., Haagsman, H. P., and van Golde, L. M. G. (1990). Pulmonary surfactant protein A enhances the host-defence mechanism of rat alveolar macrophages. *Am. J. Respir. Cell Mol. Biol.*, **2**, 91–8.

119   van Iwaarden, J. F., van Strijp, J. A. G., Ebskamp, M. J. M., Welmers, A. C., Verhoef, J., and van Golde, L. M. G. (1991). Surfactant protein is opsonin

in phagocytosis of herpes simplex virus type 1 by rat alveolar macrophages. *Am. J. Physiol.*, **261**, 204–9.

120   Malhotra, R., Thiel, S., Jensenius, J. C., and Sim, R. B. (1991). Interaction of lung surfactant protein A with C1q receptor. *Complement and Inflammation*, **8**, 188 (abstract).

121   Rohrer, L., Freeman, M., Kodama, T., Penman, M., and Krieger, M. (1990). Coiled-coil fibrous domains mediate ligand binding by macrophage scavenger receptor type II. *Nature,* **343**, 570–2.

7 C3 and C4 as opsonins in natural immunity

M. K. HOSTETTER

1 Introduction

Since Metchnikoff defined phagocytosis in 1884, the role that he assigned to serum elements as 'modifiers' of the phagocyte has expanded considerably in the intervening 100 years. In 1903, Wright and Douglas's commanding proof that serum elements were required for phagocytosis of virulent pneumococci (1) elevated opsonins to equal status with the phagocyte and gained the notice of George Bernard Shaw: 'Opsonin is what you butter the disease germs with to make your white corpuscles eat them.' (*The Doctor's Dilemma, Act 1, 1909.*)

However, it was not until 1933 that the heat-stable components of the opsonic interaction (antibodies) were distinguished from non-specific, heat-labile serum proteins, now named complement (2). The rate of phagocytosis in the presence of antibody alone was accelerated more than seven-fold by the addition of active complement proteins in fresh human serum. At around

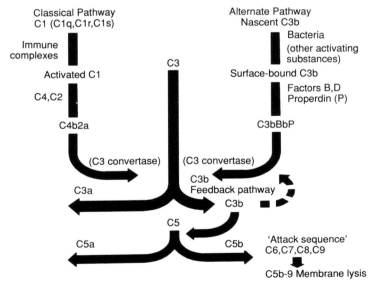

Fig. 7.1 Summary of sequential steps in the activation of complement by the classical (*left side*) or alternative (*right side*) pathways.

the same time, the 'adjuvant' action of complement was also observed to be of greater importance in non-immune serum, lacking specific antibodies to bacterial surface constituents, than in immune serum (3).

Whilst activation of the classical complement pathway can occur through antibody-independent mechanisms (see Chapter 6, Figure 6.5), studies of activation of complement in the absence of antibody have involved primarily investigation of the alternative complement pathway.

C3 is a major opsonin among the complement proteins, by virtue of its position at the junction of the classical and alternative pathways, and its functional activity even in the absence of specific antibodies (Figure 7.1 and Chapter 5). This chapter will focus on the dual aspects of the opsonic interaction: (a) the biochemical mechanisms which localize the opsonic functions of C3 and C4, and (b) the microbial components which modulate opsonic deposition, including regulation of the opsonic interaction.

Discussion of the biochemistry of opsonization will deal with the internal thiolester bond in C3 and C4. The microbiological aspects will deal predominantly with studies using virulent strains of *Streptococcus pneumoniae*.

2   Historical evidence for the role of complement in opsonization

2.1   *In vitro* studies

Certain properties of 'heat-labile opsonins'—their temperature sensitivity, their inactivation by hydrazine or ammonia, their absence in the gamma-globulin fraction of serum, their lack of specificity in cross-absorption studies (4)—were thought to resemble complement proteins. However, definitive proof of the participation of complement proteins in opsonization was first provided in 1969 in studies showing that depletion of C3 by pre-incubation of rat serum with zymosan or cobra venom factor (cobra C3b which forms a stable C3 convertase with mammalian factors B, D, and P, see Chapter 5) significantly suppressed phagocytosis of encapsulated, as opposed to unencapsulated *Streptococci pneumoniae* (5). Other experiments with heat-killed, formalinized *Streptococci pneumoniae*, sensitized with rabbit anti-capsular antibodies, demonstrated, using human serum, that C1, C4, C2, and C3 were necessary for optimal phagocytosis, but the important role of C3 as a major opsonin was illustrated by complete abolition of phagocytosis in human serum deficient in C3 (6). Subsequent investigations identified C3b, rather than C3a, as the opsonically active fragment (7).

2.2   Evidence *in vivo*

2.2.1   *Complement deficiencies in experimental animal models*

In experimental animals, congenital absence of C3 or C4 and depletion of C3 by treatment of whole animals with cobra venom factor have provided support for the role of these proteins, in particular C3, in opsonization. When normal guinea pigs were depleted of C3 by treatment with cobra venom factor, clearance of encapsulated *Streptococci pneumoniae* after intravenous injection of the bacteria, was significantly delayed in the early phases of infection. Moreover, replication of bacteria continued to the point of sustained bacteraemia and death (8).

C4 deficient guinea pigs showed little difference from normal animals in early clearance (first 2–4 hours) or in progression to bloodstream sterilization (36–48 hours). This study (8) provided definitive evidence for the central role of C3 and the alternative complement pathway in host defence against pneumococcal bacteraemia.

Similar results confirming the importance of C3 in opsonization and clearance have converged from both ends of the microbiological spectrum, including studies with enveloped viruses and fungi. When Sindbis virus was inoculated subcutaneously, mice depleted of complement proteins C3–9 by treatment with cobra venom factor exhibited a prolonged initial viraemia and a three log increase in the titre of infectious virus in the central nervous system (9). Retarded clearance was also demonstrated after intracardiac inoculation of complement-deficient mice, but not after intracerebral inoculation (10). However, after intracardiac or subcutaneous inoculation, mice genetically deficient in C5 fared no worse than normal mice. These results indicated that bloodstream clearance of Sindbis virus was complement-dependent: more precisely, C3-dependent and suggested that persistent viral infection of the CNS in C3 depleted mice was a direct result of failed bloodstream clearance.

A requirement for C3 in opsonization of pathogenic fungi has also been confirmed. In an animal model of disseminated candidiasis, normal guinea pigs and those congenitally deficient in C4 did not differ in cumulative mortality after intravenous inoculation of *Candida albicans* (11). However, C4 deficient animals pre-treated with cobra venom factor to deplete C3–9 suffered prolonged fungaemia, logarithmic increases in quantitative cultures of liver and kidney, and significantly increased rates of death.

Genetic studies of C3 and C4 deficiencies in animals have revealed distinct mechanisms by which deficiencies arise. C4 deficient guinea pigs (12) have received considerable attention since their serum is a useful reagent for quantification of C4. They have been observed to have a defect in switching from a primary to a secondary immune response which can be corrected by supplying human C4, in particular the C4A isotype (13). Opsonization of antigen (bacteriophage ϕX174) by C4A may well be important for localization of antigen in germinal centres. Studies using C4 deficient guinea pigs have suggested that there is production of C4 mRNA but pro-C4, the precursor of the native C4 molecule, does not occur. It may be that a defect in glycosylation is responsible for these guinea pigs being C4 deficient since inhibition of glycosylation of C4 has been shown to increase the rate of degradation of guinea pig pro-C4 in cultured peritoneal macrophage (14).

In contrast, C3 deficient guinea pigs produce C3 mRNA of normal size and amount in hepatocytes and peritoneal macrophage and both pro-C3 and the native protein are secreted with normal kinetics (15). However, C3 secreted by macrophage from these deficient animals lacks the reactive thiolester bond, although the nucleotide sequence from C3 cDNA clones was completely normal across the thiolester site region. These C3 deficient guinea pigs are not C4 deficient and it has been suggested that there may be a specific enzyme for formation of the thiolester in C3.

A colony of beagles completely deficient in C3 through inheritance of a defective gene has also been described (16, 17). These C3 deficient dogs have been demonstrated to have increased susceptibility to infection and these animals as well as C3 deficient guinea pigs could provide an excellent model for investigation of C3 mediated opsonization and clearance.

2.2.2   Complement deficiencies in humans (see also Chapter 5, Table 5.3)

Complete genetic deficiencies of each of the classical pathway components C1, C4, or C2 has been associated with increased susceptibility to auto-immune diseases affecting immune complex clearance. It has been suggested that the association of autoimmune disease with C4 or C2 deficiency is an indirect reflection on the inheritance of other alleles within the major histocompatibility complex in which C4 and C2 are encoded (18). However C1 is not encoded within the major histocompatibility complex and the association of immune complex disease with deficiencies of all three of these classical pathway complement proteins suggests a direct role for the classical pathway in immune complex clearance.

More compelling evidence for the primary role of C3 as an opsonin comes from rare patients with deficiencies of C3. They suffer from recurrent and severe infections with pyogenic organisms, including *Streptoccoci pneumoniae* and *Staphylococcus aureus*. C3-dependent activities including opsonization, bactericidal activity, and neutrophil chemotaxis are absent in serum from affected patients. A reduced granulocytic response to infection with Gram-positive bacteria has also been reported (19–21).

There are at least two mechanisms for human C3 deficiency: (a) homozygous inheritance of a non-expressed (null) gene on chromosome 19, and (b) deficiency of the regulatory protein factor I. A primary defect — individuals with a null C3 gene — involves decreased hepatic synthesis, which leads to concentrations of C3 in plasma that are less than 0.1 per cent of normal. Extrahepatic synthesis of C3 by cells such as macrophage from such C3 deficient individuals appears not to be severely depressed when studied *in vitro*.

Inherited deficiency of factor I leads to perpetual activation of the alternative complement pathway *in vivo* and virtually immediate degradation in plasma of secreted C3 and factor B to their by-products, C3b and Bb, respectively (compare cobra venom factor generated C3 deficiency in animals). Levels of native C3 in factor I deficient humans are barely 5 per cent of normal, while circulating native factor B is undetectable (22). The patients suffer from recurrent pneumococcal and meningococcal infections in childhood, and in adult life the author has noted an increased incidence of erysipelas due to infection with *S. pyogenes* or other streptococcal infections in these factor I deficient patients.

3   Biochemical mechanisms of opsonization

Human C3 is a two chain protein in which the alpha chain of 115 kDa is connected to the beta chain of 75 kDa by a single disulfide bond (23). The major site of C3 synthesis is the liver, where the protein appears intracellularly in precursor from (pro-C3) (24). Local sites of synthesis in tissue macrophage, epithelial, and endothelial cells may prove to be of considerable importance in tissue-specific defence (25–27 and chapter 5). Activation of C3 by the convertases of the classical or the alternative pathway is a proteolytic event in which the C3a fragment is cleaved from the amino-terminus of the alpha chain of C3 by scission of the Arg-Ser bond at residue 77. The remainder of the resulting α' chain and the uncleaved β chain constitute C3b (Figure 7.2). There is a conformational change in C3 on conversion to C3b which has been demonstrated by a range of functional and physical studies. Recent site-directed mutagenesis investigations have demonstrated that intermediate conformational states are possible and these appear to depend on the nature of the amino acids within and adjacent to the thiolester site in C3 (28).

C4, like C3, is synthesized predominantly in hepatocytes as a single chain precursor. Mature C4 is a three chain molecule and the α (93 kDa), β (78 kDa) and γ (33 kDa) chains are held together by disulfide-bridges. C4 is cleaved by C1s which removes the C4a fragment from the amino-terminus of the alpha chain and sets in motion a series of conformational changes resulting in exposure of the internal thiolester in C4b, in a similar manner to that described for C3b.

Schematic Diagram of the C3 Molecule

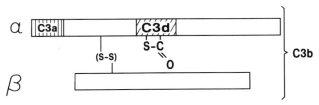

Fig. 7.2   Schematic diagram of the C3 molecule (not to scale). (Reprinted from *Rev. Infect. Dis.*, (1987), **9**, 97–109.) The interchain, but not intrachain, disulfide bridge is shown.

3.1   The labile binding site

Functional studies in the 1960s had shown that the binding of C3b to surfaces such as zymosan, sheep erythrocytes, or bacteria occurred through a labile binding site, transiently generated on cleavage of C3 to C3b (29). The nature of the interaction between C3b and activating surfaces was shown by Law and his colleagues to be an ester bond in which the carbonyl group was derived from the α chain of the C3b molecule, within the C3d region (30, 31).

Using pure human C3, studies were carried out to show that carbohydrates or amino acids could also form covalent bonds with C3 when it was activated to C3b in the presence of these compounds. Capel demonstrated that simple carbohydrates inhibited the binding of C3b to a Sepharose–trypsin matrix by serving as alternative acceptors (32). As the complexity of the carbohydrates increased from mono to tetrasaccharides, so did the affinity for the C3b binding site. Among these carbohydrates were *N*-acetylglucosamine and galactose, both components of certain pneumococcal capsular polysaccharides, as well as the complex polysaccharide of *Salmonella abortus equi*, which proved the most efficient inhibitor of all. Enlarging upon these studies, a series of papers described the binding of C3b to a wide range of acceptor molecules. Both simple and complex sugars such as mannose, glucose, galactose, or 5-thiol-D-glucose; amino acids such as threonine and lysine; and more complex amines such as putrescine were able to serve as acceptor sites for the covalent attachment of C3b (33–35).

3.2   Identification of the reactive thiolester bond

Although it was established that C3b could attach covalently to a wide variety of carbohydrates and amino groups, many of them found in nature, the active site within the C3 molecule and the biochemical mechanism directing its binding remained unknown. Janatova and colleagues showed that incubation of purified human C3 with chaotropes such as potassium bromide, or nucleophiles such as methylamine was accompanied by the expression of a single sulfhydryl group on a cysteinyl residue located on the α chain of the C3 molecule (36). After treatment with potassium bromide or methylamine, sulfhydryl expression occurred without cleavage of C3 to C3b. The resulting molecule was chemically inactive, unable to bind to the erythrocyte membrane, and incapable of supporting haemolysis (37). Methylamine bound covalently to the uncleaved α chain of C3. The methylamine which was bound and the appearance of the free sulfhydryl group were equimolar and appeared simultaneously. The site of methylamine incorporation was identified as a glutamyl residue in the C3d region (38) within three amino acid residues of the newly exposed sulfhydryl group (39). This led to the proposal of an internal thiolester bond between a Cys and a Glu residue in the labile binding site of native C3 (40, 41). Analogous sites in C4, alpha-2-macroglobulin, and pregnancy zone protein were quickly defined (42–44) (Figure 7.3). These studies have been reviewed (45, 46) and it is now clear that the Glu in the thiolester bond of C3 and C4, is encoded as a glutamine in the gene (47 for review).

3.3   Mediation of the covalent binding reaction of C3 by the reactive thiolester bond

Proof that the internal thiolester bond regulated the covalent binding reaction was soon to follow (48). When purified human C3 was cleaved to C3b in the presence of representative carbohydrates ([^{14}C] glycerol) or amino acids ([^{14}C] threonine), a 33 residue thiolester peptide was excised from the C3d subdomain and subjected to Edman degradation, after tritiation of the exposed sulfhydryl group. Tritium counts were found at residue nine of the thiolester peptide and the radiolabelled carbohydrate or amino acid was quantitatively recovered in covalent linkage with the thiolester glutamyl residue (Figure 7.4).

Thiolester Sequence Homology

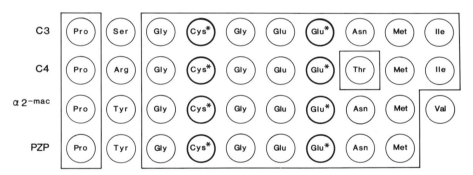

*residues of the reactive thiolester bond

Fig. 7.3   Sequence homology through the thiolester site in C3, C4, α_2-macroglobulin, and pregnancy zone protein. (Reprinted from *Rev. Infect. Dis.*, (1987), **9**, 97–109.)

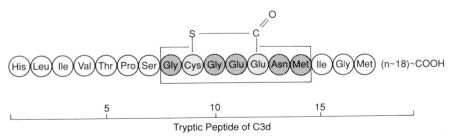

Fig. 7.4   Tryptic peptide from within the C3d subdomain which contains the C3 thiolester bond. The cysteinyl sulfhydryl group is at residue 9, with the glutamyl carbonyl at residue 12.

These experiments revealed how C3b bound covalently to small molecules with free hydroxyl or amino groups (Figure 7.5). At the labile binding site of native C3, a cysteinyl sulfhydryl group is linked in a thiolester bond with a reactive glutamyl residue. This internal thiolester bond lies protected within a hydrophobic pocket. As a result of conformational changes attendant upon cleavage of C3 to C3b, the hydrophobic pocket is breached, and the thiolester bond is labilized. In the presence of appropriate acceptor molecules, the reactive glutamyl residue may donate its carbonyl group in a transacylation reaction that results in the formation of either an ester bond with free hydroxyl groups or an amide bond with free amino groups. The transacylation reaction is limited both by the very short half-life of the labile binding site (approximately 60 microseconds) and by the concentration ($\geqslant 50$ mM) of adjacent hydroxyl or amino receptors (34, 49). The majority of activated C3 (90 per cent) binds water at the glutamyl carbonyl of the thiolester, forming a carboxylic acid and rendering the protein incapable of further covalent interaction.

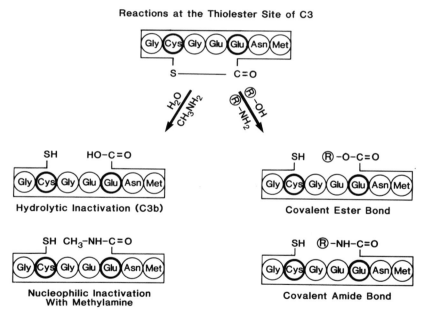

Reactions at the Thiolester Site of C3

Fig. 7.5 Diagram of the amino acid sequence of the internal thiolester bond in native C3. Species at the *lower left* represent the binding of water (*top*) or methylamine (*bottom*) to the thiolester glutamyl residue. These forms of C3 are haemolytically and opsonically inactive. Forms of C3 at the *lower right* represent the reaction of the thiolester glutamyl with a free hydroxyl group (ester bond-*top*) or a free amino group (amide bond—*bottom*). (Reprinted from the *J. Infect. Dis.*, (1984), **150**, 653–61.) R represents the complement activating surface.

It is the activated C3b which binds to a complement activating surface which is important for opsonization. C4 shows a similar mechanism of reaction to C3, although subtle differences between the two proteins will be discussed below. Once C3b and C4b are bound to a complement activating surface they (a) form part of a C3/C5 convertase, and (b) are further degraded by factor I in the presence of an appropriate cofactor (see Chapter 5). One of the cofactors is the cell surface receptor CR1 (CD35) which is present on erythrocytes and many other cell types (Chapter 5, Table 5.2) and serves to transport material opsonized with C3b and C4b to phagocytes. C3b is degraded initially to iC3b which is recognized by CR3, a member of the integrin family of receptors found on macrophage and polymorphonuclear leucocytes. iC3b is subsequently degraded to C3c and C3dg which is in turn proteolysed to form C3d. Since the thiolester site is in the C3d portion of C3, the fragments iC3b, C3dg, and C3d remain covalently bound to the complement activating surface. The interaction of C3d with the CR2 receptor on B lymphocytes may have a role in activating the specific immune response (48). In a similar manner to C3b, C4b is converted to C4c and C4d, with C4d containing the thiolester site.

4 Mechanism of C3-mediated opsonization in the non-immune host

Carbohydrates and amino acids serve as acceptors for the covalent attachment of purified C3b via the reactive glutamyl residue of the C3 thiolester bond. Free hydroxyl residues or amino groups on microbial surfaces should also function as binding sites for the opsonic deposition of C3b and the initiation of phagocytosis.

4.1 Absolute requirement for the reactive thiolester bond in opsonization

In order to assess this possibility, Hostetter and colleagues compared the opsonic efficacy of thiolester reactive and thiolester inactive forms of purified human C3 in reconstituting the alternative complement pathway in normal human serum depleted of both C3 and C4 (50). When physiological concentrations of purified human C3 with an intact thiolester were added to serum functionally deficient in C3 and C4, the alternative complement pathway was effectively reconstituted: subsequent phagocytic uptake of virulent pneumococci after opsonization in serum reconstituted with thiolester reactive C3 was not significantly different from that in normal serum. However, if C3 and C4 deficient serum was reconstituted with C3b (in which the thiolester is hydrolysed) or with C3 in which the thiolester glutamyl residue has reacted with methylamine (Figure 7.5), no opsonization or phagocytosis occurred with any of the pneumococcal serotypes. These studies thus establish that the covalent bond between the reactive glutamyl residue of the C3 thiolester and constituents of the bacterial surface was both the central mechanism of opsonization and the mediator of phagocytic recognition.

4.2   Opsonization by C4

Although C4 has been shown in functional studies to be less important as an opsonin in natural immunity, certain aspects of the binding of C4 merit attention. Unlike human C3, which is encoded by a single gene on chromosome 19, there are two separate loci for C4, lying approximately 30 kilobases from the C2 and factor B genes on the short arm of chromosome 6, within the major histocompatibility complex (47). These two C4 genes encode distinct proteins C4A and C4B of which the C4d fragments correspond to the Rodgers and Chido blood group antigens, respectively, when attached to erythrocytes. Although the overall sequence homology of C4A and C4B is 99 per cent, differences in four amino acids in a group of six, 120 amino acids on the C-terminal side of the thiolester site, give rise to distinct differences in biochemical characteristics, (e.g. electrophoretic mobility; apparent molecular weight of the α chain), and functional capabilities (51). The aspartic acid at residue 1106 in C4A, is a histidine in C4B and it is thought that these charged amino acids may explain the preference of C4A for amide linkage with proteins, while C4B binds preferentially to free hydroxyl groups in ester linkage (52). In addition, C4B is approximately four times as active haemolytically as C4A. The intriguing speculation that homozygous deficiency of C4B may lead to infection with encapsulated organisms has found initial confirmation in a prospective study of 46 children with bacterial meningitis (53), among whom 10.9 per cent were homozygous for C4B deficiency, as compared to only 3.1 per cent in uninfected children. Heterozygous deficiency for C4B (or for C4A) did not show an increased association with meningitis. A separate paediatric investigation confirmed the increased prevalence of C4B deficiency in white patients with bacteraemia (14 per cent), but not in black patients with the same infections (5 per cent) (54). Whilst these studies suggest that subtle differences in C4 may have significant implications for bacteraemic infections with *Streptococcus pneumoniae, Haemophilus influenzae*, or *Neisseria meningitidis*, it may be that inheritance of C4B null alleles in the context of different major histocompatibility haplotypes accounts for the differences in association of C4B null alleles with bacteraemia in white and black patients.

5   Role of the thiolester bond in phagocytosis

The process of opsonization, whether it proceeds via the alternative pathway or via the classical pathway, culminates in a single definitive result: the deposition of C3b on the bacterial surface. For serum-sensitive Gram-negative bacteria, covalent binding of C3b initiates the assembly of the membrane attack complex C5b, C6, C7, C8, and poly-C9, which inserts through the lipid bilayer and initiates cell lysis (see Chapter 9). For Gram-positive organisms, the thickness of the peptidoglycan layer, in some cases more than 50 times thicker than the corresponding layer on Gram-negative bacteria, prevents insertion of the membrane attack complex; opsonization of these organisms therefore serves as a signal for phagocytic attachment, ingestion, and killing. For Gram-positive organisms, then, and for serum-resistant Gram-negative organisms, covalent deposition of C3b (opsonization) is the central step in bacterial clearance via phagocytosis.

5.1   Generation of C3 ligands for phagocytosis

Once attached to bacterial surface constituents, covalently deposited C3b is converted to iC3b, C3dg, and C3d by the complement regulatory proteins, including factors H and I. C3b may also be degraded by proteases from bacteria and phagocytes.

5.2   Complement receptors

The characterization of the membrane receptors for C3 fragments on cells of the immune system has permitted not only the dissection of the cellular aspects of opsonization and phagocytosis, but has considerably enlarged our understanding of complement activation, degradation, and mediation of intracellular signalling.

Complement receptor type 1 (CR1) a single chain glycoprotein of molecular weight 190–250 kDa is present on phagocytes and other cells. These include neutrophils, monocytes, macrophages, renal podocytes, dendritic reticulum cells, B and T lymphocytes, and erythrocytes (see Table 5.2). There are between 5–30 000 CR1 receptors per unstimulated human neutrophil, with an affinity for fluid-phase C3b in the range of 5×10^7 M^{-1} (55, 56); although CR1 binds preferentially with C3b, interaction with iC3b can also occur (57). Up-regulation of CR1 expression occurs with C5a, f-Met-Leu-Phe, and at temperatures between 37–40 °C (58).

Studies on inhibition of binding of C3 fragments to CR1 using antibodies and synthetic peptides have allowed identification of the sites on C3b which interact with CR1. These include a region within C3d as well as a site at the amino-terminus of the α chain of C3b which becomes available when C3 is converted to C3b (59).

Complement receptor type 2 (CR2), a single chain polypeptide of molecular weight 145 kDa, is found primarily on B lymphocytes and, although of central importance in B cell activation and immunoglobulin synthesis, is not thought to mediate phagocytosis, because phagocytic cells does not express

CR2 (60). The preferred ligands for CR2 are C3dg and its degradation product C3d; however, CR2 also recognizes iC3b, at a considerably reduced affinity (61).

Complement receptor type 3 (CR3) is a heterodimeric structure with an α chain of 165 kDa and a β chain of 9 kDa (62). A member of the leucocyte adhesion glycoproteins within the mammalian integrin family (see Table 11.2) [CD11b/CD18], CR3 recognizes iC3b preferentially, with negligible affinity for C3dg and C3d (63). C3b is not recognized. There are approximately 65 000 CR3 receptor sites on human neutrophils with a relatively low affinity for monomeric human iC3b (2.45×10^6 M^{-1}) under isotonic conditions (64). Two distinct epitopes on CR3 function either as receptor for iC3b or as a lectin-like protein, recognizing non-complement ligands (65); these sites can be distinguished by the monoclonal antibodies OKM10 and OKM1, respectively (66). The importance of CR3 in host defence against infection has been emphasized by descriptions of patients with genetic deficiencies of CR3. Presenting in infancy or early childhood with delayed umbilical cord separation, these children developed severe periodontitis, persistent leucocytosis, and in some cases fatal bacterial infections with organisms such as *E. coli, Pseudomonas aeruginosa*, and *Salmonella* (67–70). *In vitro* defects including neutrophil chemotaxis, adherence, phagocytosis, and oxidative responses to membrane stimuli such as zymosan, are now attributed to a failure of translational processing of the CR3 β chain (71) which is common to all members of this family of integrin molecules.

Highly homologous to CR3 is complement receptor type 4 (CR4), composed of an α chain of 150 kDa and a β chain of 95 kDa (72); the α chain in CR4 is 70 per cent identical in its amino acid sequence to the corresponding structure in CR3, while the β chain is the common integrin β chain (73). Included with CR3 as a member of the integrin superfamily [CD11c/CD18], CR4 is of similar functional importance to CR3, but interacts with a larger group of C3 ligands, including iC3b, C3dg, and C3d. Despite its acknowledged participation in adhesion-dependent functions, its role in opsonization and phagocytosis remains unknown.

5.3   Ability of C3 ligands to mediate phagocytosis

Whether C3 fragments alone are sufficient to initiate phagocytosis remains an issue of some controversy. A number of early studies concluded that C3b mediates attachment without ingestion when particles such as C3-coated sheep erythrocytes are used (74–78). However, opsonization of *E. coli* and *Bacteroides fragilis* with purified complement proteins including C3 readily effected phagocytosis in the absence of immunoglobulin (79, 80), and microspheres coated with purified C3b were easily ingested by both neutrophils and monocytes (81). The outcome of the interaction with phagocytes depends on the nature of the opsonized target.

Whereas complement-coated sheep erythrocytes appear to be ineffectual in eliciting phagocytosis or the production of intracellular microbicidial mediators, C3b-coated Sepharose beads, and bacteria are potent inducers of phagocytosis and microbicidal mediators including superoxide, lysosomal enzymes, and prostaglandins, even in the absence of immunoglobulin (82, 83).

The role of iC3b as a opsonizing ligand for phagocytosis has been demonstrated with bacteria such as *Streptococcus pneumoniae*, yeast, viruses, and with neutral particles bearing covalently-bound iC3b. When C3b and iC3b have been compared directly, iC3b has consistently been more potent both in the stimulation of phagocytosis and in the release of intracellular mediators including superoxide, myeloperoxidase, and lactoferrin (84).

Thus, when purified C3b and iC3b are covalently bound to neutral microspheres in the absence of other serum proteins, phagocytic ingestion of these particles occurs (81). However, the opsonization of bacteria in serum is far more complex; plasma proteins such fibronectin (see Chapter 11) and phagocytic receptors for native bacterial constituents, (e.g. the mannose-fucose receptor) may supplement complement-mediated opsonophagocytosis.

The importance of iC3b in opsonization of yeast has also been demonstrated *in vitro* where locally synthesized C3, produced by macrophage, was covalently bound to zymosan as iC3b. Phagocytosis was shown to be iC3b-dependent (85). In other studies with West Nile virus it has been demonstrated that the virus infects macrophage cell lines through interaction between covalently bound iC3b on the flavivirus and cell surface CR3 (86). Although C3 is theoretically able to bind to a wide variety of hydroxyl or amino groups on the surface of a given micro-organism, studies with complex carbohydrates and amino acceptors (35, 87) have shown that longer chain length or the inclusion of side groups in polysaccharides, as well as the interposition of phenyl rings in simple amino compounds, substantially decreased the amount of C3b bound to these receptors. Studies have also suggested that the nucleophilicity of compounds regulates their ability to bind covalently to nascent C3b and C4b (88). However, there does appear to be a degree of specificity in the binding of nascent C4b, since the different isotypes of C4 bind to distinct groups of surface molecules on erythrocytes as the complement activating surface (89).

6   Microbiology of complement-mediated opsonization

Studies of pneumococcal opsonization have been closely linked to the epidemiology of the disease, which in turn depended upon the fundamental recognition of more than 80 distinct pneumococcal capsular polysaccharides which form the basis for serotyping. By the late 1930s, the prevalence of certain pneumococcal capsular serotypes in particular diseases was well recognized (90). Surveys of invasive pneumococcal disease among adults typically found a predominance of serotypes 1, 3, 4, and 8, while pneumococcal bacteraemia or meningitis in childhood was most often caused by serotypes 6, 14, and 18 (91, 92).

Because of the pronounced differences in pneumococcal serotypes involved in adult and childhood disease, investigators compared the ability of a variety of pneumococcal serotypes to activate the alternative or classical complement pathways. Children under two years of age are incapable of producing type-specific antibodies against most pneumococcal capsular polysaccharides after carriage, local infection, or systemic disease; and so humoral defence against pneumococcal infection is mediated by the alternative complement pathway or other antibody-independent route. Activation mechanisms for the alternative complement pathway therefore received considerable attention. Unfortunately, differences in experimental methods, including the use of immune or non-immune serum as the opsonic source, the employment of heat-killed or chemically modified organisms versus live pneumococci, and the varying methods of measuring complement activation, itself a very indirect measure of opsonization, engendered many conflicting results.

The role of bacterial surface components in pneumococcal opsonization has been investigated through determination of: (a) the relative efficacy of pneumococcal capsular polysaccharides and cell wall constituents in activating the alternative complement pathway, typically measured as C3–9 consumption. This gives no information on the quantity, site, or biochemical nature of deposited C3, and (b) the relative abilities of the pneumococcal capsule (predominantly hydroxyl groups) or cell wall components (predominantly amino groups) to serve as acceptors for covalently deposited C3b.

6.1   Activation and binding of C3 by pneumococcal capsules and cell walls

As well as activation of the alternative pathway by yeast cell walls (zymosan), activation of the alternative pathway in human serum can be triggered by a variety of bacterial capsular polysaccharides and bacterial cell walls. When pneumococcal polysaccharides purified from the capsules of different types of pneumococci were added to normal human serum in concentrations as low as 1 μg/ml, there was a marked reduction in haemolytic C3–9 titres, as well as impairment in the opsonic capacity of human serum for these and other types of bacteria (93). Because unencapsulated pneumococci also led to complement consumption (94, 95), Winkelstein and Tomasz considered that cell walls were responsible for complement activation. They showed that the techoic acid component of pneumococcal cell walls was more active than capsular polysaccharide in triggering consumption of C3–9. They used

C4 deficient guinea pig serum to show that alternative pathway activation was occurring (96–98).

Subsequent experiments have attempted to define the bacterial component to which C3b binds. Early experiments had shown that opsonization of virulent, encapsulated pneumococcae (type 25) lead to deposition of C3b on the capsule (7). Conflicting results were obtained using a series of glutaraldehyde treated *Streptococcus pneumoniae* in which no capsular deposition of C3b was measured in the absence of anti-capsular antibodies. In order to distinguish between C3b bound to capsules and to cell walls, ^{125}I-labelled guinea pig C3 was used (99). These studies (99, 100) showed that C3b was bound to cell walls in both encapsulated and unencapsulated strains: 50 per cent of total C3b which was bound to cell walls was bound to techoic acid and the rest was bound to unidentified components.

Using ^{3}H-labelled purified human C3 to reconstitute the alternative complement pathway in agammaglobulinaemic serum in which C3 and C4 had been inactivated, Hostetter quantitated covalent deposition of C3b and its degradation fragments (see Figure 7.6) on encapsulated (serotypes 3, 4, 6A, and 14) and unencapsulated (R36a) *S. pneumoniae*. The results demonstrated that unencapsulated pneumococci, as expected, bound C3b at the level of the cell wall, while deposition on encapsulated serotypes occurred on both the capsule and the cell wall, with relative distributions varying according to serotype (Table 7.1) (101).

In other experiments, hypogammaglobulinaemic serum or the cleavage of purified human C3 with trypsin in a serum-free system was used to deposit C3b on pneumococci. Electron micrographs clearly demonstrate that the capsular polysaccharide of the type 3 pneumococcus serves as an acceptor site for opsonic deposition of C3b (Figure 7.7), via ester or amide bonds.

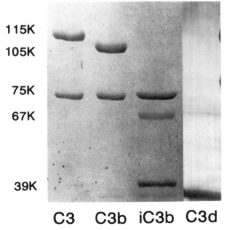

Fig. 7.6 10% SDS-PAGE gel of native C3 and its fragments—C3b, iC3b, C3d.

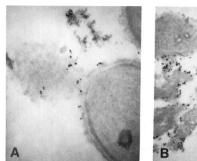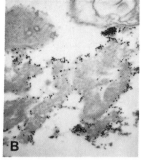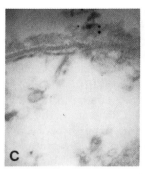

Fig. 7.7 Deposition of purified human C3 on *Streptococcus pneumoniae*, serotype 3, in a serum-free system. Site of C3 deposition is localized for electron microscopy with the use of 12 nanometer colloidal gold particles bound to goat anti-human C3. (A) Section through intact organism and extruded capsule (× 56 000). (B) Section through capsular polysaccharide (× 42 000). (C) Section showing inner plasma membrane, cell wall, and C3 on capsule (× 105 000). Electron micrographs courtesy of Elena M. Retsinas and Margaret K. Hostetter.

Table 7.1   Deposition of C3b on virulent pneumococci in non-immune serum

Serotype	Number of C3b molecules covalently attached[*]	C3b molecules on capsule (%)	C3b molecules on cell wall (%)	C3 fragments[**]	Resistance to phagocytosis
3	29 100	12	88	C3b, iC3b, C3d	++++
4	155 000	–	–	C3b, iC3b, C3d	++++
6A	53 000	22	78	iC3b	++
14	108 800	45	55	iC3b	++

[*] Per organism.
[**] Determined by SDS-polyacrylamide gel electrophoresis of radiolabelled C3 fragments released from pneumococci by treatment with hydroxylamine to cleave ester bonds (31).

6.2   The 'anti-phagocytic' effect of the pneumococcal capsule

Studies on phagocytosis of encapsulated pneumococci showed that the presence of the capsule inhibited phagocytosis (102, 103), and it was further concluded that this 'anti-phagocytic' effect was related to the complexity of the capsular polysaccharide, rather than to the amount or thickness of the capsular polysaccharide (104). A possible role of the opsonin, in addition to components of the bacterial capsule, was postulated to contribute to this effect. It was hypothesized that interactions of surface-bound C3b with the complement regulatory factors H and I, could modulate phagocytosis by controlling amplification of the alternative pathway. This latter conclusion was formed on the basis of observations on the relative rates of iC3b production from C3b deposited on surfaces which activated the alternative pathway compared with surfaces that did not lead to alternative pathway activation, e.g. sheep erythrocytes. C3b deposited on sheep erythrocytes is very rapidly degraded to iC3b and so cannot bind to factor B to amplify further C3b deposition.

Apparently contradictory results were obtained from studies with heat-killed or glutaraldehyde treated pneumococci (strains 7F and 12) which activate the alternative pathway slowly. Results showed that C3b deposited on either the cell wall or capsular polysaccharide (via the classical pathway) was resistant to degradation by factor I. However, the affinity of capsular C3b for factor B was reduced. The authors concluded that activation of the alternative complement pathway by heat-killed or gluataraldehyde treated pneumococci proceeded slowly because of the reduced affinity of C3b for factor B (105). Using monoclonal antibodies, to distinguish C3b from iC3b, Newman and Mikus, in contrast readily detected cleavage of C3b to iC3b on heat-killed *Streptococcus pneumoniae* type 3, even under conditions supporting only alternative complement activation (106). Using live patient isolates of *S. pneumoniae* (serotypes 3, 4, 6A, and 14), Hostetter also studied C3b binding, localization, and degradation in agammaglobulinaemic serum in an attempt to understand some of the determinants of serotypic virulence (101). The number of deposited C3b molecules alone does not explain serotypic variation in resistance to phagocytosis (Table 7.1); nor does the chemical nature of C3b deposition either ester or amide, as defined by the release of ester-linked C3b by nucleophiles. However, degradation of deposited C3b might well influence the interaction of the pneumococcus with membrane receptors for C3b or iC3b on the phagocytic cell. Since C3b deposited on the pneumococcal cell wall is too deep to be recognized by phagocytic cells (107), *capsule*-bound C3 fragments were structurally analysed by SDS-polyacrylamide gel electrophoresis and western blotting after hydroxylamine release. Results showed that pneumococci types 3 and 4, highly resistant to phagocytosis, bore on their capsules ester-linked C3b, iC3b, and C3d after opsonization periods of 20 and 90 minutes, while types 6A and 14, which are less resistant to phagocytosis, bore only iC3b (101). Since phagocytic cells lack receptors for C3d, (CR2) but have receptors for iC3b (CR3), these results suggested that the pattern of degradation of capsule-bound C3b to fragments inhibiting recognition by phagocytic complement receptors might explain the 'anti-phagocytic' effect.

The implication that C3 fragments could serve as ligands for complement-mediated phagocytosis was subsequently explored (108). When the iC3b receptor (CR3) on normal neutrophils was blocked by the monoclonal antibody OKM10, neutrophil phagocytosis of pneumococcal serotypes 6A and 14, which bore exclusively iC3b, was inhibited by 60–80 per cent. Blockade of the neutrophil C3b receptor (CR1) failed to inhibit phagocytosis for these iC3b-bearing serotypes. For serotype 3, which bears capsule-bound C3b, iC3b, and C3d, CR3-mediated phagocytosis accounted for only 20 per cent of the uptake and again there was no evidence for CR1-mediated phagocytosis. When purified iC3b was bound to neutral microspheres, iC3b elicited consistently greater release of neutrophil superoxide, myeloperoxidease, and lactoferrin than did C3b. These experiments proved that the iC3b/CR3 interaction was the central mechanism for phagocytosis of iC3b-bearing pneumococci and for stimulation of intracellular bactericidal processes.

6.3   Identification of covalent binding sites for C3b on other micro-organisms

Studies with a wide variety of Gram-positive and Gram-negative bacteria and parasites have demonstrated that the site of deposition of opsonically active C3b, as well as its availability for degradation to iC3b and C3d, is essential for the regulation of complement-mediated phagocytosis. C3 deposition and degradation on *Staphylococcus aureus* and *Escherichia coli* has been analysed after opsonization in varying concentrations of pooled human serum (109). C3b, iC3b, and C3d were readily detectable on both types of bacteria (Table 7.2), and identical fragmentation patterns were observed for protein A-negative, protein A-positive, and methicillin-resistant clinical isolates of *S. aureus*, as well as for K antigen-negative, and K antigen-positive clinical isolates of *E. coli*. Ester-linked C3 fragments on encapsulated *S. aureus* and *E. coli* represented 34 per cent and 82 per cent, respectively, of covalently-bound C3. For both organisms, a proportion of C3b was refractory to cleavage with purified factor I. These results suggested that covalently-bound C3b has two possible fates: it can be cleaved to iC3b, in which form it promotes phagocytosis, or it can remain as surface-bound C3b, to continue alternative pathway activation. Microbial surface constituents which influence the ultimate fate of bound C3b have not yet been identified.

Table 7.2 Deposition of C3b on *Staphylococcus aureus* and *Escherichia coli*

Organism	Percentage of bound C3b in ester linkage[**]	Degradation pattern[*]		
		C3b	iC3b	C3d
S. aureus	34%	17%	64%	19%
E. coli	82%	53%	44%	2%

[*] Determined from SDS-polyacrylamide gel electrophoretic analysis of radiolabelled C3 fragments released from bacteria after treatment with hydroxylamine.

[**] Determined from comparison with radiolabelled C3 fragments on bacteria resistant to treatment with hydroxylamine.

Deposition of C3b on group A streptococcus, e.g. Pyogenes, differs considerably. Some group A streptococcal strains are encapsulated and may or may not carry the M protein. The M protein is 'anti-phagocytic' and is accessible on the surface of the capsule. Although M-negative streptococci bind C3 more efficiently than M-positive cells, the amount of C3 deposited on M-positive cells should be adequate for ingestion by neutrophils, which is impaired with M-positive cells (110). Analysis of degradation fragments indicated that C3b and iC3b were deposited on M-positive streptococci, but predominantly in non-covalent linkage, which fails to promote phagocytosis (111). The carbohydrate of the capsule of group B streptococci differs from group A but the type III group B streptococcus is antigenically similar to that of the type 14 pneumococcus, except for the interposition of terminal sialic acid residues. Sialic acid, restricts the deposition of C3b by preventing the generation of the surface-bound and increased in deposition as the duration of opsonization lengthened (112).

Studies of covalent deposition of C3b on Gram-negative organisms have demonstrated that long chain lipopolysaccharide molecules serve as acceptor sites for C3b on strains on *Salmonella montevideo* (113) and studies of complement deposition on *Neisseria meningitidis* and *Neisseria gonorrhoeae* have been comprehensively reviewed (114).

Among eukaryotic infectious agents, covalent deposition of C3b has been identified on *Candida albicans* and on *Cryptococcus neoformans*, and subsequent cleavage to iC3b, which is the major surface-bound ligand on *C. neoformans*, occurs readily (115). A 72 kDa moiety has been identified as the covalent binding site for C3b deposition on epimastigotes of *Trypanosoma cruzi* (116). Other investigators have proposed an amide linkage between C3b and a high molecular weight fragment from *Leishmania donovani* promastigotes and cleavage to iC3b occurs with 75 per cent of deposited C3b molecules (117). With *L. major*, rapid cleavage of C3b to iC3b favours CR3-mediated phagocytosis of promatisgotes by murine macrophages. CR3-mediated phagocytosis also occurs in the absence of serum, and it is likely that the iC3b binding site and the lectin-like epitope of CR3 are involved (118). Thus, evidence for the covalent deposition of C3b and its subsequent cleavage to iC3b and other active degradation fragments has been clearly demonstrated for bacteria, fungi, and parasites. Local production of C3 by macrophage has also been shown to be adequate to promote phagocytosis of zymosan (85).

7   Other factors which enhance or impede opsonic deposition of C3b

7.1   Enhancement of opsonic deposition

7.1.1   Role of specific immunoglobulin

Antigen–antibody complexes can activate the alternative pathway and it has been demonstrated that C3b binds covalently to antibody–antigen complexes

(119). Subsequent studies using IgG and IgM antibodies to the unencapsulated, avirulent, R36a strain of *Streptococcus pneumoniae* (heat-killed) (120) clearly showed covalent deposition of C3b in both ester and amide linkage to IgG and IgM antibodies attached to this unencapsulated organism. Similar information was obtained with virulent organisms and covalent deposition of C3b was nearly four-fold greater when virulent strains (serotypes 3, 4, 6A, 14) of pneumococci were incubated in immune sera (101). Since such an increase in deposition far outstripped the surface area available for covalent attachment of this protein, the antibodies themselves are likely to provide additional sites for C3b deposition.

In addition to direct interaction of surface-bound antibodies with Fc receptors on phagocytic cells, type-specific anti-capsular antibodies promote opsonophagocytosis by acting as an acceptor site for covalent binding of C3b and by augmenting alternative pathway activation.

7.1.2   Role of cytokines

Because C3 and C4 are acute phase reactants, inflammatory mediators have long been considered to play a role in regulating their synthesis: cytokines such as IL-1, IL-6, and tumour necrosis factor increase the synthesis of C3, although the effects of these mediators are tissue-specific. Direct evidence for cytokine control of C3 synthesis arose from studies employing a construct linking 199 base pairs of the human C3 promoter to the firefly luciferase gene. A 58 base pair fragment (-127 to -70) of the promoter region was shown by deletional mutagenesis to contain *cis*-acting elements responsive to IL-1 and to a synergistic action of IL-1 plus IL-6. Although not conclusive, these results suggested that the induction of C3 synthesis may be mediated by a protein belonging to the family of enhancer-binding proteins (121). In addition, steroid hormones such as oestrogen or glucocorticoids will increase C3 synthesis by certain cells (122, 123). Although the mechanism of oestrogen's effect is not known, the effect of glucocorticoids may be in part ascribable to two regions in the 5' flanking sequence of the C3 gene which shares 80 per cent homology with the family of glucocorticoid responsive elements (124).

7.2   Factors impeding opsonic deposition

The plasma concentrations of C3 and C4 are important in determining their respective ability to serve as opsonins. The liver provides more than 90 per cent of the plasma concentration of C3 and C4, and in congenital C3 deficiency caused by the inheritance of a null gene, hepatic synthesis of the protein is the most severely affected, while monocyte synthesis is less impaired (125).

7.2.1   Age-dependent changes in C3 structure and function

A second important factor which may impose severe limitations on the opsonic capacity of C3 and C4 is age. A number of studies have demonstrated that the plasma concentration of C3 rises significantly with age in infants. The concentration of C3 in the plasma of full-term newborns may approach only 70 per cent of that in adults, and levels are even lower in premature newborns (126–129). The function of the alternative complement pathway may also be impaired in premature babies (130). However, in addition to absolute reductions in the amount of C3, Zach and co-workers have recently provided biochemical evidence for the presence of non-functional C3 in the plasma of premature newborns (131). When C3 was isolated from the plasma of full-term and premature newborns by affinity chromatography, incorporation of [^{14}C] methylamine into the C3 thiolester was markedly decreased, when compared to methylamine incorporation in C3 isolated from adult plasma by identical methods. The percentage of dysfunctional C3 correlated significantly with gestational age. Since the nucleotide sequence of human C3 codes for a glutamine residue, rather than a glutamic acid residue, at the thiolester site (132), it is possible that post-translational deamination of synthesized C3 fails to occur in the neonatal liver, thereby resulting in the synthesis of a dysfunctional C3 molecule. This could contribute to the susceptibility of newborns and premature infants to bacterial infection.

7.2.2 *Biochemical modification by ammonia or glucose*

Strong nucleophiles which are able to gain access to the thiolester site in native C3 and C4 (34, 37–39) such as hydrazine and methylamine are inherently reactive with thiolester bonds. Incubation of purified human C3 with methylamine leads to the incorporation of one mole of methylamine at the reactive glutamyl residue for each mole of thiolester disrupted (Figure 7.5, left panel). Although amide linkage of methylamine or other nucleophiles at the glutamyl carbonyl renders the protein haemolytically (and opsonically) inactive (37, 38), nucleophilic modification results in C3 which is 'C3b-like' and 'C3b-like C3' is able to bind factor B and to form an alternative pathway C3 convertase (133, 134) and to be recognized by CR1. This 'C3b-like C3' is not itself cleaved by a C3 convertase. There is now evidence to suggest that there are intermediate conformational states between C3 and C3b. A series of C3 mutants has been generated in which single amino acid residues around the thiolester region have been modified (27) and some of these amino acid substitutions, (e.g. the active site Cys changed to Ala) result in a full-length C3 molecule with no thiolester but which is cleaved by a C3 convertase.

There is one nucleophile, ammonia, which is commonly present in biological systems. Ammonia attacks the C3 thiolester and binds to the glutamyl carbonyl in amide linkage in a concentration-dependent reaction (Figure 7.8) to form amidated C3. When covalently bound to neutral microspheres, amidated C3 can trigger chemiluminescence and elicit the release of superoxide, myeloperoxidase, and lactoferrin from neutrophils or monocytes by binding to CR1 (81, 84).

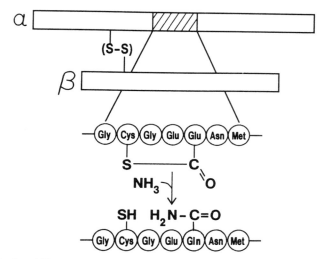

Fig. 7.8 Nucleophilic modification of the C3 thiolester bond by free base ammonia. (Reprinted from *Rev. Infect. Dis.* (1987), **9**, 97–109.)

There is now substantial evidence that ammonia genesis in human disease states has profound inflammatory consequences and bacterial ammonia genesis is particularly relevant. In the lungs of patients with cystic fibrosis, heavy colonization with *Pseudomonas aeroginosa* leads to neutrophil degranulation without phagocytosis of the organism; that is opsonic failure with phagocytic activation. *In vitro* experiments have shown that purified human C3 is amidated by supernatants of *P. aeruginosa* grown in media containing arginine or urea as nitrogen sources where ammonia is produced. Amidated C3 formed in the presence of *P. aeruginosa* is opsonically inactive but is able to trigger neutrophil degranulation through reaction with neutrophil complement receptors (CR3) (135). Evidence supporting the formation of amidated C3 and its cascade of phlogistic consequences has also accrued from studies of ammonia genesis in chronic renal failure, interstitial nephritis, and myonecrosis (84, 136).

It has recently been suggested that ammonia-treated C3 can reform a thiolester bond but it is not clear whether this can happen *in vivo* (137).

In addition to reaction of nucleophiles with intact C3 or C4, other larger soluble nucleophilic molecules have been shown to react with the thiolester site in C3 or C4 when these proteins are activated. These nucleophiles include drugs which induce immune complex disease as an adverse side effect (138). This interaction could contribute to the mechanism of immunotoxicity affecting immune complex deposition and solubilization. One of these drugs, penicillamine, is an anti-rheumatic compound and it has been proposed that the covalent binding of penicillamine to the thiolester site in C4 when C4 is activated to C4b could contribute to its anti-arthritic action (139).

Disruption of the C3 thiolester under conditions of alternative pathway activation will also permit binding of the thiolester glutamyl to free monosaccharides. To study the relevance of this reaction for opsonization, Loewenson and colleagues demonstrated that alternative pathway activation of purified human C3 in the presence of 50 mM D-glucose led to a four-fold increase in glycosylation of the molecule when compared with the same reaction in 5 mM D-glucose. Under conditions permitting alternative pathway activation, glycosylation occurred not only on the β chain, but more significantly, at the thiolester site on the α chain (140). Opsonic deposition of tritiated C3 on *Candida albicans* was significantly reduced after glycosylation in 50 mM, as opposed to 5 mM D-glucose. Thus, amidation and glycosylation of the thiolester glutamyl carbonyl of C3 impair opsonic deposition of C3. Ammonia genesis and hyperglycaemia, whether occurring in a physiological state or as a result of infection or other disease process, may constitute a significant impediment to C3-mediated opsonization.

7.2.3   Inhibition of opsonization by micro-organisms

Mechanisms whereby organisms subvert C3-mediated opsonization have been identified for herpes simplex viruses and for *Candida albicans* and related species. When expressed on the surface of infected cells, HSV-1 glycoproteins gC-1 and gC-2 function as C3b receptors (CR1-like function) and bind C3b non-covalently, with resultant inhibition of viral neutralization (141, 142).

A similar mechanism for inhibition of opsonophagocytosis has been observed in *C. albicans* and related species, which express a surface protein that is antigenically, structurally, and functionally related to the mammalian integrins CR3 and p150,95 (143–145). This protein functions as a receptor for iC3b and its expression can be increased four to six-fold by growth of the yeast in the presence of high concentrations of glucose ($\geqslant 10$ mM) or by transformation to the mycelial form (146). The protein also serves as an important adhesin, mediating the attachment of *C. albicans* to human epithelium and endothelium alike by recognition of the tripeptide sequence R-G-D in surface constituents of host cells (147, 148) (see Chapter 11). For both of these organisms, an understanding of this molecular mimicry should lead to a greater appreciation of the subtle struggle between host and pathogen in the process of complement-mediated opsonization in natural immunity.

Acknowledgements

We thank Doreen Bower for excellent secretarial assistance. This work was supported by NIH grants AI 24162 and 25827.

References

1 Wright, A. E., and Douglas, S. R. (1903). An experimental investigation of blood fluids in connection with phagocytosis. *Proc. Roy. Soc. Lond. B. Biol. Sci.*, **72**, 357–70.

2 Ward, H. K. and Enders, J. F. (1933). An analysis of the opsonic and tropic action of normal and immune sera based on experiments with pneumococcus. *J. Exp. Med.*, **57**, 527–47.

3 Tokley, W. W. C. and Wilson, G. S. (1929). The principles of bacteriology and immunity. Vol. 1, p.176. New York, William Hood and Co.

4 Hirsch, J. D., and Strauss, B. (1964). Studies on heat-labile opsonins in rabbit serum. *J. Immunol.*, **92**, 145–54.

5 Smith, M. R. and Wood Jr, W. B. (1969). Heat labile opsonins to pneumococcus. I. Participation of complement. *J. Exp. Med.*, **129**, 1209–25.

6 Johnston, R. B., Klemperer, M. R., Alper C. A., and Rosen F. S. (1969). The enhancement of bacterial phagocytosis by serum. *J. Exp. Med.*, **129**, 1275–90.

7 Shin, H. S., Smith, M. R., and Wood Jr, W. B. (1969). Heat labile opsonins to pneumococcus. II. Participation of C3 and C5. *J. Exp. Med.*, **130**, 1229–40.

8 Hosea, S. W., Brown, E. J., and Frank, M. M. (1980). The critical role of complement in experimental pneumococcal sepsis. *J. Infect Dis.*, **142**, 903–9.

9 Hirsch, R. L., Griffin, D. E., and Winkelstein, J. A. (1978). The effect of complement depletion on the course of Sindbis virus infection in mice. *J. Immunol.*, **121**, 12760–80.

10 Hirsch, R. L., Griffin, D. E., and Winkelstein, J. A. (1980). The role of complement in viral infections. II. The clearance of Sindbis virus from the blood stream and central nervous system of mice depleted of complement. *J. Infect. Dis.*, **141**, 212–17.

11 Gelfand, J. A., Hurley, D. L., Fauci, A. S., and Frank, M. M. (1978). Role of complement in host defence against experimental disseminated candidiasis. *J. Infect. Dis.*, **138**, 9–16.

12 Ochs, H. D., Wedgewood, R. J., Frank, M. M., Heller, S. R., and Hosea, S. W. (1983). The role of complement in the induction of antibody responses. *Clin. Exp. Immunol.*, **53**, 208–17.

13 Finco, O., Li, S., Cuccia, M., Rosen, F. S., and Carroll, M. C. (1992). Structural differences between the two human C4 isotypes affect the humoral immune response. *J. Exp. Med.*, **175**, 537–43.

14 Matthews, W. J., Goldberger, G., Marino, J. T., Einstein, L. P., Gash, D. J., and Colten, H. R. (1982). Complement proteins C2, C4, and factor B. Effect of glycosylation on their secretion and metabolism. *Biochem. J.*, **204**, 839–46.

15 Auerbach, H. S., Burger, R., Dodds, A., and Colten, H. R. (1990). Molecular basis of complement C3 deficiency in guinea pigs. *J. Clin. Invest.*, **86**, 96–106.

16 Winkelstein, J. A., Cork, L. C., Griffin, D. E., Adams, R. J., and Price, D. L. (1981). Genetically determined efficiency of the third component of complement in the dog. *Science*, **212**, 1169–73.

17 O'Neil, K. M., Ochs, H. D., Heller, S. R., Cork, L. C., Morris, J. M., and Winkelstein, J. A. (1988). Role of C3 in humoral immunity. *J. Immunol.*, **140**, 1939–45.

18 Carroll, M. C., Campbell, R. D., Bentley, D. R., and Porter, R. R. (1984). The Class III region of the human major histocompatibility complex. *Nature*, **307**, 237–41.

19 Alper, C. A., Colten, H. R., Rosen, F. S., Rabson, A. R., MacNab, G. M., and Gear, J. S. S. (1972). Homozygous deficiency of C3 in a patient with repeated infections. *Lancet*, **2**, 1179–81.

20 Ballow, M., Shira, J. E., Harden, L., Yang, S. Y., and Day, N. K. (1975). Complete absence of the third component of complement in man. *J. Clin. Invest.*, **56**, 703–10.

21 Alper, C. A, Colten, H. R., Gear, J. S. S., Rabson, A. R., and Rosen, F. S. (1976). Homozygous human C3 deficiency: the role of C3 in antibody production, C2s-induced vasopermeability, and cobra venom-induced passive hemolysis. *J. Clin. Invest.*, **57**, 222–9.

22 Alper, C. A., Abramson, N., Johnston Jr, R. B., Jandel, J. H., and Rosen, F. S. (1970). Increased susceptibility to infection associated with abnormalities of complement-mediated functions and of the third component of complement (C3). *N. Engl. J. Med.*, **282**, 349–54.

23 Tack, B. F. and Prah, J. W. (1976). Third component of human complement: purification from plasma and physiochemical characterization. *Biochemistry*, **15**, 4513–21.

24 Brade, V., Hall, R. E., and Colten, H. R. (1977). Biosynthesis of pro-C3, a precursor of the third component of complement. *J. Exp. Med.*, **146**, 759–65.

25 Beatty, D. W., Davis, A. E., Cole, F. S., Einstein, L. P., and Colten, H. R. (1981). Biosynthesis of complement by human monocytes. *Clin. Immunol. Immunopathol.*, **18**, 334–43.

26 Strunk, R. C., Eidlen, D. M., and Mason, R. J. (1988). Pulmonary alveolar type II epithelial cells synthesize and secrete proteins of the classical and alternative complement pathways. *J. Clin. Invest.*, **81**, 1419–26.

27 Warren, H. B., Panzaris, P., and Davis, P. F. (1987). The third component of complement is transcribed and secreted by cultured human endothelial cells. *Am. J. Pathol.*, **129**, 9–13.

28 Isaac, L. and Isenman, D. E. (1992). Structural requirements for thiolester bond formation in human complement component C3. *J. Biol. Chem.*, **207**, 10062–9.

29 Müller-Eberhard, H. J., Dalmasso, A. P., and Calcott, M. A. (1966). The reaction mechanism of β_{1C}-globulin (C'3) in immune homolysis. *J. Exp. Med.*, **123**, 33–54.

30 Law, S. K. and Levine, R. P. (1977). Interaction between the third complement protein and cell surface macromolecules. *Proc. Natl. Acad. Sci. U.S.A.*, **74**, 2701–5.

31 Law, S. K., Lichtenberg, N. A., and Levine, R. P. (1979). Evidence for an ester-linkage between the labile binding site of C3b and receptive surfaces. *J. Immunol.*, **123**, 1388–94.

32 Capel, P. J. A., Groeneboe, R. O., Grosveld G., and Pondman, K. W. (1978). The binding of activated C3 to polysaccharides and immunoglobulins. *J. Immunol.*, **121**, 2566–72.

33 Law, S. K., Minich, T. M., and Levine, R. P. (1981). The binding reaction between the third human complement protein and small molecules. *Biochemistry*, **20**, 7457–63.

34 Sim, R. B., Twose, T. M., Patterson D. S., and Sim, E. (1981). The covalent-binding reaction of complement component C3. *Biochem. J.*, **193**, 115–27.

35 Mann, J., O'Brien, R., Hostetter, M. K., Alper, C. A., Rosen, S. F., and Babior, B. M. (1981). The third component of complement: covalent attachment

of a radioactive sugar to the labile binding site of C3 via the alternative pathway. *J. Immunol.*, **126**, 2370–2.

36 Janatova, J., Lorenz, P. E., Schechter, A. N., Prahl, J. W., and Tack, B. F. (1980). Third component of human complement: appearance of a sulfhydryl group following chemical or enzymatic inactivation. *Biochemistry*, **19**, 4471–8.

37 Janatova, J., Tack, B. F., and Prahl, J. W. (1980). Third component of human complement: structural requirements for its function. *Biochemistry*, **19**, 4479–85.

38 Howard, J. B. (1980). Methylamine reaction and denaturation-dependent fragmentation of complement component C3 *J. Biol. Chem.*, **255**, 7082–4.

39 Tack, B. F., Harrison, R. A., Janatova, J., Thomas, M, L., and Prahl, J. W. (1980). Evidence for presence of an internal thiolester bond in third component of human complement. *Proc. Natl. Acad. Sci. U.S.A.*, **77**, 5764–8.

40 Thomas, M. L., Janatova, J., Gray, W. R., and Tack, B. F. (1982). Third component of human complement: localization of the internal thiolester bond. *Proc. Natl. Acad. Sci. U.S.A.*, **79**, 1054–8.

41 Thomas, M. L., Davidson, F. F., and Tack, B. F. (1983). Reduction of the β-Cys-γ-Glu thiolester bond of human C3 with sodium borohydride. *J. Biol. Chem.*, **258**, 13580–6.

42 Harrison, R. A., Thomas, M. L., and Tack, B. F. (1981). Sequence determination of the thiolester site of the fourth component of human complement. *Proc. Natl. Acad. Sci. U.S.A.*, **78**, 7388–92.

43 Sottrup-Jensen, L., Peterson, T. E., and Magnusson, S. (1980). A thiolester in α_2-macroglobulin cleaved during proteinase complex formation. *FEBS Lett.*, **121**, 275–9.

44 Sand, O., Folkersen, J., Westergaard, J. G., and Sottrup-Jensen, L. (1985). Characterization of human pregnancy zone protein: comparison with human α2-macroglobulin. *J. Biol. Chem.*, **260**, 15723–35.

45 Tack, B. F. (1983). The β-Cys-γ-Glu thiolester bond in human C3, C4, and α2-macroglobulin. *Springer Semin. Immunol. Pathol.*, **6**, 259–82.

46 Hostetter, M. K. and Gordon, D. L. (1987). Biochemistry of C3 and related thiolester proteins in infection and inflammation. *Rev. Infect. Dis.*, **9**, 97–108.

47 Campbell, R. D., Law, S. K. A., Reid, K. B. M., and Sim, R. B. (1988). The structure, organization, and regulation of the complement genes. *Annu. Rev. Immunol.*, **6**, 161–85.

48 Uher, F., Rajnavolgyi, E., and Erdei, A. (1992). Novel regulators of the humoral immune response. *Immunol. Today*, **13**, A4–A5.

49 Hostetter, M. K., Thomas, M. L., Rosen, F. S., and Tack, B. F. (1982). Binding of C3b proceeds by a transesterification reaction at the thiolester site. *Nature*, **298**, 72–5.

50 Hostetter, M. K., Krueger, R. A., and Schmeling, D. J. (1984). The biochemistry of opsonization: central role of the reactive thiolester of the third component of complement. *J. Infect. Dis.*, **150**, 653–61.

51 Yu, C. Y., Belt, K. T., Giles, C. M., Campbell, R. D., and Porter, R. R. (1986). Structural basis of the polymorphism of human complement components C4A and C4B: gene size, reactivity, and antigenicity. *EMBO J.*, **5**, 2873–81.

52 Carroll, M. C., Fathallah, D. M., Bergamaschini, L., Alicot, E. M., and Isenman, D. E. (1990). Substitution of a single amino acid (aspartic acid for histidine) converts the functional activity of human C4B to C4A. *Proc. Natl. Acad. Sci. U.S.A.*, **87**, 6868–72.

53 Rowe, P. C., McLean, R. H., Wood, R. A., Leggiadro, R. J., and Winkelstein, J. A. (1989). Association of homozygous C4B deficiency with bacterial meningitis *J. Infect. Dis.*, **160**, 448–51.

54 Bishof, N. A., Welch, T. R., and Beischel, L. S. (1990). C4B deficiency: a risk factor for bacteraemia with encapsulated organisms. *J. Infect. Dis.*, **162**, 248–50.

55 Fearon, D. T. (1980). Identification of the membrane glycoprotein that is the C3b receptor of the human erythrocyte, polymorphonuclear leucocyte, B lymphocyte, and monocyte. *J. Exp. Med.*, **152**, 20–30.

56 Arnaout, M. A., Melamed, J., Tack, B. F., and Colten, H. R. (1981). Characterization of the human complement (C3b) receptor with the fluid-phase C3b dimer. *J. Immunol.*, **127**, 1348–54.

57 Ross, G. D., Newman, S. L., Lambris, J. D., Devery-Pocius, J. E., Cain, J. A., and Lachmann, P. J. (1983). Generation of three different fragments of bound C3b with purified factor I or serum. II. Location of binding sites in the C3 fragments for factors B and H, complement receptors, and bovine conglutinin. *J. Exp. Med.*, **158**, 334–52.

58 Kay, A. B. (1982). Complement receptor enhancement by chemotactic factors. *Mol. Immunol.*, **19**, 1307–11.

59 Becherer, J. D., Alsenz, J., Esparza, I., Hack, C. E., and Lambris, J. D. (1992). Segment spanning residues 727–768 of the complement C3 sequence contains a neoantigenic site and accommodates the binding of CR1, factor H, and factor B. *Biochemistry*, **31**, 1787–94.

60 Iida, K., Nadler, L., and Nussenzweig, V. (1983). Identification of the membrane receptor for the complement fragment C3d by means of a monoclonal antibody. *J. Exp. Med.*, **158**, 1021–33.

61 Kalli, K. R., Ahern, J. M., and Fearon, D. T. (1991). Interaction of iC3b with recombinant isotypic and chimeric forms of CR2. *J. Immunol.*, **147**, 590–4.

62 Sanchez-Madrid, F., Nagy, J. A., Robbins, E., Simon P., and Springer T. A. (1983). A human leucocyte differentiation antigen family with distinct α-subunits and a common β-subunit: the lymphocyte function associated antigen (LFA-1), the C3bi complement receptor (OKM1/Mac-1), and the p150,95 molecule. *J. Exp. Med.*, **158**, 1785–803.

63 Ross, G. D. and Lambris, J. D. (1982). Identification of a C3bi specific membrane complement receptor that is expressed on lymphocytes, monocytes, neutrophils, and erythrocytes. *J. Exp. Med.*, **155**, 96–110.

64 Gordon, D. L., Johnson, G. M., and Hostetter, M. K. (1987). Characteristics of iC3b binding to polymorphonuclear leucocytes. *Immunology*, **60**, 553–8.

65 Ross, G. D., Cain, J. A., and Lachmann, P. J., (1985). Membrane complement receptor type 3 (CR3) has lectin-like properties analogous to bovine conglutinin and functions as a receptor for zymosan and rabbit erythrocytes as well as a receptor for iC3b. *J. Immunol.*, **134**, 3307–15.

66 Wright, S. D., Rao, P. E., Van Voorhis, W. C., Craigmyle, L. S., Iida, K., Talle, M. A., Westberg, E. F., Goldstein, G., and Silverstein, S. C. (1983). Identification of the C3bi receptor of human monocytes and macrophages by using monoclonal antibodies. *Proc. Natl. Acad. Sci. U.S.A.*, **80**, 5699–703.

67 Crowley, C. A., Curnutte, J. T., Rosin, R. E., André-Schwartz, J., Gallin, J. I., Kiemphar, M., Snyderman, R., Southwick, F., Stossel, T. P., and Babior, B. M. (1980). An inherited abnormality of neutrophil adhesion: its

genetic transmission and its association with the missing protein. *N. Engl. J. Med.*, **302**, 1163–8.

68   Bowen, T. J., Ochs, H. D., Altman, L. C., Price, H. C., VanEpps, D. E., Brautigan, D. C., Rosin, R, E., Perkins, W. D., Babior, B. M., Klebanoff, S. J., and Wedgwood, R. J. (1982). Severe recurrent bacterial infections associated with defective adherence and chemotaxis in two patients with neutrophils deficient in a cell-associated glycoprotein. *J. Pediatr.*, **101**, 932–40.

69   Arnaout, M. A., Pitt, J., Cohen, H. J., Melamed, J., Rosen, F. S., and Colten, H. R. (1982). Deficiency of a granulocyte-membrane glycoprotein (gp150) in a boy with recurrent bacterial infections. *N. Engl. Med.*, **306**, 693–9.

70   Anderson, D. C., Schmalsteig, F. C., Kohl, S., Arnaout, M. A., Hughes, B. J., Towse, M. F., Bafoney, G. J., Brinkley, B. R., Dickey, W. D., Abramson, J. S., Springer, T. A., Boxer, L. A., Hollers, J. M., and Smith, C. W. (1984). Abnormalities of polymorphonuclear leucocyte function associated with a heritable deficiency of a high molecular weight surface glycoprotein (gp138): common relationship to diminished cell adherence. *J. Clin. Invest.*, **74**, 546–55.

71   Springer, T. A., Thompson, W. S., Miller, L. J., Schmalstieg, F. C., and Anderson, D. C. (1984). Inherited deficiency of the Mac-1, LFA1, p150,95 glycoprotein family and its molecular basis. *J. Exp. Med.*, **160**, 1901–18.

72   Vik, D. P. and Fearon, D. T. (1985). Neutrophils express a receptor for iC3b, C3dg, and C3d that is distinct from CR1, CR2, and CR3. *J. Immunol.*, **134**, 2571–9.

73   Corbi, A. L., Miller, T. J., O'Connor, K., Larson, R. S., and Springer, T. A. (1987). cDNA cloning and complete primary structure of the α-subunit of a leucocyte adhesion glycoprotein, p150,95 *EMBO J.*, **6**, 4023–8.

74   Mantovani, B. (1975). Different roles of IgG in complement receptors and phagocytosis by polymorphonuclear leucocytes. *J. Immunol.*, **115**, 15–17.

75   Scribner, D. J. and Fahrney, D. (1976). Neutrophil receptors for IgG in complement: their roles in the attachment and the ingestion phases of phagocytosis. *J. Immunol.*, **116**, 892–7.

76   Ehlenberger, A, G. and Nussenzweig, V. (1977). The role of membrane receptors for C3b and C3d in phagocytosis. *J. Exp. Med.*, **145**, 357–71.

77   Newman, S. L. and Johnston, R. B. (1976). Role of binding through C3b and IgG in polymorphonuclear neutrophil function: studies with trypsin generated C3b. *J. Immunol.*, **123**, 1839–46.

78   Wright, S. D. and Silverstein, S. C. (1983). Receptors for C3b and C3bi promote phagocytosis but not the release of toxic oxygen from human phagocytes. *J. Exp. Med.*, **158**, 2016–23.

79   Schreiber, R. D., Morrison, D. C., Podack, E. R., and Müller-Eberhardt, H. J. (1979). Bactericidal activity of the alternative complement pathway generated from 11 isolated plasmid proteins. *J. Exp. Med.*, **149**, 870–82.

80   Bjornson, A. B., Magnafichi, P. I., Schreiber, R. D., and Bjornson, H. S. (1987). Opsonization of bacteroides by the alternative complement pathway reconstructed from isolated plasma proteins. *J. Exp. Med.*, **165**, 777–98.

81   Gordon, D. L., Krueger, R. A., Quie, P. G., and Hostetter, M. K. (1985). Amidation of C3 at the thiolester site: stimulation of chemiluminescence and phagocytosis by a new inflammatory mediator. *J. Immunol.*, **134**, 3339–45.

82   Rutherford, B. and Schenkein, H. A. (1983). C3 cleavage products stimulate release of prostaglandins by human mononuclear phagocytes *in vitro*. *J. Immunol.*, **130**, 874–7.

83 Melamed, J., Medicus, R. G., Arnaout, M. A., and Colten, H. R. (1983). Induction of granulocyte histaminase released by particle-bound complement C3 cleavage products (C3b, C3bi) and IgG. *J. Immunol.*, **131**, 439–44.

84 Hostetter, M. K. and Johnson, G. M. (1989). The erythrocyte as instigator of inflammation. *J. Clin. Invest.*, **84**, 665–71.

85 Ezekowitz, A. R., Sim, R. B., Hull, M., and Gordon, S. (1984). Local opsonization by secreted macrophage complement components. Role of receptors for complement in uptake of zymosan. *J. Exp. Med.*, **159**, 244–60.

86 Cardosa, M. J., Porterfield, J. S., and Gordon, S. (1983). Complement receptor mediates enhanced flavivirus replication in macrophage. *J. Exp. Med.*, **158**, 258–63.

87 Pangburn, M. K. (1989). Analysis of recognition in the alternative complement pathway of complement. Effect of polysaccharide size. *J. Immunol.*, **142**, 2766–70.

88 Sim, E., Parker, K. E., and Jones, A. (1993). Effects of nucleophiles on complement proteins C3 and C4. In *Activators and inhibitors of the complement system* (ed. R. B. Sim), pp. 107–25. Kluwer, Dordrecht.

89 Dodds, A. W., Law, S. K., and Porter, R. R. (1985). The origin of the very variable haemolytic activities of the common human complement component C4 allotypes including C4-A6. *EMJO J.*, **4**, 2239–44.

90 Finland, M. (1937). The significance of specific pneumococcus types in disease including types IV to XXII. *Ann. Int. Med.*, **10**, 1531–43.

91 Mufson, M. A., Kruss, D. M., Wasil, R. E., and Metzger, W. I. (1974). Capsular types and outcome of bacteraemic pneumococcal disease in the antibiotic era. *Arch. Int. Med.*, **134**, 505–10.

92 Bratton, L., Teele, D. W., and Klein, J. O. (1977). Outcome of unsuspected pneumoccaemia in children not initially admitted to the hospital. *J. Pediatr.*, **90**, 703–6.

93 Giebink, G. S., Grebner, J. V., Kim, Y., and Quie, P. G. (1978). Serum opsonic deficiency produced by *Streptococcus pneumoniae* and by capsular polysaccharide antigens. *Yale J. Biol. Med.*, **51**, 527–38.

94 Winkelstein, J. A., Boccini, J. A., and Schiffman, G. (1976). The role of the capsular polysaccharide in the activation of the alternative pathway by the *Pneumococcus*. *J. Immunol.*, **116**, 367–70.

95 Edwards, M. and Stark, J. M. (1977). The ability of smooth and rough strains of *Streptococcus pneumoniae* to activate human complement by the alternative pathway. *J. Med. Microbiol.*, **11**, 7–14.

96 Winkelstein, J. A. and Tomasz, A. (1977). Activation of the alternative pathway by pneumococcal cell walls. *J. Immunol.*, **118**, 451–4.

97 Winkelstein, J. A. and Tomasz, A. (1978). Activation of the alternative complement pathway by pneumococcal cell wall teichoic acid. *J. Immunol.*, **120**, 174–8.

98 Winkelstein, J. A., Abramovitz, A. S., and Tomasz, A. (1980). Activation of C3 via the alternative complement pathway results in fixation of C3b to the pneumococcal cell wall. *J. Immunol.*, **124**, 2502–6.

99 Brown, E. J., Joiner, K. A., Cole, R. M., and Beryer, U. (1983). Localization of complement component 3 on *Streptococcus pneumoniae*: anti-capsular antibody causes complement deposition on the pneumococcal capsule. *Infect. Immun.*, **39**, 403–9.

100 Hummell, D. S., Berninger, R. W., Tomasz, A., *et al.* (1981). The fixation of C3b to pneumococcal cell wall polymers as a result of activation of the alternative complement pathway. *J. Immunol.*, **127**, 1287–9.

101   Hostetter, M. K. (1986). Serotypic variations among virulent pneumococci in deposition and degradation of covalently bound C3b. Implications for phagocytosis and antibody production. *J. Infect. Dis.*, **153**, 682–93.

102   Ward, H. K. (1930). Observations on the phagocytosis of the pneumococcus by human whole blood. I. The normal phagocytic titre, and the anti-phagocytic effect of the specific soluble substance. *J. Exp. Med.*, **51**, 675–84.

103   Wood Jr, W. B. and Smith, M. R. (1949). The inhibition of surface phagocytosis by the capsular 'slime layer' of pneumococcus type III. *J. Exp. Med.*, **90**, 85–99.

104   Knecht, J. C., Schiffman, G., and Austrian, R. (1970). Some biological properties of *Pneumococcus* type 37 and the chemistry of its capsular polysaccharide. *J. Exp. Med.*, **132**, 475–87.

105   Brown, E. J., Joiner, K. A., Gaither, T. A., Hummer, C. U., and Frank, M. M. (1983). The interaction of C3b bound to pneumococci with factor H (α1H globulin), factor I (C3b/C4b an activator), and prepared in factor B of the human complement system. *J. Immunol.*, **131**, 409–15.

106   Newman, S. L. and Mikus, L. K. (1985). Deposition of C3b and iC3b on to particulate activators of the human complement system. Quantitation with monoclonal antibodies to human C3. *J. Exp. Med.*, **161**, 1414–31.

107   Brown, E. J., Hosea, S. W., Hammer, C. H., Burch, C. G., and Frank, U. H. (1982). A quantitative analysis of the interactions of anti-pneumococcal antibody and complement in experimental pneumococcal bacteraemia. *J. Clin. Invest.*, **69**, 85–98.

108   Gordon, D. L., Johnson, G. M., and Hostetter, M. K. (1986). Ligand–receptor interactions in the phagocytosis of virulent *Streptococcal pneumoniae* by polymorphonuclear leucocytes. *J. Infect. Dis.* **154**, 619–26.

109   Gordon, D. J., Rice, J., Finlay-Jones, J., McDonald, P., and Hostetter, M. K. (1988). Analysis of C3 degradation patterns on bacterial surfaces after opsonization. *J. Infect. Dis.*, **157**, 697–704.

110   Jacks-Weis, J., Kim, Y. K., and Cleary, P. P. (1981). Restricted deposition of C3 on M+ group A streptococci: correlation with resistance to phagocytosis. *J. Immunol.*, **128**, 1897–902.

111   Weiss, J. J., Law, S. K., Levine, R. P., and Cleary, P. P. (1985). Resistance to phagocytosis by group A streptococci: failure of deposited complement opsonins to interact with cellular receptors. *J. Immunol.*, **134**, 500–5.

112   Campbell, J. R., Baker, C. J., and Edwards, M. S. (1991). Deposition and degradation of C3 on type III group B streptococci. *Infect. Immun.*, **59**, 1978–83.

113   Joiner, K. A., Grossman, N., Schmetz, M., and Leive, L. (1986). C3 binds preferentially to long chain lipopolysaccharide during alternative pathway activation by *Salmonella montevideo*. *J. Immunol.*, **136**, 710–15.

114   Densen, P. (1989). Interaction of complement with *Neisseria meningitidis* and *Neisseria gonorrhoeae*. *Clin. Micro. Rev.*, **S1**, 11–7.

115   Kozel, T. R., Brown, R. B., and Pfrommer, G. S. T. (1987). Activation and binding of C3 by *Candida albicans*. *Infect. Immun.*, 1890–4.

116   Joiner, K. A., Hieny, S., Kirchhoff, L. V., and Sher, A. (1985). gp72, the 72 kilodalton glycoprotein, is the membrane acceptor site for C3 on *Trypanosoma cruzi* epimastigotes. *J. Exp. Med.*, **161**, 1196–212.

117   Puentes, S. M., Dwyer, D. M., Bates, P. A., Joiner K. A. (1989). Binding and release of C3 from *Leishmania donovani* promastigotes during incubation in normal human serum. *J. Immunol.*, **143**, 3743–9.

118   Mosser, D. M. and Edelson, P. J. (1985). The mouse macrophage receptor for C3bi (CR3) is a major mechanism in the phagocytosis of *Leishmania* promastigotes. *J. Immunol.*, **135**, 2785–9.

119   Gadd, K. J. and Reid, K. B. M. (1981). The binding of complement component C3 to antibody-antigen aggregates after activation of the alternative pathway in human serum. *Biochem. J.*, **195**, 471–80.

120   Brown, E. J., Berger, M., Joiner, K. A., Frank, M. M. (1983). Classical complement pathway activation by anti-pneumococcal antibodies leads to covalent binding of C3b to antibody molecules. *Infect. Immun.*, **42**, 594–8.

121   Wilson, D. R., Juan, TS.-C., Wilde, M. D., Fey, G. H., and Darlington G. J. (1990). A 58 base-pair region of the human C3 gene confers synergistic inducibility by interleukin-1 and interleukin-6. *Molec. Cell Biol.*, 6181–91.

122   Sundstron, S. A., Komm, B. S., Ponce-de-Leon, H., Yi, Z., Teuscher, C., and Lyttle, C. R. (1989). Estrogen regulation of tissue-specific expression of complement C3. *J. Biol. Chem.*, **264**, 16941–7.

123   Zach, T. L., Herrman, V. A., Nelson, R. M., and Hostetter, M. K. (1991). C3 gene expression in pulmonary epithelial cells is enhanced by glucocorticoids. *Ped. Res.*, **29**, 165A.

124   Vik, D. P., Amiguet, P., Moffat, G. J., Fey, M., Amiguiet-Barras, F., Wetsel, R. A., and Tack, B. F. (1990). Structural features of the human C3 gene: intron/exon organization, transcriptional start site, and promoter region sequence. *Biochemistry*, **30**, 1080–7.

125   Colten, H. R., Alper, C. A., and Rosen, S. F. (1981). Genetics and biosynthesis of complement proteins. *N. Eng. J. Med.*, **304**, 653–6.

126   Ballow, M., Fang, F., Good, R. A., and Day, N. K. (1974). Developmental aspects of complement components in the newborn. *Clin. Exp. Immunol.*, **18**, 257–66.

127   Johnson Jr, R. B., Altenburger, K. M., Atkinson, A. W., and Curry, R. H. (1979). Complement in the newborn infant. *Pediatrics*, **64S**, 781–5.

128   Adamkin, D., Stitzel, A., Urmson, J., Farnett, M. L., Post, E., and Spitzer, R. (1978). Activity of the alternative pathway of complement in the newborn infant. *J. Pediatr.*, **93**, 604–8.

129   Edwards, M. S., Buffone, G. J., Fuselier, P. A., Weeks, J. I., and Baker, C. J. (1983). Deficient classical complement pathway activity in newborn sera. *Pediatr. Res.*, **17**, 685–8.

130   Winkelstein, J. A., Kurlandsky, L. E., and Swift, A. J. (1979). Defective activation of the third component of complement in the sera of newborn infants. *Pediatr Res.*, **13**, 1093–6.

131   Zach, T. L. and Hostetter, M. K. (1989). Biochemical abnormalities of the third component of complement in neonates. *Pediatr. Res.*, **26**, 116–20.

132   De Bruijn, M. H. L. and Fey, G. H. (1985). Human complement component C3: cDNA coding sequence and derived primary structure. *Proc. Natl. Acad. Sci. U.S.A.*, **82**, 708–2.

133   Isenman, D. E., Kells, D. I., Cooper, N. R., Müller-Eberhard, H. J., and Pangburn, M. K. (1981). Nucleophilic modification of human complement protein C3. Correlation of conformational changes with acquisition of C3b-like functional properties. *Biochemistry*, **20**, 4458–67.

134   Von Zabern, I., Nolte, R., and Vogt, W. (1981). Treatment of human complement components C4 and C3 with amines or chaotropic ions. *Scand. J. Immunol.*, **13**, 413–31.

135 Hostetter, M. K., Johnson, G. M., and Retsinas, E. M. (1986). Amidation of C3 by mucoid *Pseudomonas aeruginosa*: a mechanism for opsonic failure and phagocytic activation in the cystic fibrosis lung. *Clin. Res.*, **34**, 520A.

136 Nath, K. A., Hostetter, M. K., and Hostetter, T. H. (1985). Pathophysiology of chronic tubulo-interstitial disease in rats: interactions of dietary acid load, ammonia, and complement component C3. *J. Clin. Invest.*, **76**, 667–75.

137 Pangburn, M. K. (1992). Spontaneous reformation of the intra-molecular thiolester in complement protein C3 and low temperature capture of a conformational intermediate capable of reformation. *J. Biol. Chem.*, **267**, 8584–90.

138 Sim, E., Gill, E. W., and Sim, R. B. (1984). Drugs that induce systemic lupus erythematosus inhibit complement component C4. *Lancet*, **2**, 422–4.

139 Edmonds, S., Gibb, A., and Sim, E. (1993). Effect of thiol compounds on human complement component C4. *Biochem. J.*, **289**, 801–5.

140 Loewenson, P. M. and Hostetter, M. K. (1987). Functional implications of site-specific glycosylation of human C3 in hyperglycaemia. *Clin. Res.*, **35**, 858A.

141 Friedman, H. M., Cohen, G. H., Eisenberg, R. J., Seidel, C. A., and Cines, D. B. (1984). Glycoprotein C of herpes simplex virus 1 acts as a receptor for the C3b complement component on infected cells. *Nature*, **309**, 633–5.

142 McNearney, T. A., Odell, C., Holers, V. M., Spear, P. G., and Atkinson, J. P. (1987). Herpes simplex glycoproteins gC-1 and gC-2 bind to the third component of complement and provide protection against complement-mediated neutralization of viral infectivity. *J. Exp. Med.*, **166**, 1525–35.

143 Heidenreich, F. and Dierich, M. P. (1985). *Candida albicans* and *Candida stellatoidea*, in contrast to other Candida species, bind iC3b and C3d but not C3b. *Infect. Immun.*, **50**, 598–600.

144 Edwards Jr, J. E., Gaither, T. A., O'Shea, J. J., Rotrosen, D., Lawley, T. J., Wright, S. A., Frank, M. M., and Green. (1986). Expression of specific binding sites on Candida with functional and antigenic characteristics of human complement receptors. *J. Immunol.*, **137**, 3577–83.

145 Gilmore, B. J., Retsinas, E. M., Lorenz, J. S., and Hostetter, M. L. (1988). An iC3b receptor on *Candida albicans*: structure, function, and correlates for pathogenicity. *J. Infect. Dis.*, **157**, 38–46.

146 Hostetter, M. K., Lorenz, J. S., Preus, L., and Kendrick, K. E. (1990). The iC3b receptor on *Candida albicans* subcellular localization and modulation of receptor expression by glucose. *J. Infect. Dis.*, **161**, 761–8.

147 Gustafson, K. S., Vercellotti, G. M., Bendel, C. M., and Hostetter, M. K. (1991). Molecular mimicry in *Candida albicans:* role of an integrin analogue in adhesion of the yeast to human endothelium. *J. Clin. Invest.*, **87**, 1896–902.

148 Bendel, C. M. and Hostetter, M. K. (1991). Correlation of adhesion and pathogenic potential in yeast. *Pediatr. Res.*, **29**, 167A.

8 Complement-derived anaphylatoxins in natural immunity

R. BURGER AND G. ZILOW

1 Introduction

The complement system is a major element of the humoral defence reaction. This group of plasma proteins contributes to non-specific host defence and to the inflammatory response. In addition, complement-dependent mechanisms are involved in the induction and also the effector phase of the specific immune response. Therefore, complement might be classified as an endogenous immunoregulatory system. The complement proteins circulate in the body in native configuration. The native proteins are biologically inactive. An activation step via the classical or the alternative pathway is required to generate biological activity. In the course of this cascade-like activation sequence, specific proteolytic cleavage leads to the formation of defined complement fragments. These biologically active fragments are able to bind to specific cellular receptors and thereby trigger subsequent cellular reactions (1–8).

One group of highly active mediators generated as activation products during the activation process are the anaphylatoxins C3a, C4a, and C5a (1–3). They are structurally similar fragments of the complement proteins C3, C4, and C5 and have a molecular weight of about 10 kDa. The anaphylatoxins have recently attracted increasing interest not only from immunologists but also from clinicians, because it was recognized that these proteins contribute to the pathogenesis of dysfunctions of the lung and a series of other diseases (9).

Anaphylatoxins were first identified at the beginning of this century. The terminus 'toxin' was used because of their toxin-like effect in guinea pigs. This animal species is particularly sensitive to anaphylatoxin action and shows symptoms resembling an anaphylactic shock. A lethal shock associated with a marked bronchospasm was observed in guinea pigs when fresh serum was incubated with aggregated immunoglobulin and injected intravenously. It took several decades, until the end of the 1950s, to realize that anaphylatoxins are derived from the complement proteins C3 and C5 and—even later—C4. It is since the 1970s that it has been known that there are three different complement-derived anaphylatoxins C3a, C4a, and C5a.

Advances in protein chemistry allowed the isolation of C3a, C4a, and C5a in highly purified form. The amino acid sequence was determined at the protein level and recently at the cDNA level. By X-ray crystallography, the three-dimensional structure of C3a was elucidated. There are marked sequence homologies amongst C3a, C4a, and C5a. Purified C3a, C4a, and C5a and synthetic peptides corresponding to defined molecular sites were used successfully in various *in vitro* systems for analysis of anaphylatoxin function in host defence, inflammation, and immune reaction. Recombinant anaphylatoxins have become available and facilitate these studies. Some of the present highlights of anaphylatoxin research are identification of specific receptors on cells and signal transduction, pharmacological modulation of anaphylatoxin functions, their role in pathogenesis of pulmonary dysfunction and other diseases involving complement activation, and, finally, the involvement of C3a, C4a, and C5a in defined steps of the humoral or cellular immune reaction. Most reports describe C3a and C5a; much less is known about C4a. The following overview summarizes the general properties of the three polypeptides (see also 1–5, 10) and reviews recent studies on clinical aspects of anaphylatoxins (AT).

2   General properties of anaphylatoxins

2.1   Generation of anaphylatoxins

C3a, C4a, and C5a are generated either specifically through the enzymes formed during classical or alternative pathway activation, (e.g. the classical pathway C3 convertase), or through direct proteolytic attack by proteases released from tissues or cells upon local damage (see Chapter 5). Cleavage of the parent proteins occurs at a defined site (11). Based on the concentration of the native precursor protein in plasma, a maximal concentration of about 2×10^{-6} M to 5×10^{-7} M might be obtained. However, anaphylatoxin activity extends to a far lower range (to about 10^{-9} M for C5a). The generation of AT is therefore a sensitive indicator of complement activation. In the absence of specific C3 or C5 convertases or of other proteases, only trace concentrations of AT are observed in the circulation (for C3a about 100–200 ng/ml, i.e. 10^{-8} M).

2.2   Structure of anaphylatoxins

The anaphylatoxins (AT) consist of 77 (human C3a and C4a) or 74 amino acids (C5a). The structure of the AT, particularly of C3a, is well elucidated (3, 4, 12). The single polypeptide chain contains intramolecular disulfide bridges forming a relatively compact core-like structure. The corresponding six half-cysteine residues are highly conserved in C3a C4a, and C5a from different species. All three AT contain a proportion of basic amino acids and behave as polycations. The AT are remarkably stable over a wide range of temperature and pH. Alpha-helical structure is present in 40–45 per cent of the AT polypeptide chain. The C-terminus forms a wobbly tail consisting of the last 10–12 amino acids which has no defined structure (13–15). A common feature of all three AT is the presence of the amino acid arginine at the C-terminus, i.e. at the cleavage site from the parent protein. This C-terminal Arg in position 77 or 74, respectively, is essential for the biological activity (see Section 2.4), and after its removal by carboxypeptidase N in blood most biological activities are lost. The des-arginated AT variants are designated as C3a-desArg, C5a-desArg and C4a-desArg and are no longer able to interact with cellular anaphylatoxin receptors. However, C5a-desArg also has chemotactic activity for neutrophils which is unaffected by removal of the C-terminal Arg residue. The desArg forms of C3a, C4a, and C5a have extended half-lives *in vivo*. In contrast to C3a and C4a, C5a bears a substantial carbohydrate moiety (about 3 kDa) at position 64 (4). The three AT are antigenically quite different and no cross-reaction of antisera or monoclonal antibodies has been observed.

Improvement in purification methods allowed the isolation of individual AT on a preparative scale, which in turn was the pre-requisite for partial or complete amino acid sequencing and for X-ray crystallographic analysis (13, 17). The crystal structure deduced for C3a has been used for modelling C5a and C4a. The interior residues are particularly highly conserved whereas the external surface residues differ considerably (18). The early X-ray diffraction studies of C3a-desArg crystals were extended by one- or two-dimensional NMR spectroscopy for analysis of C3a secondary structure in solution (14, 15). In soluble C3a, a shorter helical portion was found and the C-terminus shows a flexible and dynamic random coil conformation (14). The removal of Arg 77 does not cause major alterations of C3a conformation. A solution structure for C5a has also been determined and serves to emphasize the flexibility of the C-terminus (16).

A large variety of synthetic peptides was synthesized which corresponded to individual sites or domains of the AT. The peptides were used to define the functionally relevant sites. Structural data of the three AT from various species are summarized in several recent, excellent articles in the literature and are therefore omitted from this overview (3, 17, 18).

2.3 Biological functions of anaphylatoxins

The anaphylatoxins, especially C3a and C5a, are functionally highly active (2–4, 6, 19). Biological activity is detectable down to below the nanomolar range corresponding to concentrations of nanogram or even picogram per millilitre depending on the assay system. In general, the specific activity of C5a is higher than C3a which in turn more active than C4a. This high specific activity requires extensive purification for functional studies in order to exclude interference by minor, but highly active contaminants. AT are able to induce a wide variety of release reactions, some of which are useful for measuring AT *in vitro*. The AT affect various tissues. Release reactions and metabolic or morphologic alterations are induced by AT with different cell populations.

AT induce the release of several mediators which are highly active and influence the local environment. In general, the AT-induced release reaction contribute to the inflammatory response. The major target cells for AT are polymorphonuclear neutrophils, mast cells, basophils, monocytes, macrophages, and platelets, and, in addition, T cells and eosinophils. The classical AT functions include the contraction of smooth muscle, observed for example in the AT-induced bronchospasm in the guinea pig, and the release of histamine from mast cells or basophils. AT cause vasoconstriction and increased vasopermeability and have the ability to cause neutropaenia and thrombocytopaenia. AT induce an aggregation of platelets and also of granulocytes, and the release of lysosomal enzymes or reactive oxygen derivatives from this cell population. The release of serotonin or, similary, ATP from guinea pig platelets is useful for the measurement of human or guinea pig AT (20). Despite single contrary reports, human platelets do not respond to C3a and obviously do not express the corresponding C3a receptor (21). C5a and C5a-desArg have chemotactic activity whereas C3a is inactive. C5a enhances the expression of complement receptors CR1 and CR3 for C3b/iC3b (22) (see Chapter 5). C3a induces the release of IL-1 (Chapter 2) and of thromboxane, prostaglandins, and leukotrienes (see Chapter 13) (19, 23). Additional functions of AT are discussed in Section 2.9.

2.4   Control of anaphylatoxin functions

There are at least two efficient and independent control mechanisms of AT activity under physiological conditions as summarized in Figure 8.1. The

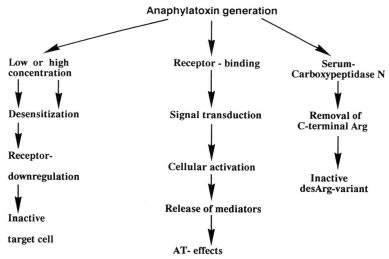

Fig. 8.1   Control mechanisms of anaphylatoxin action.

well known serum carboxypeptidase N (AT inhibitor) rapidly removes the C-terminal Arg of the AT which is essential for most of its biological activities (16). This ubiquitous enzyme thereby converts active AT into the desArg variants. A second, independent and perhaps even more rapid control mechanism is receptor down-regulation (see Section 2.10). Incubation with either high or with sub-threshold concentrations of AT render responding cells refractory (specific desensitization or tachyphylaxis). Through this de-activation mechanism, an inefficient or detrimental AT response might be prevented (4). The deactivation process is reversible. A further possible control mechanism has been described in peritoneal and synovial fluid where an inhibitor of C5a chemotactic function has been found (24) which causes limited proteolysis of C5a.

2.5   Measurement of anaphylatoxins

Haemolytic complement tests and measurement of concentration of intact components cannot provide accurate information about the extent of complement activation: activation cannot be distinguished from reduced synthesis or increased catabolism. An acute phase reaction (see Chapters 1–4) leading to increased synthesis could compensate for even extensive activation (8, 10, 25). A direct approach to detecting complement activation is measurement of cleavage products such as C3a, C4a, and C5a. The measurement of these activation products has several advantages. AT are only produced as a consequence of activation and they are produced on cleavage of the parent molecules on an equimolar basis (Figure 8.2). A series of assays systems are available for measurement of AT, including functional and serological

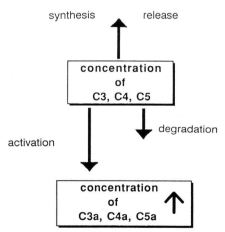

Fig. 8.2 Concentration of anaphylatoxins as a direct parameter of complement activation. In contrast, the concentration of the circulating native molecule is influenced by additional factors.

assays. Functional assays use measurement of increased vasopermeability, contraction of guinea pig ileum, and serotonin or ATP release from platelets (20). AT are also measured by their capacity to cause platelet or granulocyte aggregation. Functional assays have the major disadvantage that they detect only the active AT variant but not the desArg form present in the circulation. Analysis of clinical specimens therefore requires serological assays. Radioimmunoassays (26, 27), as well as enzyme-linked immunoassays using monoclonal antibodies (28–30), have depended on removal of the uncleaved components, C3, C4, or C5 from the sample, since antisera to the fragments also recognize the native, uncleaved parent molecule. To overcome this problem, monoclonal antibodies reacting with neo-determinants of C3a (31) and C5a (32) have been produced and methods were established which detect AT via neoantigenic epitopes (25, 33–36) (Figure 8.3).

2.6   Analysis with synthetic analogues of anaphylatoxins

Synthetic peptides have facilitated the analysis of AT function considerably and provided information on essential structural elements and the role of individual amino acids (3, 4). Whilst this has been useful with C3a analogues (37–41), C5a peptides were inactive. These studies suggest that a single linear sequence of amino acids in C5a is unlikely to be sufficient to promote interaction of C5a with its receptor. For C3a these experiments revealed that the C-terminus is crucial for receptor-binding and therefore for AT activity.

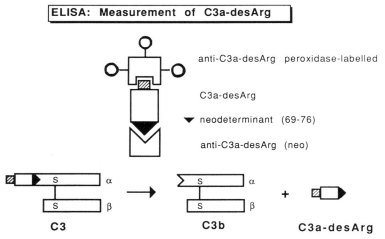

Fig. 8.3 Anaphylatoxins measured by ELISA to detect 'neoantigenic determinants'. Monoclonal antibodies to neoantigenic determinants exposed only after cleavage of the AT from the parent molecule (shown here for the AT C3a-desArg, 25, 31). This assay does not require radioactive material or precipitation steps for removal of the native protein.

Model peptides corresponding to the C-terminus of C3a are able to trigger qualitatively the same functions as the intact AT although the peptides are usually less efficient by a factor of 100–1000. Even a short C-terminal synthetic pentapeptide (LGLAR) of C3a was able to elicit C3a functions *in vitro* (41). An extension in length from the C-terminal pentapeptide to a 21 residue fragment increased biological function on a molar basis to almost the same level as the natural ligand. Sites in C3a in addition to the C-terminal pentapeptide obviously contribute to receptor-binding. This might be an indirect effect, e.g. by influencing the conformation of the C-terminus. Alternatively, the binding to the receptor might involve more than one AT site, i.e. an additional site distinct from the C-terminus. The formation of an alpha-helical conformation might determine the potency of an analogue. (1). Recently, a series of analogues with defined substitutions, (e.g. attachment of hydrophobic groups) were reported which had a higher activity (10–100 times higher) than the natural peptides (37–40) probably because of an improved, non-specific interaction with the cell membrane since tripeptides were generated which still had AT activity (40).

2.7   Inhibitors of anaphylatoxin generation or function

Specific inhibitors of AT activity are obviously of importance both for therapeutic purposes and for experimental studies. They might allow inhibition of undesired complement function in patients. There are several principal approaches to interfere with AT action. (a) Synthetic analogues corresponding to the active site, e.g. the C-terminus of the AT, might be used as competitive inhibitors to prevent binding to receptors. This would require analogues which are by themselves inactive and have a reasonable half-life *in vivo*. Recombinant AT analogues with modified structure might also be used (42). (b) Antibodies to the AT receptors which block AT-binding but do not elicit a response would provide an efficient tool. (c) Specific inhibitors of the AT generating enzymes should prevent AT formation. However, peptides corresponding to the vicinity of the cleavage site proved to be poor inhibitors (43) whereas other synthetic or natural protease inhibitors were partially effective *in vitro* and in experimental animals, e.g. FUT-175. (44, 45). (d) Antibodies to neoantigens expressed selectively on the AT but not on the parent molecule should block AT function. (e) Application of physiological inhibitors might be an alternative (24). (f) Finally, AT cleaving proteases, identified for example in group B streptococci, might potentially be applied (46). To date, no efficient and reliable inhibitors of AT function with therapeutic application have been identified.

2.8   Anaphylatoxins and immune response

A number of *in vitro* studies have suggested that AT (C3a and C5a) modulate the specific immune response (47–49). Non-specific stimulation (Fc fragment induced antibody production) and the antibody response to sheep red blood cells was initially studied. C3a had an inhibitory effect whereas C5a (and also C5a-desArg) enhanced the ongoing immune reaction. CD8 positive T cells were suggested to be the target cell affected by the AT. No unequivocal effect on T helper cell function was observed although the addition of IL-2 did partially reverse the inhibitory effect of C3a on the immune response to T cell-dependent antigens. The response to T-independent antigens was not affected. The exact mode of AT action within these complex systems requiring cellular interaction and in addition the release and signalling by soluble cytokines remains to be identified. The selective effect of C5a on antigen-induced T cell response and its failure to influence the mitogen response also requires further studies.

For both C5a and C3a, the cells of the monocyte/macrophage lineage might represent the major elements for modulation of immune reactivity (23). C5a and C3a stimulate the production of IL-1 known to influence T cell responses and to affect many other cellular functions. The desArg variants of C3a and C5a also have IL-1 inducing capacity. Therefore, an effect on T cells might occur not only at the site of complement activation, i.e. in the vicinity of foreign antigen or other stimuli, but the desArg variants might also exert their effect at a distinct site.

2.9   Interaction of anaphylatoxins with other systems

The generation of anaphylatoxins influences several other humoral and cellular immune mechanisms through a network of interactions supporting host defence reactions. Anaphylatoxins cause the release of histamine from mast cells and basophils and are potent inducers of degranulation. One particularly interesting control element for this reaction are cytokines. After pre-treatment of basophils with IL-3, C5a and C3a are able to induce the production of leukotrienes (Chapters 12 and 13) whereas C3a or C5a alone have no effect. IL-3 also enhances AT-induced degranulation (50, 51). Similarly, GM-CSF enhanced the C3a response of basophils (51). The cytokines might induce AT receptor expression.

Purified or recombinant C5a stimulates the secretion of TNF (Chapter 4) and IL-1 (Chapter 2) (52, 53). Both cytokines are pluripotent mediators which affect a variety of other cell populations and contribute to the septic shock syndrome (Chapter 5). This C5a effect is dependent on previous activation of monocytes or macrophage with LPS. Also the 'inactive' C3a-desArg variant, which has no biological activity in most other biological systems, was able to induce IL-1 production and to enhance LPS-induced IL-1 release (53, 54), even at a concentration of C3a-desArg of 10^{-8} M. Through this cytokine-inducing capacity, the AT have the ability to influence not only local reactions but also to trigger a systemic response including the acute phase reaction.

It should be emphasized that the results from some of these *in vitro* studies differed substantially and might depend on the nature and quantity of LPS contamination of the anaphylatoxin preparation. Highly purified, LPS depleted AT preparations were not able to stimulate IL-1 synthesis or secretion (55). In addition, more subtle regulatory mechanisms at the transcriptional or translational level might be involved. In the absence of LPS, C5a was shown to stimulate transcription of IL-1 and TNF production. LPS or IL-1 itself provides a translational signal (Chapter 2) (56).

Recombinant C5a causes the release of IL-6 by human monocytes (Chapter 3) and the C5a-desArg variant was active (57). IL-6 in turn has multiple activities and might therefore influence B cell differentiation, T cell response, or differentiation from progenitor cells via this pleiotropic cytokine. The ability of AT to induce the production of prostaglandins known to regulate MHC Class II expression might affect the capacity of accessory cells for antigen presentation (19, 23).

2.10   Anaphylatoxin receptors

The existence or presence of specific receptors for anaphylatoxins on a given cell population is suggested either by functional studies or from binding studies. Alteration of cellular function after incubation with AT or their synthetic analogues is taken as an indication for the expression of a functional receptor on the cell surface. Based on functional assays, neutrophils, basophils, eosinophils, mast cells, a T cell subpopulation, monocytes, macrophages, and —at least in the guinea pig but not in the human—platelets express AT receptors (3, 4). C3a/C4a and C5a bind to two distinct, specific receptors which regulate cell function independently, (e.g. deactivation in tachyphylaxis). The fact that extremely low concentrations of AT are sufficient to trigger a cellular response indicate the presence of AT receptors with high affinity for its ligand. So far, only a few cell lines have been shown to express the C3a receptor. The HL-60 line expresses the C3a receptor as revealed by binding studies and by demonstration of C3a-induced cellular functions. The cell lines U937, HL-60, and P388D1 respond to C5a. AT receptors have also been characterized in more detail by binding or cross-linking studies (21, 58–60).

2.10.1   C5a receptor

Most information is available on the C5a receptor on neutrophils and eosinophils. In SDS-PAGE, it is a single band with an apparent molecular weight of 52–55 kDa and an additional solubilized molecular variant of 95 kDa was identified (61–63). The C5a receptor on U937 cells consisted of a 41 kDa band. On PMN and U937 cells, up to 100 000 high affinity binding sites were measured. Recombinant C5a variants proved to be useful tools for C5a receptor analysis (42). The addition of an extension peptide recognized by monoclonal antibodies allowed detection of receptor-bound C5a and permitted analysis of cell populations, e.g. by FACS.

Recently, the C5a receptor was cloned (and encodes a protein of 350 amino acids) from U937 and HL-60 cell lines, and after expression in COS cells had the capacity to bind its ligand C5a with high affinity and to mediate signal transduction via G proteins which are associated with the C5a receptor (59, 64a, 64b). For C5a, receptor-mediated endocytosis was described leading to internalization and finally degradation.

2.10.2   C3a receptor

On platelets, two proteins of 95 kDa and 105 kDa were initially identified by cross-linking experiments. They bound C3a but not C3a-desArg (60). Subsequently, similar photoaffinity labelling showed additional proteins in a molecular weight range of 85–114 kDa (21). The number of binding sites varied in these studies between 200–1200 per platelet. The C3a-binding elements differed in affinity (low and high affinity binding sites). The mast cell proved to be a difficult cell type for AT receptor studies because binding was not saturable. Degradation of C3a prevented a definitive receptor identification and obscured the specific binding reaction (65). In guinea pigs, a genetic C3a receptor deficiency was identified (21, 66). These animals responded *in vivo* and *in vitro* to C5a but not C3a.

2.11   Recombinant anaphylatoxins

The production of recombinant C5a and, more recently, C3a was achieved by chemical synthesis of the corresponding DNA sequence (67, 68). After cloning and expression in *E.coli*, the recombinant anaphylatoxins were reactive in the conventional radioimmunoassay and were functionally active, e.g in ileum contraction or platelet aggregation, including the capacity to induce tachyphylaxis. Through the availability of recombinant AT many difficulties and problems in AT preparation and supply are avoided. In addition, site-directed mutagenesis allows the production of defined molecular variants for structural analysis or for studies of receptor–ligand interaction as shown for C5a (69). In agreement with earlier findings using synthetic peptides these studies revealed that three or more discontinuous regions of C5a are involved in receptor-binding and AT function. The fact that non-glycosylated C5a produced in bacteria is active demonstrates that the carbohydrate moiety has no major role in C5a function although stability, aggregation, or absorption phenomena might be affected.

3   Anaphylatoxins and disease

The complement system is involved in human disease on two main fronts. Several diseases are a direct or indirect consequence of a selective deficiency of one complement component or a regulatory protein (see Table 5.3). Numerous diseases result from inflammation and tissue damage initiated or perpetuated by complement activation. Information about activation of the complement system might be of use in a clinical setting. The known role of complement in inducing tissue damage implies that the degree of activation should reflect the intensity of the inflammatory process. The nature of the stimulus determines the pathway of activation. Information about route, extent, and course of complement activation helps to predict the immunopathological mechanisms of a disease.

A quantitative assessment of complement activation should give an index of disease activity in those cases in which products of the complement cascade play a role in the mediation of tissue damage and clinical manifestation. Complement activation, without the need for specific antibodies, occurs through both the classical and alternative pathways (Chapters 5–7). Both of these pathways result in production of the most potent anaphylatoxin, C5a.

3.1 Anaphylatoxin formation in extracorporeal circuits

Beginning in the 1970s, clinical and laboratory studies revealed that transient but profound leukopaenia developed during the first few minutes of haemodialysis (70) resulting from complement activation (71, 72). Cellophane membranes in dialysers activated complement during haemodialysis and low molecular weight components of the complement system induced sequestration of granulocytes and monocytes within the pulmonary vasculature (71). This sequestration accounted for the transient leukopaenia and correlated with the development of hypoxia and pulmonary dysfunction (73). During this period of haemodialysis C5a is generated and C5a is responsible for granulocyte aggregation and sequestration (74). These observations during haemodialysis were similarly observed in another extracorporeal perfusion technique, namely during cardiopulmonary bypass (72, 75).

More recent studies confirmed and extended the initial clinical findings by employing radioimmunoassay techniques to quantitate anaphylatoxins in extracorporeal circuits. Extensive complement activation was shown to be very similar, with only temporal and quantitative differences, during haemodialysis and cardiopulmonary bypass. There was a dramatic increase in C3a-desArg levels and an often brief duration of granulocytopaenia, while changes in C4a-desArg or C5a-desArg concentrations were only modest or non-existent (75). Administration of protamine sulfate following cardiopulmonary bypass produced an additional increase of C4a-desArg indicating classical pathway activation. In patients with immediate adverse reactions after protamine administration, a statistically significant increase in C4a-desArg compared with non-reactor patients was found. Therefore, it was suggested that activation was caused by protamine–heparin complexes or protamine–anti-protamine complexes (76).

In a recent study it was demonstrated that despite intense complement and PMN activation there was no alteration or damage to the alveolar component of the pulmonary alveolar capillary membrane assessed by radioaerosol lung clearance (77). One possible explanation for the lack of demonstrable acute lung injury may be the brief duration of complement activation, leading to more benign and reversible episodes of lung dysfunction, in contrast to severe cases of adult respiratory distress syndrome (ARDS) and multi-system organ failure (MOF).

3.2   Anaphylatoxin formation in ARDS and MOF

AT formation has been intensively studied in patients with sepsis syndrome (78–80). Sepsis is one of the most frequent conditions associated with ARDS and the development of MOF (Table 8.1). ARDS and MOF are also known to develop in patients with acute pancreatitis, burn, or severe trauma (81, 82). Complement activation and AT formation was observed in burnt and severely traumatized patients (79) and in patients with severe pancreatitis (83–86). C3a-desArg and C5a-desArg plasma concentrations were elevated during attacks of acute pancreatitis and correlated significantly with the severity of the disease. In patients recovering from the disease, C3a-desArg levels rapidly declined, whereas in cases with a fatal outcome, C3a-desArg levels remained elevated. C5a-desArg concentration in plasma did not correlate with the severity of disease at admission. Differences in AT elimination from the circulation and in metabolism might account for these findings.

In one study, C3a-desArg levels were significantly higher in patients with septic shock than in patients without septic shock (87). In contrast to our own (88, 89) and other investigations (79, 90–93) Hack and his colleagues found no difference in C3a-desArg or C4a-desArg levels in patients with or without ARDS. The reason for the discrepancies between these studies may be caused by differences in the study design. In cases of severely traumatized patients,

Table 8.1   Diagnostic relevance of anaphylatoxins C3a, C4a, and C5a

Patients at risk for ARDS and MOF
   Severe trauma
   Pancreatitis
   Severe (abdominal) infection
   Severe burns

Extracorporeal perfusion
   Haemodialysis
   Cardiopulmonary bypass

Systemic lupus erythematosus

Rheumatoid arthritis

the time of initiation of the trauma can be exactly defined, while there is no defined onset of sepsis or acute pancreatitis. The significant difference in C3a-desArg concentration between ARDS and non-ARDS patients in the early post-trauma phase in our own study was limited to a few hours, because the initial rise in C3a-desArg levels was transient. When blood samples are taken only once a day, this time point is easily missed. Elevated levels of C3a-desArg and C4a-desArg are associated with a fatal outcome in sepsis (87, 94). 92 per cent of the patients with C3a-desArg levels higher than a critical value at admission died, suggesting that complement activation is involved in the development of lethal complications in sepsis.

C3a-desArg can be easily detected in the circulation by serological AT assays, but it must not necessarily be considered to cause the fatal complications occurring after polytrauma, burn, or sepsis. More likely, it is the second more potent AT, C5a, which—in contrast to C3a—is not easily detected in the circulation (95, 96). The reason is apparently that the majority of C5a binds rapidly and irreversibly to its receptors on neutrophils and monocytes (61, 62, 97). Alternatively, conventional assays for detection of C5a-desArg might not be sensitive enough. Therefore, C5a-desArg might only be detectable in plasma upon excessive C5 activation. However, a recently developed specific and highly sensitive ELISA with a detection limit of 20 pg C5a-desArg/ml plasma allowed determination of normal plasma levels of C5a/C5a-desArg in healthy blood donors (35). Studies with this novel method demonstrated that C5a/C5a-desArg is released in patients undergoing cardiopulmonary bypass indicating that previous assays for measurement C5a/C5a-desArg were not sensitive enough (98).

Although there are some controversial results and opinions on the role of AT in the pathogenesis of various diseases, there seems to be a general agreement that a central target of AT is the neutrophil. According to the 'complement hypothesis' (9), AT are generated by complement activation triggered through an initial stimulus, (e.g. Gram-negative bacteria) and cause an aggregation of neutrophils and their sequestration in the lung. The AT induce cellular activation processes. The cells locally release mediators, including toxic oxygen derivates, lysosomal enzymes, and lipid derived mediators (Chapters 12 and 13), which cause massive tissue damage. An increase in vasopermeability occurs leading to frequently fatal oedema.

3.3   Anaphylatoxin generation in inflammatory fluids (Table 8.2)

Local complement activation in the lower respiratory tract of patients with ARDS has been demonstrated. Chemotactically active C5a (95) as well as C3a-desArg (88, 99) was found in epithelial lining fluid. The presence of C5a correlated with the presence of neutrophils. Neutrophil proteases such as elastase which are present in bronchoalveolar lavage fluid (100) are able

Table 8.2 Anaphylatoxin generation in inflammatory fluids

Epithelial lining fluid

Peritoneal fluid

Pleural fluid

Pericardial fluid

Burn bullae fluid

Cerebrospinal fluid
   Guillain–Barré syndrome
   Bacterial meningitis
   Viral menigitis

Ovarian follicular fluid

to cleave C3 (101) and might contribute to the generation of AT. Accumulation of C3a and C5a was found in several other inflammatory fluids such as peritoneal (102), pleural, pericardial, or burn bullae fluid (103) in concentrations comparable with plasma (104). High C3a-desArg levels were found in all these fluids and the concentration did not depend on high plasma concentrations of C3a-desArg. In peritoneal or burn bullae fluid, no concomitant increase of C5a was detected, despite high concentrations of the terminal complement complex indicating that the cascade has been fully activated. This demonstrates again that measurement of C5a cannot be considered as an optimal parameter for complement activation.

C3a and C5a concentrations were significantly elevated in the cerebrospinal fluid from patients suffering from acute monophasic Guillain–Barré syndrome compared with samples from a control group of patients with non-inflammatory neurologic diseases. Plasma concentrations, however, were within the normal range (105). In addition, elevated C3a levels were observed in cerebrospinal fluid from patients with bacterial and, to a lesser degree, with viral meningitis (106, 107). In experimental meningitis, intracisternally administered C5a caused in rabbits a rapid early influx of leucocytes into the cerebrospinal fluid. Prostaglandin E_2 given simultaneously decreased leucocytosis in cerebrospinal fluid in a dose-dependent manner (108). The anti-inflammatory effect was thought to be due to alteration of receptor-binding of C5a or to alteration of cyclic adenosine monophosphate levels in neutrophils (109).

Synovial fluids of patients with rheumatoid arthritis contain high levels of C3a and C5a compared with synovial fluids from patients with degenerative joint disease or with traumatic arthritis (110, 111). It has been assumed that C3 cleavage occurred through activation of the complement cascade by immune complexes containing rheumatoid factors. The result of C3a measurement was in substantial agreement with measurements of the C3 fragments C3c and

C3d (112–117), which were also elevated. In ovarian follicular fluid obtained during the pre-ovulatory period, high amounts of C3a and C5a were found (118). Urokinase led in follicular fluid to the formation of plasmin, which in turn generates C3a and C5a. This *in vitro* activation of the complement cascade might indicate a possible role of complement in the multi-factorial mechanism of ovulation.

3.4 Complement activation in systemic lupus erythematosus (SLE)

To define the role of complement activation with respect to the activity of SLE, circulating levels of complement activation products were measured (119–121), since conventional measures of complement activation had only limited value as predictors of disease activity (122). An increase in plasma C3a-desArg levels occurred one to two months prior to clinical evidence of SLE disease flare and increased markedly during a disease flare (123). In addition, patients with acute CNS lupus had significantly higher levels of circulating C3a-desArg and C5a-desArg than patients with active disease but without CNS involvement. The significance of this increase in cases of CNS lupus was indicated in histopathologic findings (123). In contrast, significantly higher C4a-desArg levels, indicative of classical pathway activation, were found in patients with aggressive disease by Wild *et al.* whereas C3a-desArg did not differ from control values. In this study C4a-desArg appeared to be a sensitive indicator of severity, however, it remains to be shown that the observed increase of C4a-desArg is not a consequence of the therapeutic procedures (124).

3.5 Additional diseases associated with anaphylatoxin generation

A significant increase in circulating AT peptides was demonstrated in cases of pre-eclampsia (125), after wasp-sting challenge in patients with severe anaphylactic reactions (126), in aspirated blood collected for autologous transfusion (104, 127), in cytapheresis (128), after surgery (129–131), after therapy with IL-2 (132), and after short-term aerobic exercise (133). In most of these observations, the meaning and importance of the increased AT level remains to be clarified.

4 Summary

The anaphylatoxins C3a, C5a, and C4a are biologically highly active mediators of known structure. They are generated during activation of the complement system. The measurement of AT concentration provides therefore a parameter for complement activation. A new generation of AT assays based on detection via neoantigenic epitopes facilitates AT measurement. The function of AT is controlled by enzymatic inactivation (serum carboxypeptidase N) or by receptor down-regulation. The anaphylatoxin receptor for C5a has been cloned and the site of interaction with C5a has been identified. There are no efficient inhibitors of AT available for therapeutic use. Synthetic analogues and recombinant AT facilitated analysis of structure, function, and receptor interaction. Depending on the site of AT generation and AT concentration, the various AT have either a beneficial effect supporting host defence or, alternatively, cause inflammatory reactions and have a detrimental function. Increased levels of AT were observed in many clinical conditions associated with complement activation. AT generation might contribute to the pathogenesis of various diseases and influence disease activity. AT are obviously responsible for tissue damage and eventually for organ failure, particularly in pulmonary dysfunctions. AT influence the clinical manifestations observed during extracorporeal circulation and various inflammatory reactions including neurological diseases.

References

1   Hugli, T. E. (1984). Structure and function of the anaphylatoxin. *Springer Seminar Immunopathol.*, **7**, 193–219.
2   Hugli, T. E. (1986). Biochemistry and biology of anaphylatoxins. *Complement*, **3**, 111–27.
3   Hugli, T. E. (1990). Structure and function of C3a anaphylatoxins. Curr. Top. Microbiol. Immunol. **153**, 181–208.
4   Bitter-Suermann, D. (1988). The anaphylatoxins. In *The complement system* (ed. K. Rother and G. Till), pp. 367–95. Springer, New York.
5   Damerau, B. (1987). Biological activities of complement-derived peptides. *Rev. Physiol. Biochem. Pharmacol.*, **108**, 152–91.
6   Burger, R. (1987). The complement component C3 as a mediator of the inflammatory reaction. *Prog. appl. Microcirc.*, **12**, 108–23.
7   Lambris, J. D. (ed.) (1990). The third component of complement—chemistry and biology. Springer, Berlin.
8   Dalmasso, A. P. (1986). Complement in the pathophysiology and diagnosis of human diseases. *Crit. Rev. Clin. Lab. Sci.*, **24**, 123–83.
9   Rinaldo, J. E. (1986). Mediation of ARDS by leucocytes. *Chest*, **89**, 590–3.
10 Hammerschmidt D. E. (1986). Clinical utility of complement anaphylatoxin. *Complement*, **3**, 166–78.
11 Müller-Eberhard, H. J. (1988). Molecular organization of the complement system. *Annu. Rev. Biochem.*, **57**, 321–52.
12 Hugli, T. E. (1975). Human anaphylatoxin (C3a) from the third component of complement: primary structure. *J. Biol. Chem.*, **250**, 8293–8.
13 Huber, R., Scholze, H., Paques, E. P., and Deisenhofer, J. (1980). Crystal structure analysis and molecular model of human C3a anaphylatoxin. *Hope-Seyle's Z Physiol. Chem.*, **361**, 1389–99.

14 Nettesheim, D. G., Edalji, R. P., Mollison, K. W., Greer, J., and Zuiderweg, E. R. P. (1988). Secondary structure of complement component C3a anaphylatoxin in solution as determined by NMR spectroscopy: differences between crystal and solution conformations. *Proc. Natl. Acad. Sci. U.S.A.*, **85**, 5036–40.

15 Muto, Y., Fukumoto, Y., and Arata, Y. (1987). Solution conformation of carboxy-terminal fragments of the third component of human complement C3: proton nuclear magnetic resonance study of C3a, desArg-C3a and C3a Arg[69]. *J. Biochem.*, **102**, 635–41.

16 Williamson, M. P. and Madison, V. S. (1990). Solution structure of the C5a anaphylatoxin using ^{1}H-NMR. *Biochemistry*, **29**, 2895–990.

17 Hugli, T. E., Gerard, C., Kawahara, M., Scheetz, M. E., Barton, R., Brigs, S., Koppel, G., and Russel, S. (1981). Isolation of three separate anaphylatoxins from complement-activated human serum. *Mol. Cell Biochem.*, **41**, 59–66.

18 Greer, J. (1986). Comparative structural anatomy of the complement anaphylatoxin proteins C3a, C4a, and C5a. *Enzyme*, **36**, 150–63.

19 Hartung, H. P., Bitter-Suermann, D., and Hadding, U. (1983). Induction of thromboxane release from macrophages by anaphylatoxic peptide C3a of complement and synthetic hexapeptide C3a 72–77. *J. Immunol.* **130**, 1345–9.

20 Meuer, S., Ecker, U., Hadding, U., and Bitter-Suermann, D. (1981). Platelet-serotonin release by C3a and C5a two independent pathways of activation. *J. Immunol.* **126**, 1506–9.

21 Gerardy-Schahn, R., Ambrosius, D., Saunders, D., Casaretto, M., Mittler, C., Karwarth, G., Görgen, S., and Bitter-Suermann, D. (1989). Characterization of C3a receptor-proteins on guinea pig platelets and human polymorphonuclear leucocytes. *Eur. J. Immunol.*, **19**, 1095–102.

22 Berger, M., O'Shea, J., Cross, A. S., Folks, T. M., Chused, T. E., Brown, E. J., and Frank, M. M. (1984). Human neutrophils increase expression of C3bi as well as C3b receptors upon activation. *J. Clin. Invest.* **74**, 1566–71.

23 Hartung, H. P. and Hadding, U. (1983). Synthesis of complement by macrophages and modulation of their functions through complement activation. *Springer Semin. Immunopathol.* **6**, 283–326.

24 Ayesh, S. K., Ferne, M., Flechner, I., Babior, B., and Matzner, Y. (1990). Partial characterization of a C5a-inhibitor in peritoneal fluid. *J. Immunol.* **144**, 3066–70.

25 Zilow, G., Naser, W., Rutz, R., and Burger, R. (1989). Quantitation of the anaphylatoxin C3a in the presence of C3 by a novel sandwich ELISA using a monoclonal antibody to a C3a-neoepitope. *J. Immunol. Methods*, **121**, 261–8.

26 Hugli, T. E. and Chenoweth, D. E. (1980). Biologically active peptides of complement: techniques and significance of C3a and C5a measurements. In *Future perspectives in clinical laboratory immunoassays* (ed. R. M. Nakamura), pp. 443–59. Alan R. Liss, New York.

27 Lamche, H. R., Paul, E., Schlag, G., Redl, H., and Hammerschmidt, D. E. (1988). Development of a simple radioimmunoassay for human C3a. *Inflammation*, **12**, 265–77.

28 Burger, R., Bader, A., Kirschfink, M., Rother, U., Schrod, L., and Zilow, G. (1987). Functional analysis and quantification of the complement C3 derived anaphylatoxin C3a with a monoclonal antibody. *Clin. Exp. Immunol.*, **68**, 703–11.

29 Klos, A., Ihrig, V., Messner, M., Grabbe, J., and Bitter-Suermann, D. (1988). Detection of native human complement components C3 and C5 and their primary

activation peptides C3a and C5a (anaphylatoxic peptides) by ELISA's with monoclonal antibodies. *J. Immunol. Methods*, **111**, 241–52.

30 Schulze, M. and Götze, O. (1986). A sensitive ELISA for the quantitation of human C5a in blood plasma using a monoclonal antibody. *Complement*, **3**, 25–39.

31 Burger, R., Zilow, G., Bader, A., Friedlein, A., and Naser, W. (1988). The C-terminus of the anaphylatoxin C3a generated upon complement activation represents a neoantigenic determinant with diagnostic potential. *J. Immunol.*, **141**, 553–8.

32 Oppermann, M., Fuhrmann, A., Schulze, M., Werfel, T., and Götze, O. (1989). A monoclonal antibody with specificity for a C5a-neoepitope is an inhibitor of C5a-mediated biological functions and allows the quantitation of C5a in human EDTA-plasma. *Complement Inflamm.*, **6**, 382–3 (abstract).

33 Takeda, J., Kinoshita, T., Takata, Y., Kozono, H., Tanaka, E., Hong, K., and Inoue, K. (1987). Rapid and single measurement of human C5a-desArg level in plasma or serum using monoclonal antibodies. *J. Immunol. Methods*, **101**, 265–70.

34 Nilsson, B., Svensson, K. E., Inganäs, M., and Nilsson, U. R. (1988). A simplified assay for the detection of C3a in human plasma employing a monoclonal antibody raised against denatured C3. *J. Immunol. Methods*, **107**, 281–7.

35 Oppermann, M., Schulze, M., and Götze, O. (1991). A sensitive enzyme immunoassay for the quantitation of human C5a/C5a(desArg) anaphylatoxin using a monoclonal antibody with specificity for a neoepitope. *Complement Inflamm.*, **8**, 13–24.

36 Mollnes, T. E. (1989). Antigenic changes associated with complement activation. *Complement Inflamm.*, **6**, 133–41.

37 Gerardy-Schahn, R., Ambrosius, D., Casaretto, M., Grötzinger, J., Saunders, D., Wollmer, A., Brandenburg, D., and Bitter-Suermann, D. (1988). Design and biological activity of a new generation of synthetic C3a analogues by combination of peptidic and non-peptidic elements. *Biochem. J.*, **255**, 209–16.

38 Ambrosius, D., Casaretto, M., Gerady-Schahn, R., Saunders, D., Brandenburg, D., and Zahn, H. (1989). Peptide analogues of the anaphylatoxin C3a; synthesis and properties. *Hoppe-Seyler's Z. Biol. Chem.*, **370**, 217–27.

39 Ember, J. A., Johansen, N. L., and Hugli, T. E. (1991). Designing synthetic superagonists of C3a anaphylatoxin. *Biochemistry*, **30**, 3603–12.

40 Köhl, J., Casaretto, M., Gier, M., Karwath, G., Gietz, C., Bautsch, W., Saunders, D., and Bitter-Suermann, D. (1990). Re-evaluation of the C3a active site using short synthetic C3a analogues. *Eur. J. Immunol.* **20**, 1463–8.

41 Caporale, L. H., Tippett, P. S., and Erickson, B. W. (1980). The active site of C3a anaphylatoxin. *J. Biol. Chem.*, **235**, 10758–63.

42 Gerard, N. P. and Gerard C. (1990). Construction and expression of a novel recombinant anaphylatoxin, C5a-N19, as a probe for the human C5a receptor. *Biochemistry*, **29**, 9274–81.

43 Peake, P., Szelke, M., Singleton, A, Sueiras-Diaz, J., and Lachmann, P. J. (1990). Peptide inhibitors of C3 breakdown. *Clin. Exp. Immunol.*, **79**, 454–8.

44 Inagi, R., Miyata, T., Maeda, K., Sugiyama, S., Miyama, A., and Nakashima, I. (1991). Fut-175 as a potent inhibitor of C5/C3 convertase activity for production of C5a and C3a. *Immunol. Lett.*, **27**, 49–52.

45 Issekutz, C. A., Roland, D. M., and Patrik, R. A. (1990). The effect of Fut-175 (Nafamstat Mesilate) on C3a, C4a, and C5a generation *in vitro* and inflammatory reactions *in vivo*. *Int. J. Immunopharmacol.*, **12**, 1–9.

46 Bohnsack, J. F., Mollison, K. W., Buko, A. M., Ashworth, J. C., and Hill, H. R. (1991). Group B streptococci inactivate complement component C5a by enzymic cleavage at the C-terminus. *Biochem. J.*, **273**, 635–40.

47 Morgan, E. L., Weigle, W. O., and Hugli, T. E. (1982). Anaphylatoxin-meditated regulation of the immune response. I. C3a-meditated suppression of human and murine humoral immune responses. *J. Exp. Med.*, **155**, 1412–26.

48 Weigle, W. O., Goodman, M. G., Morgan E. L., and Hugli, T. E. (1983). Regulation of immune response by components of the complement cascade and their activated fragments. *Springer Semin. Immunopathol.*, **6**, 173–94.

49 Böttger, E. C. and Bitter-Suermann, D. (1987). Complement and the regulation of humoral immune response. *Immunol. Today*, **8**, 261–4.

50 Kurimoto, Y., de Weck, A. L., and Dahinden, C. A. (1989). Interleukin-3-dependent mediator release in basophils triggered by C5a. *J. Exp. Med.*, **170**, 467–79.

51 Bischoff, S. C., de Weck, A. L., and Dahinden, C. A. (1990). Interleukin-3 and granulocyte/macrophage colony-stimulating factor render human basophils responsive to low concentrations of complement component C3a. *Proc. Natl. Acad. Sci. U.S.A.*, **87**, 6813–17.

52 Okusawa, S., Yancey, K. B., van der Meer, J. W. M., Endres, S., Lonnemann, G., Hefter, K., Frank, M. M., Burke, J. F., Dinarello, C. A., and Gelfand, J. A. (1988). C5a stimulates secretion of tumour necrosis factor from human mononuclear cells *in vitro*. *J. Exp. Med.*, **168**, 443–8.

53 Cavaillon, J. M., Fitting, C., and Haeffner-Cavaillon, N. (1990). Recombinant C5a enhances interleukin-1 and tumour necrosis factor release by lipopolysaccharide-stimulated monocytes and macrophages. *Eur. J. Immunol.*, **20**, 253–7.

54 Haeffner-Cavaillon, N., Cavaillon, J. M., Laude, M., and Kazatchkine, M. D. (1987). C3a (C3a-desArg) induces production and release of interleukin-1 by cultured human monocytes. *J. Immunol.*, **139**, 794–9.

55 Arend, W. P., Massoni, J. R., Niemann, M. A., and Giclas, P. C. (1989). Absence of induction of IL-1 production in human monocytes by complement fragments. *J. Immunol.*, **142**, 173–8.

56 Schindler, R., Gelfand, A. J., and Dinarello, C. A. (1990). Recombinant C5a stimulates transcription rather than translation of interleukin-1 (IL-1) and tumour necrosis factor: translational signal provided by lipopolysaccharide or IL-1 itself. *Blood*, **76**, 1631–8.

57 Scholz, W., McClurg, M. R., Cardenas, G. J., Smith, M., Noonan, D. J., Hugli, T. E., and Morgan, E. L. (1990). C5a-mediated release of interleukin-6 by human monocytes. *Clin. Immunol. Immunopathol.*, **57**, 297–307.

58 Gerard, N. P., Hodges, M. K., Drazen, J. M., Weller, P. F., and Gerard, C. (1989). Characterization of a receptor for C5a anaphylatoxins on human eosinophils. *J. Biol. Chem.*, **264**, 1760–6.

59 Gerard, N. P. and Gerard, C. (1991). The chemotactic receptor for human C5a anaphylatoxin. *Nature*, **349**, 614–17.

60 Fukuoka, Y. and Hugli, T. E. (1988). (1988). Demonstration of a specific C3a receptor on guinea pig platelets. *J. Immunol.*, **140**, 3496–501.

61 Huey, R. and Hugli, T. E. (1985). Characterization of a C5a receptor on human polymorphonuclear leucocytes (PMN). *J. Immunol.*, **135**, 2063–8.

62 Rollins, T. E. and Springer, M. S. (1985). Identification of the polymorphonuclear leucocyte C5a receptor. *J. Biol. Chem.*, **260**, 7157–60.

63 Rollins, T. E., Siciliano, S., and Springer, M. (1988). Solubilization of the functional C5a receptor from human polymorphonuclear leucocytes. *J. Biol. Chem.*, **263**, 520–6.

64a Rollins, T. E., Siciliano, S., Kobayashi, S., Cianciarulo, D. N., Bonilla-Argudo, V., Collier, K., and Springer, M. S. (1991). Purification of the active C5a receptor from human polymorphonuclear leucocytes as a receptor-Gi complex. *Proc. Natl. Acad. Sc. U.S.A.*, **88**, 971–75.

64b Boulay, F., Mery, L., Tardif, M., Brouchon, L., and Vignais, P. (1990). Expression cloning of a receptor for C5a anaphylatoxin on differentiated HL-60 Cells. *Biochemistry*, **30**, 2993–9.

65 Fukuoka, Y. and Hugli, T. E. (1990). Anaphylatoxin binding and degradation by rat peritoneal mast cells—mechanims of degranulation and control. *J. Immunol.*, **145**, 1851–8.

66 Bitter-Suermann, D. and Burger, R. (1986). Guinea pigs deficient in C2, C4, C3, or the C3a receptor. *Prog. Allergy*, **39**, 134–58.

67 Mandecki, W., Mollison, K. W., Bolling, T. J., Carter, G. W., and Fox, J. L. (1985). Chemical synthesis of a gene encoding the human complement fragment C5a and its expression in *Escherichia coli*. *Proc. Natl. Acad. Sci. U.S.A.*, **82**, 3543–7.

68 Fukuoka, Y., Yasui, A., and Tachibana, T. (1991). Active recombinant C3a of human anaphylatoxin produced in *Escherichia coli*. *Biochem. Biophys. Res. Commun.*, **175**, 1131–8.

69 Mollison, K. W., Mandecki, W., Zuiderwed, E. P. R., Fayer, L., Fey, T. A., Krause, R. A., Conway, R. G., Miller, L., Edalji, R. P., Shallcross, M. A., Lane. B., Fox, L. J., Greer, J., and Carter, G. W. (1989). Identification of receptor-binding residues in the inflammatory complement protein C5a by site-directed mutagenesis. *Proc. Natl. Acad. Sci. U.S.A.*, **86**, 292–6.

70 Kaplow, L. S. and Goffinet, J. A. (1968). Profound neutropaenia during the early phase of haemodialysis. *JAMA*, **203**, 1135–40.

71 Craddock, P. R., Fehr, J., Brigham, K. L., Kronenberg, R. S., and Jacob, H. S. (1977). Complement and leucocyte-mediated pulmonary dysfunction in haemodialysis. *N. Engl. J. Med.*, **296**, 769–74.

72 Craddock, P. R., Fehr, J., Dalmasso, A. P., Brigham, K. L., and Jacob, H. S. (1977). Haemodialysis leukopaenia. Pulmonary vascular leukostasis resulting from complement activation by dialyser cellophane membranes. *J. Clin. Invest.*, **59**, 879–88.

73 Hammerschmidt, D. E., Harris, P. D., Wayland, H., Craddock, P. R., and Jacob, H. S. (1981). Complement-induced granulocyte aggregation *in vivo*. *Am. J. Pathol.*, **102**, 146–50.

74 Craddock, P. R., Hammerschmidt, D., White, J. G., Dalmasso, A. P., and Jacob, H. S. (1977). Complement (C5a-)induced granulocyte aggregation *in vitro*: a possible mechanism of complement-mediated leukostasis and leukopaenia. *J. Clin. Invest.*, **60**, 260–4.

75 Chenoweth, D. E. (1986). Anaphylatoxin formation in extracorporeal circuits. *Complement*, **3**, 152–65.

76 Weiler, J. M., Gellhaus, M. A., Carter, J. G., Meng, R. L., Benson, P. M., Hottel, R. A., Schilling, K. B., Vegh, A. B., and Clarke, W. R. (1990). A prospective study of the risk of an immediate adverse reaction to protamine sulfate during cardiopulmonary bypass surgery. *J. Allergy Clin. Immunol.*, **85**, 713–19.

77 Tennenberg, S. D., Clardy, C. W., Bailey, W. W., and Solomkin, J. S. (1990). Complement activation and lung permeability during cardiopulmonary bypass. *Ann. Thorac Surg.*, **50**, 597–601.

78 Bengtsson, A. and Heideman, M. (1988). Anaphylatoxin formation in sepsis. *Arch. Surg.*, **123**, 645–9.

79 Heideman, M. and Hugli, T. E. (1984). Anaphylatoxin generation in multi-system organ failure. *J. Trauma*, **24**, 1038–43.

80 Heideman, M., Norder-Hansson, B., Bengtsson, A., and Rollnes, T. E. (1988). The terminal complement complexes and anaphylatoxins in septic and ischaemic patients. *Arch. Surg.*, **123**, 188–92.

81 Goris, R. J. A. (1987). The adult respiratory distress syndrome and multiple organ failure. *Intense Care*, **1**, 1–7.

82 Goris, R. J. A. (1990). Mediators of multiple organ failure. *Intensive Care Med.*, **16**, S193–6.

83 Goldstein, I. M., Cala, D., Radin, A., Kaplan, H. B., Horn, J., and Ranson, J. (1978). Evidence of complement catabolism in acute pancreatitis. *Am. J. Med. Sci.*, **275**, 257–64.

84 Horn, J. K., Ranson, J. H. C., Goldstein, I. M., Weissler, J., Curatola, D., and Taylor, R. (1980). Evidence of complement catabolism in experimental acute pancreatitis. *Am. J. Pathol.* **101**, 205–16.

85 Roxvall, L., Bengtsson, A., and Heideman, M. (1989). Anaphylatoxin generation in acute pancreatitis. *J. Surg. Res.*, **47**, 138–43.

86 Whicher, J. T., Baenes, M. P., Brown, A., *et al.* (1982). Complement activation and complement control proteins in acute pancreatitis. *Gut*, **23**, 944–50.

87 Hack, C. E., Nuijens, J. H., Felt-Bersma, R. J. F., Schrender, W. O., Eerenberg-Belmer, A. J. M., Paardekooper, J., Bronveld, W., and Thijs, L. G. (1989). Elevated plasma levels of the anaphylatoxins C3a and C4a are associated with a fatal outcome in sepsis. *Am. J. Med.*, **86**, 20–6.

88 Zilow, G., Joka, T., Rother, U., and Kirschfink, M. (1988). Anaphylatoxin generation in plasma and bronchoalveolar lavage fluid (BAL) in polytrauma patients. *Complement*, **5**, 200–8.

89 Zilow, G., Sturm, J. A., Rother, U., and Kirschfink, M. (1990). Complement activation and the prognostic value of C3a in patients at risk of adult respiratory distress syndrome. *Clin. Exp. Immunol.*, **79**, 151–7.

90 Hosea, S., Brown, E., Hammer, C., and Frank, M. (1980). Role of complement activation in a model of adult respiratory distress syndrome. *J. Clin. Invest.*, **66**, 375–82.

91 Jacob, H. S. (1980). Complement-induced vascular leukostasis—its role in tissue injury. *Arch. Pathol. Lab. Med.*, **104**, 617–20.

92 Slotman, G. J., Burchard, K. W., Yelling, S. A., and Williams, J. J. (1986). Prostaglandin and complement interaction in clinical acute respiratory failure. *Arch. Surg.*, **121**, 271–4.

93 Solomkin, J. S., Cotta, L. A., Satoh, P. S., Hurst, J. M., and Nelson, R. D. (1985). Complement activation and clearance in acute illness and injury: evidence for C5a as a cell-directed mediator of ARDS in man. *Surgery*, **97**, 668–78.

94 Hack, C. E., Nuijens, J. H., Strack van Schijndel, R. J. M., Abbink, J. J., Eerenberg, A. J. M., and Thijs, L. G. (1990). A model for the interplay of inflammatory mediators in sepsis—a study in 48 patients. *Intensive Care Med.*, **16**, 187–92.

95 Robbins, P. A., Russ, W. D., Rasmussen, J. K., and Clayton, M. M. (1987). Activation of the complement system in the adult respiratory distress syndrome. *Am. Rev. Respir. Dis.*, **135**, 651–8.

96 Gardinali, M., Cicardi, M., Frangi, D., Bergamaschini, L., Gallazzi, M., Gattinoni, L., and Agostoni, A., (1985). Studies of the complement activation in ARDS patients treated by long-term extracorporeal CO_2 removal. *Int. J. Artif. Organs*, **8**, 135–40.

97 Chenoweth D. E. and Hugli T. E. (1978). Demonstration of specific C5a receptor on intact human polymorphonuclear leucocytes. *Proc. Natl. Acad. Sci. U.S.A.*, **75**, 3943–7.

98 Mollnes, T. E., Videm, V., Götze, O., Harboe, M., and Oppermann, M. (1991). Formatation of C5a during cardiopulmonary bypass: inhibition by pre-coating with heparin. *Ann. Thorac. Surg.*, **52**, 92–7.

99 Zilow, G., Joka, T., Obertacke, U., Rother, U., and Kirschfink, M. (1992). Generation of anaphylatoxin C3a in plasma and bronchoalveolar lavage in trauma patients at risk of adult respiratory distress syndrome. *Critical Care Med.*, **20**, 468–73.

100 Lee, C. T., Fein, A. M., Lippmannm, M., Holtzman, H., Kimbel, P., and Weinbaum, G. (1981). Elastolytic activity in pulmonary lavage fluid from patients with adult respiratory distress syndrome. *N. Engl. J. Med.*, **304**, 192–6.

101 McGuire, W. W., Spragg, R. G., and Cohen, A. B. (1982). Studies on the pathogenesis of the adult respiratory distress syndrome. *J. Clin. Invest.*, **69**, 543–53.

102 Roxvall, L., Bengtsson, A. W., and Heideman, M. (1990). Anaphylatoxins and terminal complement complexes in pancreatitis. *Arch. Surg.*, **125**, 918–21.

103 Bengtsson, A., Larsson, M., Gammer, W., and Heideman, M. (1987). Anaphylatoxin release in association with methylmethacrylate fixation of hip protheses. *J. Bone. Jt. Surg.*, **69**, 46–9.

104 Bengtsson, A. and Lisander, B. (1990). Anaphylatoxin and terminal complement complexes in red cell salvage. *Acta Anaesthesiol. Scand.*, **34**, 339–41.

105 Hartung, H. P., Schwenke, C., Bitter-Suermann, D., and Toyka, K. V. (1987). Guillain–Barre syndrome: activated complement components C3a and C5a in CSF. *Neurology*, **37**, 1007–9.

106 Zilow, G., Burger, R., Naser, W., and Kleine, T. (1989). Indication for activation of the complement system in CSF during inflammation or haemorrhages of the CNS. *J. Clin. Chem. Clin. Biochem.*, **27**, 929–30.

107 Zilow, G., Burger, R., and Kleine, T. O. (1991). Aktivierung des Komplement-systems in Liquor cerebrospinalis bei verschiedenen Erkrankungen des Zentral-nervensystems. *Lab. Med.*, **15**, 95–8.

108 Kadurugamuwa, J. L., Hengstler, B., Bray, M. A., and Zak, O. (1989). Inhibition of complement factor C5a-induced inflammatory reactions by prostaglandin E_2 in experimental meningitis. *J. Infect. Dis.*, **160**, 715–9.

109 Fantone, J. C., Kunkel, S. L., and Zurier, R. B. (1985). Effects of prosta-glandins on *in vitro* immune and inflammatory reactions. In *Prostaglandins and immunity* (ed. J. S. Goodwin), pp. 123–46. Martinus Nijhoff, Boston.

110 Moxley, G. and Ruddy, S. (1985). Elevated C3a anaphylatoxin levels in syn-ovial fluids from patients with rheumatoid arthritis. *Arthritis Rheum.*, **28**, 1089–95.

111 Jose, P. J., Moss, I. K., Maini, R. N., and Williams, T. J. (1990). Measurement of the chemotactic complement fragment C5a in rheumatoid synovial fluids by

radioimmunoassay: role of C5a in the acute inflammatory phase. *Ann. Rheum. Dis.*, **49**, 747–52.

112 Lambert, P. H., Nydegger, U. E., Perrin, L. H., McCormick, J., Fehr, K., and Miescher, P. A. (1975). Complement activation in seropositive and seronegative rheumatoid arthritis. In *Rheumatology* Vol. 6 (ed. J. Rotstein), pp. 52–9. S. Karger, Basel.

113 Zvaifler, N. J. (1969). Breakdown products of C3 in human synovial fluids. *J. Clin. Invest.*, **48**, 1532–42.

114 Hunder, G. G., McDuffie, F. C., and Clark, R. J. (1979). Consumption of C3 via the classical and alternative complement pathway by sera and synovial fluids from patients with rheumatoid arthritis. *J. Clin. Lab. Immunol.*, **2**, 269–73.

115 Berkowicz, A., Kappelgaard, E., Peterson, J., Nielson, H., Ingemann-Hansen, T., Halkjaer-Kristensen, J., and Sorensen, H. (1983). Complement C3c and C3d in plasma and synovial fluid in rheumatoid arthritis. *Acta Pathol. Microbiol. Immunol. Scand.*, **91**, 397–402.

116 Nydegger, U. E., Zubler, R. H., Gabay, R., Joliat, G., Karagevrekis, C., Lambert, P. H., and Miescher, P. A. (1977). Circulating complement breakdown products in patients with rheumatoid arthritis: correlation between plasma C3d, circulating immune complexes, and clinical activity. *J. Clin. Invest.*, **59**, 862–8.

117 Hedberg, H., Lundh, B., and Laurell, A. B. (1970). Studies of the third component of complement in synovial fluid from arthritic patients. *Clin. Exp. Immunol.*, **6**, 707–12.

118 Perricone, R., De Carolis, C., Moretti, C., Santuari, E., De Sanctis, G., and Fontana, L. (1990). Complement, complement activation, and anaphylatoxins in human ovarian follicular fluid. *Clin. Exp. Immunol.* **82**, 359–62.

119 Belmont, H. M., Hopkins, P., Edelson, H. S., Kaplan, H. B., Ludewig, R., Weissmann, G., and Abramson, S. (1986). Complement activation during systemic lupus erythematosus: C3a and C5a anaphylatoxins circulate during exacerbations of disease. *Arthritis Rheum.*, **19**, 1085–9.

120 Falk, R. J., Dalmasso, A. P., Kim, Y., Lam, S., and Michael, A. (1985). Radioimmunoassay of the attack complex of complement in serum from patients with systemic lupus erythematosus. *N. Engl. J. Med.*, **312**, 1594–9.

121 Kerr, L. D., Adelsberg, B. R., Schulman, P., and Spiera, H. (1989). Factor B activation products in patients with systemic lupus erythematosus. A marker of severe disease activity. *Arthritis Rheum.*, **32**, 1406–13.

122 Valentijn, R. M., van Overhagen, H., Hazevret, H. M., Hermans, J., Cats, A., Daha, M. R., and van Es, L. A. (1985). The value of complement and immune complex determinations in monitoring disease activity in patients with systemic lupus erythematosus. *Arthritis Rheum.*, **28**, 904–13.

123 Hopkins, P., Belmont, H. M., Buyon, J., Philips, M., Weissmann, G., and Abramson, S. B. (1988). Increased levels of plasma anaphylatoxins in systemic lupus erythematosus predict flares of the disease and may elicit vascular injury in lupus cerebritis. *Arthritis Rheum.*, **31**, 632–41.

124 Wild, G., Watkins, J., Ward, A. M., Hughes, P., Hume, A., and Rowell, N. R. (1990). C4a anaphylatoxin levels as an indicator of disease activity in systemic lupus erythematosus. *Clin. Exp. Immunol.*, **80**, 167–70.

125 Haeger, M., Bengtson, A., Karlsson, K., and Heideman, M. (1989). Complement activation and anaphylatoxin (C3a and C5a) formation in pre-eclampsia and by amniotic fluid. *Obstet. Gynecol.*, **73**, 551–6.

126 Van der Linden, P. W. G., Hack, C. E., Kerckhaert, J. A. M., Struyvenberg, A., and van der Zwan, J. C. (1990). Preliminary report: complement activation in wasp-sting anaphylaxis. *Lancet*, **336**, 904–6.

127 Bengtsson, J. P., Backman, L., Stenqvist, O., Heideman, M., and Bengtsson, A. (1990). Complement activation and reinfusion of wound drainage blood. *Anaesthesiology*, **73**, 376–80.

128 Kretschmer, V., Söhngen, D., Göddecke, W., Kadar, J. G., Pelzer, H., Prinz, H., and Eckle, R. (1989). Biocompatibility and safety of cytapheresis. *Infusionstherapie*, **16**, 10–20.

129 Bengtsson, A. and Heideman, M. (1987). Anaphylatoxin formation in plasma and burn bullae fluid in the terminally injured patient. *Burns*, **13**, 185–9.

130 Mikawa, K, Ikegaki, J., Maekawa, N., Hoshina, H., Tanaka, O., Goto, R., Obara, H., and Kusunoki, M. (1990). Perioperative effect of methylprednisolone given during lung surgery on plasma concentrations of C3a and C5a. *Scand. J. Thor. Cardiovasc. Surg.*, **24**, 229–33.

131 Hallgren, R., Samuelsson, T., and Modig, J. (1987). Complement activation and increased alveolar-capillary permeability after major surgery and in adult respiratory distress syndrome. *Crit. Care Med.*, **15**, 189–93.

132 Thijs, L. G., Hack, C. E., Strack van Schijndel, R. J. M., Nuijens, J. H., Wolbink, G. J., Eerenberg-Belmer, A. M., van der Wall, H., and Wagstaff, J. (1990). Activation of the complement system during immunotherapy with recombinant IL-2. Relation to the development of side effects. *J. Immunol.*, **144**, 2419–24.

133 Smith, J. K., Chi, D. S., Krish, G., Reynolds, S., and Cambron, G. (1990). Effect of exercise on complement activity. *Ann. Allergy*, **65**, 304–10.

9 The terminal complement sequence in natural immunity

S. BHAKDI

1 Biochemistry of the terminal complement sequence

The proteins involved in the terminal complement sequence are C5 to C9 complement components; serum S protein *alias* vitronectin and serum protein SP40–40, also designated 'clusterin' which are believed to represent inactivators; and less well characterized cell membrane proteins including homologous restriction factor-20 (HRF-20) *alias* CD59, which appear to be responsible for minimizing complement-mediated lysis of homologous cells. Table 9.1 summarizes properties of these proteins (see also Table 5.1).

The terminal sequence is initiated when C5 is cleaved to C5a and C5b by a C5 convertase of either the classical or alternative pathway. With a few exceptions, activation of either pathway probably harbours similar or identical consequences as long as the degree of activation (C5 cleavage) is equivalent. Scission of C5 is the last proteolytic step in the complement sequence. All subsequent interactions involve tight, non-covalent associations of components with each other or with their inhibitors (Figure 9.1). These interactions are not disrupted by moderate concentrations of mild (non-denaturing) detergents such as deoxycholate, so that the complexed products can be detected on cells and in tissues, and also isolated as intact moieties (1, 2, 11).

Release of C5a anaphylatoxin constitutes an integral element of terminal sequence activation. The properties of this important mediator have been reviewed (12, 13) and are discussed in Chapter 8. C5a is chemotactic and activates phagocytes via binding to cell surface receptors.

C5b associates with C6 to form a binary complex that can reversibly attach to lipid bilayers. The half-life of C5b6 complexes is usually very short because C7 quickly binds to it, forming the C5b–7 complex. At this stage, the fate of terminal complexes is determined by the environment in which they are generated because conformational changes lead to exposure of hydrophobic domains on the trimolecular complex. If C5b–7 forms on a cell surface, it may spontaneously insert into the target bilayer. If a suitable lipid bilayer is not available for insertion, the C5b–7 complex will rapidly lose its ability for cellular interaction due to binding of C8, C9, and the serum inactivators S protein and SP40–40. The amphiphilic membrane complexes are endowed with pore-forming properties, whereas SC5b–9 represents its hydrophilic, inactive serum counterpart (Figure 9.2).

Table 9.1 Properties of terminal complement components

	Molecular weight	Chain structure	Sedimentation rate (S)	Serum concentration (μg/ml)	Electrophoretic mobility
C5	196 000	α, 116 000 β, 80 000	8.7	70–160	$\beta1$
C6	120 000	single	5.7	60–70	$\beta2$
C7	110 000	single	5.6	50–60	$\beta2$
C8	151 000	α, 64 000 β, 64 000 γ, 22 000	8.0	70–90	$\gamma1$
C9	71 000	single	4.5	60–70	α
Vn	75 000	single		150–200	α
SP40-40	80 000	α, 40 000 β, 40 000		150	α

Data from references 1–10.

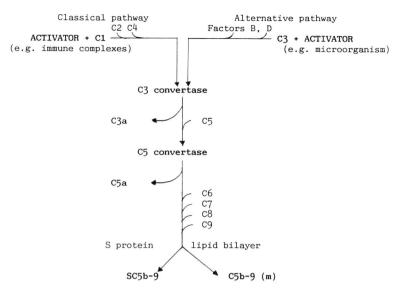

Fig. 9.1 Schematic representation of the complement activation pathways. See Figure 6.5 for antibody-independent activation of the classical pathway.

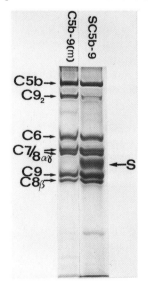

Fig. 9.2 SDS-PAGE of purified C5b–9(m) and SC5b–9. SP40–40 (clusterin) co-migrates with S protein (vitronectin).

The regulation of the terminal complement sequence takes place at two levels: (a) fluid-phase regulation by S protein (11, 14) and SP40–40 (10, 15) (see also Chapter 11), (b) regulation by cell associated components (16–20).

Originally, it was thought that vitronectin (S protein) bound to apolar regions of C5b-7, thus preventing the complex from attacking innocent bystander cells. However, more recent evidence indicates that conformational changes accompanying assembly of terminal complement complexes causes exposure of cryptic anionic sites that are contained in C7 to C9, and these associate with the heparin-binding domain of vitronectin (21). In line with this concept is the finding that proteolytic removal of vitronectin from SC5b-9 results in re-exposure of apolar domains (22). The mechanism via which SC5b-9 is rendered water soluble may therefore be more indirect. In this context, C5b-9 complexes generated on cell membranes also contain small amounts of vitronectin (23), a finding that would be explainable if the inactivators interacted with a charged domain of C5b-9 rather than with the membrane embedded, hydophobic region. In contrast to vitronectin, clusterin does contain a region that might directly interact with apolar regions in nascent terminal complexes (10).

It has long been known that homologous C5b-9 complexes are poorly haemolytic and cytotoxic, but the molecular basis for this phenomenon has only recently begun to be delineated. The best characterized and generally accepted cell associated regulatory protein is HRF-20 *alias* CD59 (17-20), which is present on blood and endothelial cells (24, 25). The protein appears to interact with C5b-8 and C5b-9 complexes to prevent insertion or pore formation by C8/C9 (26). The molecular mechanism for this is unknown, as is the basis for the species specificity of the reaction. Another 60 kDa erythrocyte and platelet protein purportedly endowed with homologous restriction activity has been described but not well characterized (16). In addition to these proteins, there may be other factors that contribute to homologous restriction which have as yet eluded discovery.

2   Properties and functions of membrane C5b-9 complexes

C5b-9 complexes forming on target membranes comprise a heterogeneous population of macromolecules each with a C5b-8 tetramer to which varying numbers of C9 molecules are bound. The structural formula of the membrane complex is thus $C5b-8_1C9_n$, whereby n apparently can range from 2-12 (11). Complex formation is paralleled by conformational changes in the C5-9 components, which in turn are reflected by changes in their antigenic properties. Novel epitopes, termed neoantigens, become exposed on the assembled macromolecules. Poly and monoclonal antibodies have been raised against such neoantigens and they can be used to detect and quantify the terminal complexes (27, 28). The molecular weight of C5b-9(m) complexes is in the range of $1-1.3 \times 10^6$. The complexes are amphiphilic and can only be extracted from membranes by the use of detergents, (e.g. deoxycholate). The complexes sediment in sucrose density gradients as a broad peak corresponding to 25–40S (11). Terminal complexes with high numbers of C9 molecules exhibit the structure of hollow cylinders, approximately 15 nm in height, containing a central channel of approximately 10 nm diameter (Figure 9.3). The cylinder is rimmed by an annulus at one end that projects into the aqueous phase. Approximately 5 nm of the opposite end carry the apolar domains that bind lipid and insert into the membrane (11, 29). C9 molecules

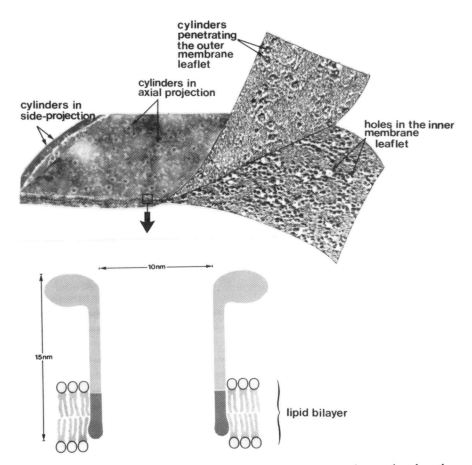

Fig. 9.3 *Top*: photomontage of electron micrographs of a complement-lysed erythrocyte membrane fragment using negative staining and freeze-fracture electron microscopy. Complement pores are seen in 'side' and 'axial' projections in the negatively stained specimen. The cylindrical structures are pulled out of the internal lipid monolayer during freeze-fracture and are seen in the outer membrane leaflet. Holes in the inner membrane leaflet can be seen in the complementary fracture face. *Bottom*: schematic presentation of a fully formed C5b–9(m) cylinder embedded in the lipid bilayer. For details, see references 11 and 29.

alone are able, under artificial conditions, to form cylindrical structures akin to C5b–9(m) complexes. It has been proposed that such 'poly-C9' aggregates also represent the dominating or even sole component of the pore-forming domain in C5b–9(m) (2). However, this view is an over-simplification. Since C6–8 all possess regions showing sequence homology to the putative intra-membrane domains of C9, it is likely that C6–8 could form the same type of structure as the C9 molecules in the genuine C5–9(m) complexes (30), compared with the poly-C9 aggregates.

Terminal complexes carrying low numbers of C9, although not visible as cylindrically structured entities in the electron microscope, can also form functional, albeit smaller, transmembrane pores (31). The question hence arises why terminal complexes containing multiple C9 molecules should have evolved in nature. One answer is that incorporation of multiple C9 molecules represents a pre-requisite for C5b–9(m) to exert bactericidal effects (32, 33). It would not be surprising if this mechanism should be found to extend to killing of protozoa and worms; the latter contention will easily be amenable to testing. C5b–9(m) pores form with high efficiency in artificial lipid bilayers and in membranes of highly susceptible cells. They have been shown to be 10–70 Å in diameter (depending on the number of C9 molecules contained in a complex), are filled with water, are essentially non-ion selective, and pore openings are generally irreversible. We have calculated that the binding of ten or fewer human C5b–9 complexes suffices to induce haemolysis of a guinea pig erythrocyte (unpublished data). Essentially, this implies that virtually every C5b–9 complex inserts to form a pore that is not repairable by these cells. The high intracellular osmotic pressure exerted by haemoglobin causes intracellular swelling, and haemolysis occurs when the membranes finally rupture. Genuine cell lysis can only be expected to occur when the intracellular osmotic pressure is exceptionally high, as in erythrocytes. In other cells, pore formation will be expected to cause cell swelling only. These cells will, of course, still die because they are unable to sustain the vitally important intracellular ionic milieu.

Not all cell-bound C5b–9 complexes necessarily form pores and cause cell death. Homologous restriction factors act to render cells relatively resistant to attack by C5b–9 of the same species. The molecular basis for the selective inhibition of homologous terminal complexes is an enigma. We have estimated that human erythrocytes can 'tolerate' deposition of 1000–2000 terminal complexes without undergoing lysis (unpublished data). However, it appears that sublytic amounts of C5b–9 cause small and perhaps transient ion fluxes that could have pathophysiological consequences for the attacked cells (34).

Further, independent of homologous restriction proteins, nucleated cells are able to repair a limited number of C5b–9 lesions, probably by endocytic uptake and exocytic shedding of afflicted membrane areas (35–37). Overall, therefore, death of nucleated cells may be a relatively rare event despite the deposition of terminal complexes *in vivo*.

Formation of transmembrane pores may be followed by diverse secondary reactions, a major trigger for which is probably the passive flux of calcium ions into the cells. Stimulation of arachidonate metabolism with release of lipid mediators has been observed in several cell systems. Depending on the localization and nature of such mediators, different pathophysiological effects may be elicited (38–40) (see Chapters 12 and 13).

Since Ca^{2+} is also a major trigger for secretory processes, it is not surprising that exocytotic liberation of vesicular components has been observed following the action of complement and other pore-formers on cells such as platelets and polymorphonuclear granulocytes. Secretion from platelets is accompanied by generation of pro-thrombinase activity, this in turn exerts a net pro-coagulatory effect (41) (see Chapter 10). It is not known whether this finding bears relevance *in vivo*; rabbits deficient in C6 display normal coagulation functions.

Finally, Ca^{2+} ions should cause activation of protein kinase C. Indeed, C5b–9 deposition appears to be accompanied by activation of this enzyme, and there are data to indicate that the latter process is important for cells to successfully repair complement lesions (42).

In summary, secondary reactions evoked by formation of complement pores in various cells may be complex and diverse. The above-mentioned processes represent some well documented examples, and there is an ongoing search for other sequelae that may be of biological relevance.

C5b–9(m) can kill a variety of Gram-negative organisms, probably by generating pores across the bacterial cell envelope (33, 43). This mechanism is directly relevant in human defence against pathogenic *Neisseria* and against some serum-sensitive Gram-negative rods. Pathogenic Gram-negative rods often display serum resistance, however (44). This may be due to expression of long polysaccharide chains in the LPS molecules that restrict diffusion of terminal complexes to the bacterial outer membrane (45, 46). In these cases, no bactericidal effects are noted despite massive complement activation on the bacterial cell surface, and terminal complexes are retrieved mainly in the form of inactive C5b–9 in the fluid-phase. A potentially promising therapeutic approach to overcome serum resistance is the use of a non-toxic peptide derived from polymyxin B, which apparently disorganizes LPS orientation in the outer membrane to render the bacteria susceptible to killing by C5b–9 (47). In addition to the direct microbicidal action of terminal complexes, there are indications that complement components augment intracellular killing of bacteria by phagocytes (48). This area merits future attention.

C5b–9 can also inactivate many enveloped viruses and kill a number of higher parasites including some forms of trypanosomes, schistosoma, cercariae, cestodes, and amoeba. The mechanisms responsible for cell death have not been studied in detail.

Finally, C5b–9(m) down-regulates complement activation by feed-back inhibition of C3 convertase formation via an unclarified mechanism (49).

This property may contribute towards preventing excessive complement activation on cell targets after effective deposition of C5b–9(m) has occurred.

3   Properties and functions of SC5b-9

Fluid-phase SC5b–9 is formed to a varying extent as a by-product during complement activation on target cells, and in larger amounts when activation takes place on non-lipid surfaces, (e.g. including polysaccharide and peptidoglycan layers surrounding serum-resistant Gram-negative bacteria and all Gram-positive organisms). SC5b–9 is also formed during complement activation in the fluid-phase, e.g. by soluble immune complexes or lectin molecules (Chapter 6) and zymosan. In the latter case, however, the efficiency of terminal complex formation relative to C3 cleavage can be particularly low (50). Hence, SC5b–9 concentrations ensuing through fluid-phase complement activation, (e.g. in diseases with complement-activating, soluble immune complexes or hereditary angio-oedema will tend to be low despite a marked turnover of C3. SC5b–9 is devoid of cytolytic potential. In addition to C5–9, it contains one to two molecules each of vitronectin and SP40–40. The molecular weight of SC5b–9 is approximately one million, and the sedimentation coefficient is approximately 23S (11). The fluid-phase complex does not present a distinct and characteristic ultrastructure visible in the electron microscope (22).

Biological functions of SC5b–9 have yet to be demonstrated. Of potential significance is its content of vitronectin. The latter is a multi-functional protein that interacts with cell surface receptors (integrins) via an RGD sequence, and with extracellular matrix molecules, thus promoting cell adhesion and spreading (51). Further, vitronectin interacts with thrombin/anti-thrombin III complexes to exert a pro-coagulatory effect in the presence of low heparin concentrations (52). The properties and function of vitronectin have been reviewed (14) and see also Chapter 11. Since SC5b–9 complexes also promote cell adhesion *in vitro* (53), deposition of this complex in tissues may affect local cell organization. The presence of vitronectin may also influence uptake and elimination of SC5b–9 in the reticuloendothelial system. A notable property of vitronectin bound to C5b–9 is its capacity to bind β-endorphin (54). The significance of this phenomenon is not known. The role of vitronectin in defence is discussed further in Chapter 11.

4   Antibody-independent pathways of terminal complement activation

4.1   Alternative pathway activation

This is the most obvious candidate for antibody-independent activation of the terminal sequence. The mechanisms and factors responsible for triggering alternative pathway activation have been reviewed (55, 56) (see also Chapter 4). The pathway is initiated by many cell wall constituents of bacteria, fungi, and higher parasites including lipopolysaccharide, yeast cell wall components (mannan, zymosan). Even certain viruses and virus-infected cells can activate the alternative pathway (57–60). In most cases, activation of the terminal sequence on bacteria and fungi leads to indirect rather than direct consequences. Most microbial activators are intrinsically resistant to C5b–9 because dense polysaccharide walls prevent diffusion of the terminal complexes to the plasma membrane. This is true of smooth, serum-resistant strains of enterobacteriacae as well as of all Gram-positive bacteria and fungi. However, generation of C5a serves to promote inflammation and recruit humoral and cellular defence components to the infected sites. SC5b–9 will be generated in quantities, and may serve hitherto undefined functions in cell organization and coagulation via interaction with vitronectin receptors.

In addition to microbial, fungal, and viral activator surfaces, the alternative pathway can be triggered by cholesterol-rich lipid particles that are present in atherosclerotic plaques (61). Complement activation at these sites may support inflammation, and generation of terminal complement complexes (Figure 9.4) may contribute to the progression of atherosclerotic lesions (61, 62). Furthermore, alternative pathway activation also occurs on certain tumour cells (63, 64), and it is conceivable that recruitment of the terminal sequence contributes to their removal.

4.2   Antibody-independent activation of C1

This may occur via interaction of C1 with the lipid A of bacterial lipopolysaccharides (65–67), lipoteichoic acids (68), mannan-binding protein (69–71), C-reactive protein (72, 73), bacterial outer membrane proteins (74), viruses (75, 76), and intracellular organelles (77–81). It has been reported that low levels of mannan-binding protein are found in approximately 5 per cent of newborns, and this may predispose them to infections (82) (see Chapter 6). Whether the terminal sequence is of importance in such cases is not known. A potentially important but generally neglected phenomenon relates to activation of C1 by cardiolipin (83, 84), which is present in mitochondria. This may be one underlying cause for complement activation occurring in necrotic tissues (85, 86). Evidence for a contributing role of complement activation to the development of reperfusion damage has indeed been obtained in experiments where a recombinant, soluble, CR1 truncate molecule was used to transiently abrogate complement activity in experimental animals (87).

4.3   Defect in regulatory membrane components

The complement system is in a dynamic state of equilibrium, activating processes being continually counterbalanced by inactivating mechanisms. Many

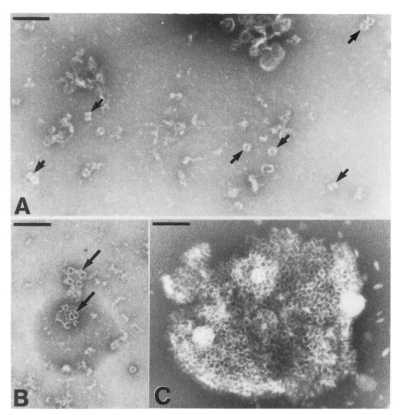

Fig. 9.4 Electron microscopic examination of C5b–9 complexes present in fractionated atherosclerotic lesion extract. (A) Negative staining of purified C5b–9 demonstrating many single copies of cylindrical complexes (*arrows*). (B) and (C). Bottom fractions from a sucrose density gradient containing many membrane fragments carrying C5b–9(m) complexes (*arrows*), sometimes in massive numbers (C). Scale bars indicate 100 nm. From (61).

of the latter take place at the level of the plasma cell membrane surface. Any defect in the membrane regulatory function may permit spontaneous deposition of complement components to occur. An extensively studied model is paroxysmal nocturnal haemoglobinuria (PNH), where multiple defects of membrane proteins that are anchored to the lipid bilayer via inositolphosphate links have been found. Among these, the defect in decay accelerating factor (DAF) appears to allow spontaneous formation of C3 convertases that ultimately trigger the terminal sequence and can lead to haemolysis (88, 89). PNH erythrocytes are particularly vulnerable to attack by C5b–9, apparently because they also lack one or several proteins that are involved in homologous restriction (19, 20). Deposition of C5b–9 on these erythrocytes is responsible for the haemolytic episodes in PNH patients, whereby the cause of the paroxysmal nature of the attacks remains an enigma. C5b–9 deposition on platelets may contribute to the pathogenesis of thrombocytopenia and thrombotic complications in these patients. The defect in PNH may also be due to a less stable lipid membrane.

Sialic acid on cell surfaces serves an anti-complementary function by promoting inactivation of C3b (90, 91). The presence of large amounts of sialic acid prevents effective alternative pathway activation and could represent a significant mechanism contributing to the pathogenesis of important infectious diseases in newborns, in particular by K1 *E.coli* and group B *Streptococci* (92).

4.4   Reactive lysis

This term has been used to designate the bystander attack of cells by C5b–9 without participation of early components (93) (up to and including C3). Reactive lysis is initiated when complement activation occurs in a C7 deficient environment. The ensuing C5b–6 complexes are stable and can attach to innocent bystander cells. If these subsequently come into contact with C7 to C9, potentially cytotoxic C5b–9 complexes are formed. Reactive lysis has hitherto only been observed *in vitro*. However, massive complement activation on artificial membranes in oxygenators (94, 95) (see also Chapter 8) appears to lead to bystander deposition of C5b–9 complexes on blood cells (95). The latter findings are significant in that they indicate that bystander attack of innocent cells is in principle possible *in vivo* (Figure 9.5). Probably, the major requirement will be that complement activation occurs in a relatively C7 deficient environment, and that cells bearing C5b–6 later acquire contact with C7 to C9.

5   Terminal complement sequence in natural immunity and summary

The possible role of the terminal complement sequence in natural immunity should be considered in several contexts. The first and most obvious relates to the part it may take in host defence against invading micro-organisms and viruses. The second pertains to its possible relevance in mediating or supporting removal of tumour cells, cell debris, and unwanted particles such as deposited cholesterol-rich lipid.

That antibody-independent activation of the terminal sequence is relevant to host defence against several infectious agents, in particular meningococci, becomes evident from several considerations. Most importantly, congenital deficiencies of properdin and factor D are associated with a high incidence of meningococcal disease, and, to a lesser extent, with infections with Gram-negative rods (*H. influenzae*, *Enterobacteriaceae*, and *Pseudomonas*) (96–105).

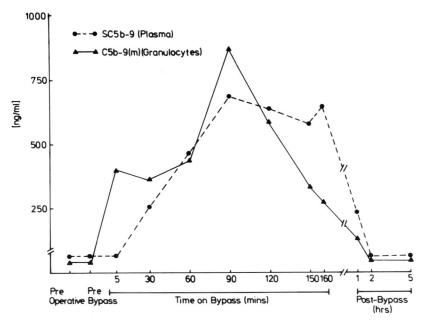

Fig. 9.5   SC5b–9 in EDTA plasma and levels of granulocyte-associated C5b–9 in a patient during cardiopulmonary bypass. One hundred microlitres of detergent extracts from 10^7 granulocytes were used in each determination; the peak value of leucocyte-associated C5b–9 observed at 90 min on bypass was equivalent to approximately 4500 C5b–9 complexes per cell. From (95). •– – –• SC5b–9 (plasma); ▲ ———— ▲ C5b–9(m) (granulocytes).

The same infectious diseases are frequently observed in individuals with congenital deficiencies in one of the terminal complement components. It is noteworthy that recurrent meningococcal infections represent a hallmark of late component, but not of properdin or factor D deficiencies (105). This could in part be explained by the fact that appearance of specific antibodies would confer resistance upon the latter individuals (but, of course, not those deficient in C5–C9). Support for this contention derives from studies in which active immunization of properdin deficient subjects led to correction of the bactericidal effect (106, 107). Together, these findings thus indicate that infectious diseases associated with defects in the alternative pathway are in fact due to failure of the immune system to recruit the terminal complement sequence.

Two further observations are worthy of note (105). Firstly, C5 deficient patients show the same disease susceptibility as do patients with deficiencies in C6–C9. Somewhat surprisingly, the additional inability to generate C5a thus does not appear to have significant consequences *in vivo* which may be due to C3a acting as an anaphylatoxin in the absence of C5a and other compounds, e.g. leukotriene B_4 (see Chapter 12) acting as a chemotactic factor. Second, the course of meningococcal diseases in C5–C9 deficient individuals tends to run a more benign course compared to infections in normal or properdin deficient individuals. The possibility that this may be due to a lower degree of endotoxin release from meningococci occurring in the absence of C5b–9 assembly on the bacteria has been discussed (105).

Although the significance of antibody-independent recruitment of the terminal sequence appears substantiated in the case of meningococcal infections, there are indications that this pathway can be qualitatively inferior to antibody-dependent activation in other instances. Thus, gonococci, although not innately resistant to the bactericidal effects of C5b–9, are apparently not killed when terminal complexes are generated via the alternative pathway, but die when activation occurs via binding of specific antibodies (108). Further, antibodies to certain surface antigens of gonococci appear to activate complement, but without exerting lethal effects. Together, these findings have been interpreted to suggest that certain (protective) antibodies may promote antibody-dependent bactericidal activity by directing C5b–9 complexes to 'correct' sites on the bacterial outer membrane (109–113). Indirect evidence that such susceptible sites exist derive from experiments in *Salmonella*, where fusion of liposomes carrying C5b–9 complexes with the bacterial outer membrane failed to result in cell death. Presumably, the terminal complexes 'planted' by membrane fusion were not deposited at the right sites (114).

With regard to infection with higher parasites, some of these infectious agents may rely on C3b inactivating (degradation) mechanisms to escape attack by C5b–9. For example, epimastigotes of *T. cruzi* are killed by C5b–9 following alternative pathway activation in non-immune sera. However, the trypomastigotes (which occur in humans) escape killing by expressing a surface glycoprotein that down-regulates C3 convertase activity (115, 116). Failure to mount a C5b–9 parasiticidal response may thus be directly related to establishment of infection in this case.

There is also some evidence that newborns with low levels of mannose-binding protein suffer more frequently from infections (82). This may be due mainly to reduced serum opsonization capacity, but an additional causative role of defective C5b–9 formation is also conceivable.

In addition to its role in host defence against infections, antibody-independent activation of the terminal complement sequence may be important in less well documented circumstances. Certain tumour cells spontaneously activate the alternative complement pathway, so that C5b–9 formation may represent an elimination mechanism of these cells. Complement activation on cell debris and cholesterol-rich lipid particles could provide an early and sustained stimulus for inflammatory reactions in necrotic tissues and atherosclerotic lesions, and promote uptake of unwanted particles via opsonization. The formation of foam cells and progression of atherosclerotic lesions may actually represent a pathological situation occurring because

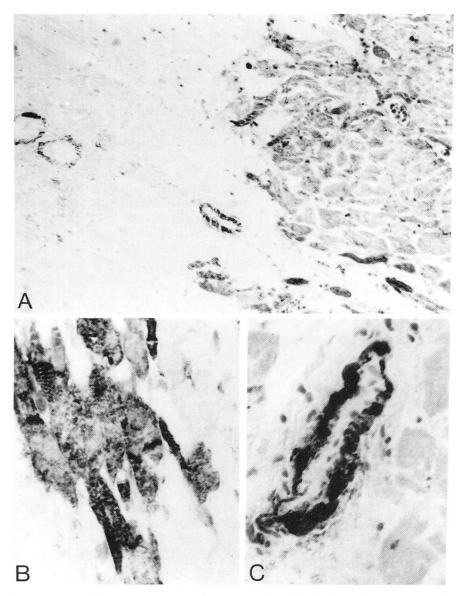

Fig. 9.6 A–C. Immunocytochemical demonstration of C5b–9 complement complex in a myocardial infarction. Frozen section from a 10 hour old myocardial infarction from autopsy material were stained with a polyclonal against C5b–9. Distinct staining of arterial walls and of areas with myocardial infarction are negative in normal myocardium. (**A**) Clear demonstration of infarcted areas even at low magnification (140 ×). (**B**) Intense cytoplasmic staining of whole necrotic cells (345 ×). (**C**) Staining of subendothelial layers in arterial walls is seen also in non-infarcted regions (345 ×). From (86).

phagocytes are unable to cope with and digest the excess of lipid that they have ingested.

It is intriguing to speculate on the possible significance of proteineous membrane inhibitors of the terminal sequence. Whatever their number and nature, these cell-bound molecules collectively act to prevent C5b–9 from successfully attacking autologous cells. The pathological situations occurring in PNH patients appears to demonstrate that these inhibitory mechanisms are important. Failure of a cell to sustain the inactivating mechanisms may result in spontaneous generation of pore-forming C5b–9 complexes. It is quite conceivable that such spontaneous attack continuously takes place as cells age or when they are dying. Should this prove true, terminal sequence activation would thus actively contribute to removal of non-functional cells. In myocardial infarctions, C5b–9 has occasionally been observed to be present on the plasma membrane of myocytes (86; Figure 9.6). In the context of immune defence against viral infections, lack of HRF on enveloped viruses that have acquired host membrane lipids (but not proteins) would render these particles vulnerable to C5b–9 attack.

In addition to protein inhibitors of C5b–9, several studies have presented evidence that intact phospholipid metabolism is required for nucleated cells to sustain optimal recovery mechanisms against C5b–9 attack (117–119). The potential significance of intact membrane phospholipid turnover also relates to the possibility that metabolic defects could become relevant in the context of elimination of diseased or dying cells.

Finally, the potentially important functions of SC5b–9 should not be neglected. These complexes mediate cell–matrix interaction, and it is quite possible that they can affect cell organization in normal and diseased tissues. SC5b–9 accumulates in an age-dependent manner in arterial walls (Figure 9.6), and it is also found in the connective matrices of renal vessels under many pathological circumstances (120, 121). These observations underline the need to consider antibody-independent activation of the terminal sequence not only in the well known context of host defence, but also in the context of tissue physiology and cell turnover. Antibody-independent activation of the terminal sequence may also emerge as a significant contributor to a variety of immunopathological reactions.

Acknowledgements

Studies conducted in the author's laboratory were supported by the Deutsche Forschungsgemeinschaft and the Verband der Chemischen Industrie. I thank Jørgen Tranum-Jensen for kindly preparing Figure 9.3, and Monika O' Malley for outstanding secretarial assistance.

References

1   DiScipio, R. G. (1987). Late-acting components of complement: their molecular biochemistry, role in the host defence, and involvement in pathology. *Pathol. Immunopathol. Res.*, **6**, 343–70.

2   Müller-Eberhard, H. J. (1988). Molecular organization and function of the complement system. *Annu. Rev. Biochem.*, **57**, 321–47.

3   DiScipio, R. G., Chakravarti, D. N., Müller-Eberhard, H. J., and Fey, G. H. (1988). The structure of human complement component C7 and C5b–7 complex. *J. Biol. Chem.*, **263**, 549–60.

4   Haefliger, J. A., Tschopp, J., Nardelli, D., Wahli, W., Kocher, H. P., Tosi, M., and Stanley, K. K. (1987). cDNA cloning of complement C8 beta and its sequence homology to C9. *Biochemistry*, **26**, 3551–6.

5   Howard, O. M. Z., Rao, A. G., and Sodetz, J. M. (1987). Complementary DNA and derived amino acid sequence of the beta subunit of human complement C8: identification of a close structural and ancestral relationship to the alpha subunit and C9. *Biochemistry*, **26**, 3565–70.

6   Stanley, K. K., Kocher, H. P., Luzio, J. P., Jackson, P., and Tschopp, J. (1985). The sequence and topology of human complement component C9. *EMBO J.*, **4**, 375–82.

7   DiScipio, R. G. and Hugli, T. E. (1989). The molecular architecture of human complement component C6. *J. Biol. Chem.*, **264**, 16197–206.

8   Jenne, D. and Stanley, K. K. (1985). Molecular cloning of S protein, a link between complement, coagulation, and cell-substrate adhesion. *EMBO J.*, **4**, 3153–7.

9   Kirzbaum, L., Sharpe, J. A., Murphy, B., d'Apice, A. J. F., Classon, B., Hudson, P., and Walker, I. D. (1990). Molecular cloning and characterization of the novel, human complement-associated protein, SP40–40: a link between the complement and reproductive systems. *EMBO J.*, **8**, 711–18.

10 Jenne, D. E. and Tschopp, J. (1989). Molecular structure and functional characterization of a human complement cytolysis inhibitor found in blood and seminal plasma: identity to sulfated glycoprotein 2, a constituent of rat testis fluid. *Proc. Natl. Acad. Sci. U.S.A.*, **86**, 7123–7.

11 Bhakdi, S. and Tranum-Jensen, J. (1987). Damage to mammalian cells by proteins that form transmembrane pores. *Rev. Physiol. Biochem. Pharmacol.*, **107**, 147–223.

12 Hügli, T. and Müller-Eberhard, H. J. (1978). Anaphylatoxins: C3a and C5a. *Adv. Immunol.*, **26**, 1–55.

13 Chenoweth, D. E. and Hugli, T. E. (1978). Demonstration of specific C5a receptor on intact human polymorphonuclear leucocytes. *Proc. Natl. Acad. Sci. U.S.A.*, **75**, 3943–7.

14 Preissner, K. T. (1989). The role of vitronectin as multi-functional regulator in the haemostatic and immune systems. *Blut*, **59**, 419–31.

15 Murphy, B. F., Kirszbaum, L. Walker, I. D., and d'Apice, J. F. (1988). SP40–40, a newly identified normal human serum protein found in the SC5b–9 complex of complement and in the immune deposits in glomerulonephritis. *J. Clin. Invest.*, **81**, 1858–64.

16 Schönermark, S., Rauterberg, E. W., Shin, M. L., Löke, S., Roelcke, D., and Hänsch, G. M. (1986). Homologous species restriction in lysis of human erythrocytes: a membrane-derived protein with C8-binding capacity functions as an inhibitor. *J. Immunol.*, **136**, 1772–6.

17 Sugita, Y., Nakano, Y., and Tomita, M. (1988). Isolation from human erythro-cytes of a new membrane protein which inhibits the formation of complement transmembrane channels. *J. Biochem.*, **104**, 633–7.

18 Davies, A., Simmons, D. L., Hale, G., Harrison, R. A., Tighe, H., Lachmann, P. J., and Waldmann, H. (1989). CD59, an Ly-6-like protein expressed in human lymphoid cells, regulates the action of the complement membrane attack complex on homologous cells. *J. Exp. Med.*, **170**, 637–54.

19 Okada, N., Harada, R., Fujita, T., and Okada, H. (1989). A novel membrane glycoprotein capable of inhibiting membrane attack by homologous complement. *Internat. Immunol.*, **1**, 205–8.

20 Holguin, M. H., Frederick, L. R., Bernshaw, N. J., Wilcox, L. A., and Parker, C. J. (1989). Isolation and characterization of a membrane protein from normal human erythrocytes that inhibits reactive lysis of the erythrocytes of paroxysmal nocturnal haemoglobinuria. *J. Clin. Invest.*, **84**, 7–15.

21 Tschopp, J., Masson, D., Schafer, S., Peitsch, M., and Preissner, K. T. (1988). The heparin binding domain of S protein/vitronectin binds to complement components C7, C8, and C9 and perforin from cytolytic T cells and inhibits their lytic activities. *Biochemistry*, **27**, 4103–9.

22 Bhakdi, S., Bhakdi-Lehnen, B., and Tranum-Jensen, J. (1979). Proteolytic transformation of SC5b–9 into an amphiphilic macromolecule resembling the C5b–9 membrane attack complex of complement. *Immunology*, **37**, 901–12.

23 Bhakdi, S., Käflein, R., Halstensen, T. S., Hugo, F., Preissner, K. T., and Mollnes, T. E. (1988). Complement S protein (vitronectin) is associated with cytolytic membrane-bound C5b–9 complexes. *Clin. Exp. Immunol.*, **74**, 459–64.

24 Nose, M., Katoh, M., Okada, N., Kyogoku, M., and Okada, H. (1990). Tissue distribution of HRF-20, a novel factor preventing the membrane attack of homologous complement, and its predominant expression on endothelial cells *in vivo. Immunology*, **70**, 145–9.

25 Hideshima, T., Okada, N., and Okada, H. (1990). Expression of HRF-20, a regulatory molecule of complement activation, on peripheral blood mononuclear cells. *Immunoloqy*, **79**, 396–401.

26 Rollins, S. A. and Sims, P. J. (1990). The complement inhibitory activity of CD59 resides in its capacity to block incorporation of C9 into membrane C5b–9. *J. Immunol.*, **144**, 3478–83.

27 Mollnes, T. E., Lea, T., Froland, S. S., and Harboe, M. (1985). Quantification of the terminal complement complex in human plasma by an enzyme-linked immunosorbent assay based on monoclonal antibodies against a neoantigen of the complex. *Scand. Immunol.*, **22**, 197–202.

28 Hugo, F., Krämer, S., and Bhakdi, S. (1987). Sensitive ELISA for quantitating the terminal membrane C5b–9 and fluid-phase C5b–9 complex of human complement. *J. Immunol. Meth.*, **99**, 243–51.

29 Tranum-Jensen, J. and Bhakdi, S. (1983). Freeze-fracture ultrastructural analysis of the complement lesion. *J. Cell Biol.*, **97**, 618–26.

30 Peitsch, M. C., Amiguet, P., Guy, R., Brunner, J., Maizel, J. V., and Tschopp, J. (1990). Localization and molecular modelling of the membrane-inserted domain of the ninth component of human complement and perforin. *Mol. Immunol.*, **27**, 589–602.

31 Bhakdi, S. and Tranum-Jensen, J. (1986). C5b–9 assembly: average binding of one C9 molecule to C5b–8 without poly-C9 formation generates a stable transmembrane pore. *J. Immunol.*, **136**, 2999–3005.

32 Joiner, K. A., Schmetz, M. A., Sanders, M. E., Murray, T. G., Hammer, C. H., Dourmashkin, R. R., and Frank, M. M. (1985). Multimeric complement component C9 is necessary for killing *Escherichia coli* J5 by terminal attack complex C5b–9. *Proc. Natl. Acad. Sci. U.S.A.*, **82**, 4808–12.

33 Bhakdi, S., Kuller, G., Fromm, S., and Muhly, M. (1987). Formation of transmural complement pores in serum-sensitive *Escherichia coli*. *Infect. Immun.*, **55**, 206–10.

34 Halperin, J. A., Nicholson-Weller, A., Brugnara, C., and Tosteson, C. (1988). Complement induces a transient increase in membrane permeability in unlysed erythrocytes. *J. Clin. Invest.*, **82**, 594–600.

35 Koski, C. L., Ramm, L. E., Hammer, C. H., Mayer, M. M., and Shin, M. L. (1983). Cytolysis of nucleated cells by complement: cell death displays multihit characteristics. *Proc. Natl. Acad. Sci. U.S.A.*, **80**, 3816–20.

36 Campbell, A. K. and Morgan, B. P. (1985). Monoclonal antibodies demonstrate protection of polymorphonuclear leucocytes against complement attack. *Nature*, **317**, 164–6.

37 Carney, D. F., Hammer, C. H., and Shin, M. L. (1986). Elimination of terminal complement complexes in the plasma membrane of nucleated cells: influence of extracellular Ca^{2+}. *J. Immunol.*, **137**, 263–70.

38 Imigawa, D. K., Osifchin, N. E., Paznekas, W. A., Shin, M. L., and Mayer, M. M. (1983). Consequences of cell membrane attack by complement: release of arachidonate and formation of inflammatory derivatives. *Proc. Natl. Acad. Sci. U.S.A.*, **80**, 6647–51.

39 Hänsch, G. M., Seitz, M., Martinotti, G., Betz, M. M., Rauterberg, E. W., and Gemsa, D. (1984). Macrophages release arachidonic acid, prostaglandin E_2, and thromboxane in response to late complement components. *J. Immunol.*, **133**, 2145–50.

40 Seeger, W., Suttorp, N., Hellwig, A., and Bhakdi, S. (1986). Non-cytolytic terminal complement complexes may serve as calcium gates to elicit leukotriene B_4 generation in human polymorphonuclear leucocytes. *J. Immunol.*, **137**, 1286–91.

41 Wiedmer, T., Esmon, C. R., and Sims, P. J. (1986). On the mechanism by which complement proteins C5b–9 increase platelet pro-thrombinase activity. *J. Biol. Chem.*, **261**, 14587–92.

42 Carney, D. F., Lang, T. J., and Shin, M. L. (1990). Terminal complement complexes generate multiple signal messengers: protein kinase C but not cAMP is involved in rapid elimination of TCC from the surface of Ehrlich cells. *J. Immunol.*, **145**, 623–9.

43 Wright, S. D. and Levine, R. P. (1981). How complement kills *E. coli* I. Location of the lethal lesion. *J. Immunol.*, **127**, 1146–51.

44 Roantree, R. and Rantz, L. (1960). A study of the relationship between the normal bactericidal activity of human serum to bacterial infection. *J. Clin. Invest.*, **39**, 72–81.

45 Joiner, K. A. (1985). Studies on the mechanism of bacterial resistance to complement-mediated killing and on the mechanism of action of bactericidal antibody. *Curr. Top. Microbiol. Immunol.*, **121**, 99–133.

46 Joiner, K. A., Grossman, N., Schmetz, M., and Leive, L. (1986). C3 bind preferentially to long-chain lipopolysaccharide during alternative pathway activation by *Salmonella montevideo*. *J. Immunol.*, **136**, 710–15.

47 Vaara, M. and Vaara, T. (1983). Sensitization of Gram-negative bacteria to antibiotics and complement by a non-toxic oligopeptide. *Nature*, **303**, 526–8.

48 Tedesco, F., Rottini, G., Roncelli, L., Basaglia, M., Menegazzi, R., and Patriarca, P. (1981). Modulating effect of the late-acting components of the complement system on the bactericidal activity of human polymorphonuclear leucocytes on *E. coli* 0111:B4. *J. Immunol.*, **127**, 1910–15.

49 Bhakdi, S., Maillet, F., Muhly, M., and Kazatchkine, M. D. (1988). The cytolytic C5b–9 complement complex: feedback inhibition of complement activation. *Proc. Natl. Acad. Sci. U.S.A.*, **85**, 1912–16.

50 Bhakdi, S., Fassbender, W., Hugo, F., Berstecher, C., Malasit, P., and Kazatchkine, M. D. (1988). Relative inefficiency of terminal complement activation. *J. Immunol.*, **141**, 3117–22.

51 Pytela, R., Pierschbacher, M. D., and Ruoslahti, E. (1985). A 125/115 kDa cell surface receptor specific for vitronectin interacts with the arginine-glycine-aspartic acid adhesion sequence derived from fibronectin. *Proc. Natl. Acad. Sci. U.S.A.*, **82**, 5766–70.

52 Preissner, K. T. and Müller-Berghaus, G. (1987). Neutralization and binding of heparin by S protein/vitronectin in the inhibition of factor Xa by anti-thrombin III. *J. Biol. Chem.*, **262**, 12174–253.

53 Biesecker, G. (1990). The complement SC5b–9 complex mediates cell adhesion through a vitronectin receptor. *J. Immunol.*, **145**, 209–14.

54 Hildebrand, A., Preissner, K. T., Müller-Berghaus, G., and Teschemacher, H. (1989). A novel β-endorphin binding protein. *J. Biol. Chem.*, **264**, 15429–34.

55 Fearon, D. T. and Austen, K. F. (1980). Current concepts in immunology: the alternative pathway of complement—a system for host resistance to microbial infection. *N. Engl. J. Med.*, **303**, 259–63.

56 Kazatchkine, M. D. and Nydegger, U. E. (1982). The human alternative complement pathway. *Prog. Allergy*, **30**, 193–222.

57 Okada, H., Tanaka, H., and Okada, N. (1983). Cytolysis of Sendai virus infected guinea pig cells by homologous complement. *Immunology*, **49**, 29–35.

58 Ramos, O. F., Kai, C., Yefenof, E., and Klein, E. (1988). The elevated natural killer sensitivity of targets carrying surface-attached C3 fragments require the availability of the iC3b receptor (CR3) on the effectors. *J. Immunol.*, **140**, 1239–43.

59 Solder, B. M., Schultz, T. F., Hengster, P., Lower, J., Larcher, C., Bitterlich, G., Kurth, R., Wachter, H., and Dierich, M. P. (1989). HIV and HIV-infected cells differentially activate the human complement system independent of antibody. *Immunol. Lett.*, **22**, 135–45.

60 Kurakata, S., Ramos, O. F., Klein, G., and Klein, E. (1989). Lysis of P3HR-1 cells induced to enter the viral cycle by antibody-dependent and independent immunological mechanisms. *Cell Immunol.*, **123**, 134–47.

61 Seifert, P. S., Hugo, F., Tranum-Jensen, J., Zähringer, U., Muhly, M., and Bhakdi, S. (1990). Isolation and characterization of a complement activating lipid extracted from human atherosclerotic lesions. *J. Exp. Med.*, **172**, 547–57.

62 Seifert, P. S., Hugo, F., Hansson, G. K., and Bhakdi, S. (1989). Pre-lesional complement activation in experimental atherosclerosis. *Lab. Invest.*, **60**, 747–54.

63 Seya, T., Hara, T., Matsumoto, M., and Akedo, H. (1990). Quantitative analysis of membrane cofactor protein (MCP) of complement. High expression of MCP on human leukaemia cell lines, which is down-regulated during cell differentiation. *J. Immunol.*, **145**, 238–45.

64 Mold, C., Nemerow, G. R., Bradt, B. M., and Cooper, N. R. (1988). CR2 is a complement activator and the covalent binding site for C3 during alternative pathway activation by Raji cells. *J. Immunol.*, **140**, 1923–9.

65   Loos, M. (1982). Antibody-independent activation of C1, the first component of complement. *Ann. Immunol.*, (Institut Pasteur) **133C**, 165–79.

66   Cooper, N. R. (1985). The classical complement pathway: activation and regulation of the first complement component. *Adv. Immunol.*, **37**, 151–207.

67   Loos, M. (1990). The complement system and natural resistance to bacteria. In *Natural Resistance to Infection* (ed. C. Sorg). Gustav Fischer Verlag, Stuttgart, New York, pp. 111–35.

68   Loos, M., Clas, F., and Fischer, W. (1986). Interaction of purified lipoteichoic acid with the classical complement pathway. *Infect. Immun.* **53**, 595–9.

69   Kuhlman, M., Joiner, K., and Ezekowitz, R. A. B. (1989). The human mannose-binding protein functions as an opsonin. *J. Exp. Med.*, **169**, 1733–45.

70   Lu, J., Thiel, S., Wiedemann, H., Timpl, R., and Reid, K. B. M. (1990). Binding of the pentamer/hexamer forms of mannan-binding protein to zymosan activates the pro-enzyme $C1r_2C1s_2$ complex of the classical pathway of complement without involvement of C1q. *J. Immunol.*, **144**, 2287–94.

71   Ohta, M., Okada, M., Yamashina, I., and Kawasaki, T. (1990). The mechanism of carbohydrate mediated complement activation by the serum mannan-binding protein. *J. Biol. Chem.*, **265**, 1980–4.

72   Volonakis, J. E. and Kaplan, M. H. (1974). Interaction of C-reactive protein complexes with the complement system. *J. Immunol.*, **113**, 9–17.

73   Claus, D. R., Siegel, J., Petras, K., Osmand, A. P., and Gewurz, H. (1977). Interactions of C-reactive protein with the first component of human complement. *J. Immunol.*, **119**, 187–92.

74   Stemmer, F. and Loos, M. (1985). Evidence for direct binding of the first component of complement, C1, to outer membrane proteins from *Salmonella minnesota*. *Curr. Top. Microbiol. Immunol.*, **121**, 73–84.

75   Cooper, N. R., Jensen, F. C., Welsh, R. M., and Oldstone, M. B. A. (1976). Lysis of RNA tumour viruses by human serum: direct antibody-independent triggering of the classical complement pathway. *J. Exp. Med.*, **144**, 970–84.

76   Bartholomew, R. M., Esser, A. F., and Müller-Eberhard, H. J. (1978). Lysis of oncornaviruses by human serum: isolation of the viral complement (C1) receptor and identification as p15E. *J. Exp. Med.*, **147**, 844–53.

77   Pinckard, R. N., Olson, M. S., Kelley, R. E., DeHeer, D. H., Palmer, J. D., O'Rourke, R. A., and Goldfein, S. (1973). Antibody-independent activation of human C1 after interaction with heart subcellular membranes. *J. Immunol.*, **110**, 1376–82.

78   Pinckard, R. N., Olson, M. S., Giclas, P. C., Terry, R., Boyer, J. T., and O'Rourke, R. A. (1975). Consumption of classical complement components by heart subcellular membranes *in vitro* and in patients after acute myocardial infarction. *J. Clin. Invest.*, **56**, 740–50.

79   Giclas, P. C., Pinckard, R. N., and Olson, M. S. (1979). *In vitro* activation of complement by isolated human heart subcellular membranes. *J. Immunol.*, **122**, 146–51.

80   Storrs, S. B., Kolb, W. P., Pinckard, R. N., and Olson, M. S. (1981). Characterization of the binding of purified human C1q to heart mitochondrial membranes. *J. Biol. Chem.*, **256**, 10924–9.

81   Storrs, S. B., Kolb, W. P., and Olson, M. S. (1983). C1q binding and C1 activation by various isolated cellular membranes. *J. Immunol.*, **131**, 416–22.

82 Super, M., Thiel, S., Lu, J., Levinsky, R. J., and Turner, M. W. (1989). Association of low levels of mannan-binding protein with a common defect of opsonization. *Lancet*, **2**, 1236–9.

83 Kovacsovics, T., Tschopp, J., Kress, A., and Isliker, H. (1985). Antibody-independent activation of C1, the first component of complement, by cardiolipin. *J. Immunol.*, **135**, 2695–700.

84 Kovacsovics, T. J., Peitsch, M. C., Kress, A., and Isliker, H. (1987). Antibody-independent activation of C1. I. Differences in the mechanism of C1 activation by non-immune activators and by immune complexes: C1r-independent activation of C1s by cardiolipin vesicles. *J. Immunol.*, **138**, 1864–70.

85 Engel, A. G. and Biesecker, G. (1982). Complement activation in muscle fibre necrosis: demonstration of the membrane attack complex of complement in necrotic fibres. *Ann. Neurol.*, **12**, 289–96.

86 Schäfer, H., Mathey, D., Hugo, F., and Bhadki, S. (1986). Deposition of the terminal C5b–9 complement complex in infarcted areas of human myocardium. *J. Immunol.*, **137**, 1945–9.

87 Weisman, H. F., Bartow, T., Leppo, M. K., Marsh Jr, H. C., Carson, G. R., Concino, M. F., Boyle, M. P., Roux, K. H., Weisfeldt, M. L., and Fearon, D. T. (1990). Soluble human complement receptor type 1: *in vivo* inhibitor of complement suppressing post-ischaemic myocardial inflammation and necrosis. *Science*, **249**, 146–51.

88 Nicholson-Weller, A., March, J. P., Rosenfeld, S. I., and Austen, K. F. (1983). Affected erythrocytes of patients with paroxysmal nocturnal haemoglobinuria are deficient in the complement regulatory protein decay accelerating factor. *Proc. Natl. Acad. Sci. U.S.A.*, **80**, 5066–70.

89 Medof, M. E., Walter, E. I., Roberts, W. L., Haas, R., and Rosenberg, T. L. (1986). Decay accelerating factor of complement is anchored to cells by a C-terminal glycolipid. *Biochemistry*, **25**, 6740–7.

90 Fearon, D. T. (1978). Regulation by membrane sialic acid of β1H-dependent decay-dissolution of amplification C3 convertase of the alternative complement pathway. *Proc. Natl. Acad. Sci. U.S.A.*, **75**, 1971–5.

91 Kazatchine, M. D., Fearon, D. T., and Austen, K. F. (1979). Human alternative complement pathway: membrane-associated sialic acid regulates the competition between B and β1H for cell bound C3b. *J. Immunol.*, **122**, 75–81.

92 Edwards, M. S., Kasper, D. L., Jennings, H. J., Baker, C. J., and Nicholson-Weller, A. (1982). Capsular sialic acid prevents activation of the alternative complement pathway by type II, group B *streptococci*. *J. Immunol.*, **126**, 1275–87.

93 Thompson, R. A. and Lachmann, P. J. (1970). Reactive lysis: the complement-mediated lysis of unsensitized cells. I. The characterization of the indicator factor and its identification of C7. *J. Exp. Med.*, **131**, 629–43.

94 Fosse, E., Mollnes, T. E., and Ingvaldsen, B. (1987). Complement activation during major operations with or without cardiopulmonary bypass. *J. Thor. Cardiovasc. Surg.*, **93**, 860–6.

95 Salama, A., Hugo, F., Heinrich, D., Höge, R., Müller, R., Kiefel, V., Mueller-Eckhardt, C., and Bhakdi, S. (1988). Deposition of terminal C5b–9 complement complexes on erythrocytes and leucocytes during cardiopulmonary bypass. *N. Engl. J. Med.*, **318**, 408–13.

96 Sjöholm, A. G., Braconier, J. H., and Söderstrom, C. (1982). Properdin deficiency in a family with fulminant meningococcal infections. *Clin. Exp. Immunol.*, **50**, 291–7.

97   Söderstrom, C., Braconier, J. H., Danielsson, D., and Sjöholm, A. G. (1987). Bactericidal activity for *Neisseria meningitidis* in properdin-deficient sera. *J. Infect. Dis.*, **156**, 107–12.

98   Nielsen, H. E. and Koch, C. (1987). Congenital properdin deficiency and meningococcal infection. *Clin. Immunol. Immunopathol.*, **44**, 134–9.

99   Nielsen, H. E., Koch, C., Magnussen, P., and Lind, I. (1989). Complement deficiencies in selected groups of patients with meningococcal disease. *Scand. J. Infect. Dis.*, **21**, 389–96.

100 Nielsen, H. E., Koch, C., Mansa, B., Magnussen, P., and Bergmann, O. J. (1990). Complement and immunoglobulin studies in 15 cases of chronic meningococcaemia: properdin deficiency and hypoimmunoglobulinaemia. *Scand. J. Infect. Dis.*, **22**, 31–6.

101 Kluin-Nelemans, J. C., van Velzen-Blad, H., van Helden H. P. T., and Daha, M. R. (1984). Functional deficiency of complement factor D in a monozygous twin. *Clin. Exp. Immunol.*, **58**, 724–30.

102 Hiemstra, P. S., Langeler, E., Compier, B., Keepers, Y., Leijh, P. C., van den Barselaar, M. T., Overbosch, D., and Daha, M. R. (1989). Complete and partial deficiencies of complement factor D in a Dutch family. *J. Clin. Invest.*, **84**, 1957–61.

103 Söderstrom, C., Sjöholm, A. G., Svensson, R., and Ostenson, S. (1989). Another Swedish family with complete properdin deficiency: association with fulminant meningococcal disease in one male family member. *Scand. J. Infect. Dis.*, **21**, 259–65.

104 Schlesinger, M., Nave, Z., Levy, Y., Slater, P. E., and Fishelson, Z. (1990). Prevalence of hereditary properdin, C7, and C8 deficiencies in patients with meningococcal infections. *Clin. Exp. Immunol.*, **81**, 423–7.

105 Figueroa, J. E. and Densen, P. (1991). Infectious diseases associated with complement deficiencies. *Clin. Microbiol. Rev.*, **4**, 359–95.

106 Densen, P., Weiler, J. M., Griffiss, J. M., and Hoffmann, L. G. (1987). Familial properdin deficiency and fatal meningococcaemia: correction of the bactericidal defect by vaccination. *N. Engl. J. Med.*, **316**, 922–6.

107 Söderstrom, C., Braconier, J. H., Kähty, H., Sjöholm, A. G., and Thuresson, B. (1989). Immune response to tetravalent meningococcal vaccine: opsonic and bactericidal functions of normal and properdin deficient sera. *Eur. J. Clin. Microbiol. Infect. Dis.*, **8**, 220–4.

108 Rice, P. A. and Kasper, D. L. (1977). Characterization of gonococcal antigens responsible for induction of bactericidal antibody in disseminated infection. *J. Clin. Invest.*, **60**, 1149–58.

109 Rice, P. A. and Kasper, D. L. (1982). Characterization of serum resistance of *Neisseria gonorrhoeae* that disseminate. Roles of blocking antibody and gonococcal outer membrane. *J. Clin. Invest.*, **70**, 157–67.

110 Harriman, G. R., Podack, E. R., Braude, A. I., Corbeil, L. C., Esser, A. F., and Curd, J. G. (1982). Activation of complement by serum-resistant *Neisseria gonorrhoeae*. Assembly of the membrane attack complex without subsequent cell death. *J. Exp. Med.*, **156**, 1235–49.

111 Joiner, K. A., Warren, K. A., Brown, E. J., Swanson, J., and Frank, M. M. (1983). Studies on the mechanism of bacterial resistance to complement-mediated killing. IV. C5b–9 forms high molecular weight complexes with bacterial outer membrane constituents on serum-resistant but not serum-sensitive *Neisseria gonorrhoeae*. *J. Immunol.* **131**, 1443–51.

112 Joiner, K. A., Scales, R., Warren, K. A., Frank, M. M., and Rice, P. A. (1985). Mechanism of action of blocking immunoglobulin G for *Neisseria gonorrhoeae*. *J. Clin. Invest.*, **76**, 1765–72.

113 Rice, P. A., Vayo, H. E., Tam, M. R., and Blake, M. S. (1986). Immunoglobulin G antibodies directed against protein III block killing of serum-resistant *Neisseria gonorrhoeae* by immune serum. *J. Exp. Med.*, **164**, 1735–48.

114 Tomlinson, S., Taylor, P. W., and Luzio, J. P. (1990). Transfer of pre-formed terminal C5b–9 complement complexes into the outer membrane of viable Gram-negative bacteria: effect on viability and integrity. *Biochemistry*, **29**, 1852–60.

115 Joiner, K., Sher, A., Gaither, T., and Hammer, C. (1986). Evasion of alternative complement pathway by *Trypanosoma cruzi* results from inefficient binding of factor B. *Proc. Natl. Acad. Sci. U.S.A.*, **83**, 6593–7.

116 Joiner, K. A., Dias da Silva, W., Rimoldi, M. T., Hammer, C. H., Sher, A., and Kipnis, T. L. (1988). Biochemical characterization of a factor produced by trypomastigotes of *Trypanosoma cruzi* that accelerates the decay of complement C3 convertases. *J. Biol. Chem.*, **263**, 11327–35.

117 Schlager, S. I., Ohanian, S. H., and Borsos, T. (1978). Correlation between the ability of tumour cells to resist humoral immune attack and their ability to synthesize lipid. *J. Immunol.*, **120**, 463–71.

118 Ohanian, S. H. and Schlager, S. I. (1981). Humoral immune killing of nucleated cells: mechanisms of complement-mediated attack and target cell defence. *CRC Crit. Rev. Immun.*, **1**, 165–209.

119 Papadimitriou, J. C., Carney, D. F., and Shin, M. L. (1991). Inhibitors of membrane lipid metabolism enhance complement-mediated nucleated cell killing through distinct mechanisms. *Mol. Immunol.*, **28**, 803–9.

120 Falk, R. J., Podack, E., Dalmasso, A. P., and Jennette, J. C. (1987). Localization of S protein and its relationship to the membrane attack complex of complement in renal tissue. *Am. J. Pathol.*, **127**, 182–90.

121 Bariety, J., Hinglais, N., Bhakdi, S., Mandet, C., Bouchon, M., and Kazatchkine, M. D. (1989). Immunohistochemical study of complement S protein (vitronectin) in normal and diseased human kidneys; relationship to neoantigens of the C5b–9 terminal complex. *Clin. Exp. Immunol.*, **75**, 76–81.

10 Blood coagulation, inflammation, and defence

D. P. O' BRIEN AND J. H. McVEY

1 Introduction

Blood coagulation is a defence system that assists in maintaining the integrity of the mammalian circulation after blood vessel injury. In this process a series of enzymes and cofactors interact to produce a polymerized fibrin mesh at the wound site (1, 2). Apart from its role in maintaining the integrity of the vasculature a link also exists between blood coagulation, inflammation, and defence. It has been recognized for some years that fibrin deposition is a feature of many inflammatory reactions, including delayed-type hypersensitivity reactions (3), glomerular nephritis (4), allograft rejection (5), murine viral hepatitis (6), and rheumatoid arthritis (7). In addition, the disseminated intravascular coagulation observed in septic shock results from the induced expression of pro-coagulant stimuli by endotoxins (8, 9). A number of cell types are able to participate in the activation of the coagulation cascade, including monocytes (10), endothelial cells (11), and neoplastic cells (12). Inflammatory mediators stimulate the coagulation cascade by promoting the expression of pro-coagulant reaction complexes on the surface of activated monocytes and endothelial cells, and by down-regulating proteins involved in anti-coagulant pathways (9).

The process leading to clot formation is highly regulated. A series of zymogens are converted sequentially to serine proteases, which act in a co-ordinated amplification reaction to generate the enzyme thrombin, which causes soluble fibrinogen to clot. Thrombin not only proteolyses fibrinogen to form fibrin but also activates an anti-coagulant pathway. Two cell surface receptor proteins are pivotal in these reactions. These are tissue factor (TF), a receptor located on the surface of perivascular cells which initiates blood coagulation on contact with flowing blood, and thrombomodulin, an endothelial cell receptor that alters thrombin action from the pro- to an anti-coagulant pathway. Both these proteins are regulated by mediators of the inflammatory response. It is principally the effect of cytokines and endotoxin on the expression of these two receptor molecules which provides the link between blood coagulation and defence. This chapter will concentrate on the roles of these two receptor proteins in the pro- and anti-coagulant pathways, and the regulation of their cellular expression in response to inflammatory mediators.

2 The regulation of the blood coagulation cascade

2.1 The initiation of the blood coagulation cascade by tissue factor

Modern techniques of molecular biology and biochemistry have revolutionized understanding of blood coagulation and its regulation. The structural analysis of coagulation factors has been greatly enhanced by the isolation and characterization of cDNAs encoding the principal proteins of the cascade. It is now possible to study wild-type and recombinant coagulation factors, and to introduce specific sequence changes in functionally critical regions of these molecules by site-directed mutagenesis, in order to investigate the mechanics of this complex process. These developments have led to a fundamental reappraisal of the coagulation cascade, in particular of its initiation and regulation, over the last decade (13).

Formerly blood coagulation was seen as a unidirectional sequence of pro-enzyme conversions to serine proteases, each enzyme activating another in an amplifier cascade leading to the formation of fibrin (14, 15). The initiation of these events was thought to begin with factor XII and pre-kallikrein, based on *in vitro* studies. It is now widely accepted that FXII and pre-kallikrein do not play a physiological role in haemostasis, and that coagulation is initiated *in vivo* by the exposure of flowing blood to TF, a receptor expressed on the surface of many extravascular cells, but not normally expressed by cells in contact with the circulation. FVII, a zymogen for a protease, binds to this receptor and is very rapidly activated (Figure 10.1). FVIIa and TF form a potent catalytically active complex which converts zymogen FIX, a single chain glycoprotein, into the two chain active enzyme, FIXa. Since the TF–FVIIa complex is membrane-bound the activation of FIX takes place on a surface (Figure 10.2). This complex of a cofactor or receptor (in this case TF), a serine protease (FVIIa), and a substrate (FIX) assembled on a phospholipid surface for maximal catalysis, serves as a paradigm for several of the reaction complexes in the pro- and anti-coagulant pathways (1). The TF/FVIIa complex is also capable of directly converting FX to FXa in what may be an accessory pathway *in vivo*.

FIXa forms a catalytic complex with another cofactor, FVIIIa, a large (300 kDa) non-proteolytic multi-domain protein which itself requires prior activation by limited proteolysis. FVIIIa orientates the enzyme (FIXa) substrate (FX) complex for maximal catalysis on the phospholipid surface. Deficiency of FVIII causes a severe bleeding disorder in man (Haemophilia A) showing that this is probably the principal route to FXa generation *in vivo* (Figure 10.1). FXa activates FVII in a back-activation step, promoting further FIXa generation. FXa also forms a complex with FVa, a non-proteolytic cofactor homologous to FVIII, on a phospholipid surface, orienting pro-thrombin for efficient catalysis. The product of pro-thrombin activation by FXa is throm-

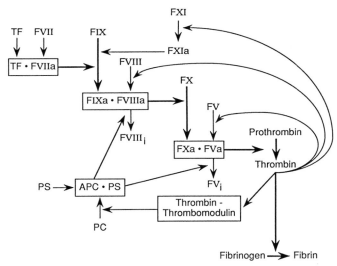

Fig. 10.1 Pathways of the blood coagulation cascade. TF forms a complex with FVII to initiate the coagulation cascade. Thrombomodulin binds to thrombin and initiates the anti-coagualant activated protein C pathway. *Boxed* reaction complexes assemble on phospholipid surfaces. FVIII$_i$ and FV$_i$ denote inactivated cofactors.

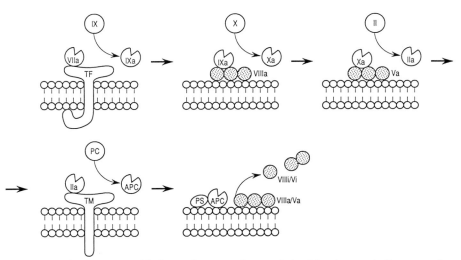

Fig. 10.2 Surface-assembled reaction complexes of the blood coagulation cascade. Several of the reaction complexes in blood coagulation assemble on phospholipid surfaces provided by endothelium, leucocytes, platelets, and extravascular tissues. The cofactors FV and FVIII are shown as lipid-bound multi-domain proteins which are inactivated by activated protein C through limited proteolysis. TM is thrombomodulin. II is pro-thrombin and IIa is thrombin.

bin, a multi-potent enzyme whose substrates include circulating fibrinogen which it cleaves to form an insoluble fibrin clot. Thrombin also proteolytically activates the pro-cofactors VIII and V in a positive feedback loop (16). Purified FXa is also capable of effecting these cleavages *in vitro*, but thrombin is the only enzyme that activates these cofactors in TF-activated human plasma (17). A second route to FIX activation is through the action of FXIa. Recently it has been shown that FXI can be activated by thrombin to FXIa (18) thus providing an explanation for the absence of abnormal bleeding in individuals totally deficient in FXII or pre-kallikrein. FXI is a homodimeric 160 kDa serine protease belonging to the trypsin superfamily of proteases and has sequence homology to the pro-enzyme pre-kallikrein. Once activated by thrombin, FXIa converts FIX to FIXa in the central reaction of the cascade (Figure 10.1). FXI deficiency is associated with a mild bleeding disorder in man (19) and it is therefore likely that FXI plays an accessory role in FIX activation *in vivo*, perhaps only called into play if there is severe injury.

Blood coagulation is not, therefore, a linear sequence of pro-enzyme conversions but rather, a series of interrelated phospholipid-bound reaction complexes comprising cofactors, enzymes, and substrates which are assembled on cell membranes, activated platelet surfaces, or leucocytes for maximal substrate catalysis leading to localized fibrin formation.

2.2   The initiation of the anti-coagulant pathway by thrombomodulin

A second receptor, thrombomodulin, is expressed on the surface of endothelial cells and platelets and plays a role in activating the anti-coagulant pathway in response to thrombin generation. Thrombomodulin binds to thrombin generated in the TF initiated coagulation cascade and, by an allosteric mechanism, alters its substrate specificity (20). The pro-coagulant substrates of thrombin, including FV, FVIII, and fibrinogen are no longer efficiently proteolysed once the thrombin–thrombomodulin complex is formed on endothelial cells. The substrate of this surface-bound catalytic complex is protein C, a zymogen which is proteolysed to activated protein C (APC) (21). This enzyme requires a cofactor, protein S, with which it forms a non-covalent complex capable of proteolytically inactivating the pro-coagulant cofactors FVa and FVIIIa. This is an important anti-coagulant pathway *in vivo* since protein C deficiency is associated with a thrombotic tendency in man (22). Catalytic concentrations of APC proteolyse specific peptide bonds in FV and FVIII, irreversibly inactivating them, thereby limiting the extent of coagulation (Figure 10.1). For full expression of anti-coagulant activity APC must bind to protein S, a non-proteolytic cofactor. All the reaction complexes of the anti- and pro-coagulant pathways assemble on membrane surfaces enabling the reactions to proceed at maximal rates in a localized fashion (Figure 10.2).

3   The structure and function of the TF/FVII complex

3.1   The structure of TF

The cloning of TF cDNAs was achieved by several groups simultaneously in 1987 (23–26). The predicted primary translation product is a 295 residue polypeptide which is processed to remove a secretory leader peptide of 32 residues. A hydrophilic extracellular domain extends from the mature N-terminus to residue 219. There follows a 23 residue hydrophobic sequence which represents the transmembrane spanning segment (Figure 10.3). A small cytoplasmic tail of 21 residues contains a cysteine which is acylated to palmitate or stearate on the inner leaflet of the membrane helping to anchor the receptor in the cell. Two disulfide-loops have been identified in the TF extracellular domain (27). An N-terminal loop is formed by Cys 49 and Cys 57. Mutation of these residues to serine in recombinant TF does not significantly impair receptor function, while the second loop formed by Cys 186 and Cys 209 has been shown to be essential for TF activity (28). The extracellular domain is glycosylated with predicted N-linked consensus sequences at position Thr 13 and Thr 126, however, the significance of this is unclear since *E. Coli*-derived, and therefore non-glycosylated recombinant TF is fully functional *in vitro* (29). There is little sequence identity between human TF and other receptors in currently available data-bases. Based on conservation of cysteine residues there appears to be homology with the cytokine receptors (28). Tissue factor acts as a cellular receptor for FVII

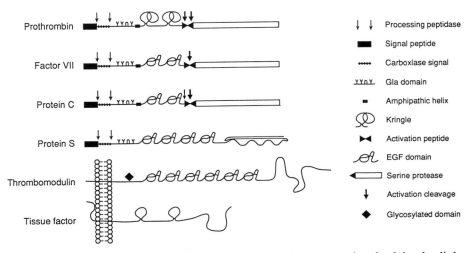

Fig. 10.3 Domain structures of the zymogens and receptors involved in the link between coagulation and defence. Modified from an original diagram by Furie and Furie 1988 (2).

and direct evidence of the binding of receptor and ligand came from affinity chromatography studies utilizing FVII coupled to a solid support which bound to, and purified, detergent solubilized TF (30). The expression of a mutant form of TF lacking the transmembrane and cytoplasmic domains demonstrated that the extracellular domain alone was sufficient for FVII/FVIIa binding (31). This mutant was secreted from transfected mammalian cells in culture and bound to FVIIa, greatly enhancing the enzyme's catalytic activity toward FX. These results indicated that the binding of TF to FVIIa has two consequences: (a) it localizes the activator complexes on the phospholipid surface, markedly increasing the local concentration of the reactants, and lowering the Km for FIX and FX activation, and (b) it alters the catalytic efficiency of the enzyme exposing recognition sites for the substrates FIX and FX.

3.2   The structure of FVII

FVII is synthesized in the liver as a single chain glycoprotein with a relative molecular mass of 50 kDa (Figure 10.3) (32). It is converted into an enzyme by proteolysis of a single peptide bond with the generation of a two chain disulphide-linked active species. Activated FVIIa has virtually no catalytic activity toward its substrates FX and FIX in the absence of TF. FVII is structurally and functionally related to FX, protein C, pro-thrombin, and FIX; they are all members of a family of proteases which require vitamin K-dependent post-translational γ-carboxylation of glutamic acid (Gla) residues in their N-terminal regions (33). These structural elements are called Gla-domains. The cluster of negative charge that results from this modification enables these proteins to bind calcium in a conformation-inducing process forming a membrane-binding module (34). The members of this family of vitamin K-dependent enzymes are secreted as single or two chain disulfide-linked pro-enzymes which are activated by limited proteolysis. The serine protease domains of these enzymes belong to the trypsin superfamily. The N-terminal light chain of FVII has ten γ-carboxylated glutamic acid residues in the Gla-domain, followed by a conserved amphipathic helical region and two domains with sequence homology to epidermal growth factor (EGF-like domains). These domains, which are found in a variety of proteins including the blood clotting proteases, bind calcium with high affinity, and are thought to be responsible for protein–protein interactions (2). The FVII light chain is disulfide-bridged to the C-terminal protease domain.

Currently an attempt is being made in several laboratories to identify the binding sites on FVII/FVIIa for TF. At least two distinct domains have been implicated: the Gla-domain may be required since the binding is calcium-dependent (35), and peptidyl inhibition studies have indicated that residues 40–50 are important for the interaction of receptor and ligand (36). There is also strong evidence for the interaction of the FVII protease domain with TF from peptide inhibition studies, which implicate residues 195–206 (37) and from a naturally occurring variant molecule which binds TF inefficiently and has a glutamine residue in place of an arginine residue at position 304 in the heavy chain (38).

3.3   The function of the FVIIa–TF complex

FVIIa must bind to TF in order to activate FIX and FX. It binds to the receptor in a 1:1 stoichiometric complex and is thought to undergo a conformational change that results in the creation of recognition sites for these substrates. This is referred to as an ordered addition, essential activation model in which neither FVIIa nor TF alone interact with FX or FIX (39). FVII and FVIIa bind to TF with equal affinity (13) and there are several schools of thought as to how the enzyme is initially activated. Originally it was thought that single chain FVII was not a true zymogen in that it had intrinsic enzymatic potential. This hypothesis was based on the observation that zymogen FVII reacted with DFP, an active site inhibitor (40). If the zymogen FVII had pro-coagulant activity it would follow that the initiation of coagulation would be effected by the breaking of the physical barrier that normally separates FVII from TF. Recent studies however, suggest that the single chain (zymogen) form of FVII does not bind to chloromethylketone active site fluoroprobes (41). In addition, oligonucleotide-directed mutagenesis was used to generate a mutant form of FVII, which could not be cleaved to the two chain enzyme. This uncleaved variant zymogen had no intrinsic activity, suggesting that FVII must be proteolytically activated to act as a catalyst (42). The proteolytic event which generates FVIIa *in vivo* is therefore not clear but it may be attributable to trace amounts of FXa normally present in plasma (43). Furthermore, trace amounts of FVIIa may circulate in plasma since the enzyme has an unusually long plasma half-life of approximately 2.5 hours (44) and is not inhibited by the serpins such as anti-thrombin III that inactivate other circulating proteases (45). It is clear however, that FVII is extremely sensitive to proteolysis when complexed with TF (46) and so trace quantities of circulating FXa in plasma could be sufficient to initiate the activation of FVII once TF and FVII have formed a complex. Thus, when TF is exposed to blood following vessel injury it forms a complex with plasma FVII which is rapidly activated and initiates the cascade through FIX activation. In this model it is clear that the expression of TF by cells in contact with the circulation, (i.e. endothelial cells and leucocytes), would be a strong procoagulant stimulus. As will be discussed later in this chapter the induction of TF on leucocyte and endothelial cell surfaces occurs following exposure of these cells to agonists associated with inflammation and defence and it is through this mechanism that the coagulation cascade and inflammation are connected.

4   The structure and function of the thrombomodulin/ thrombin complex

4.1   The structure of thrombomodulin

Thrombomodulin is a 105 kDa receptor on endothelial cells. cDNAs for human thrombomodulin have been isolated and sequenced (47). The structure of human thrombomodulin resembles the low density lipoprotein receptor. The amino-terminal portion of the molecule comprises an 18 residue hydrophobic secretory leader peptide which is removed from the protein by signal peptidase. The N-terminus of the mature protein contains sequences that are homologous to the lectin-like regions of other proteins such as the asialoglycoprotein receptor (48). The function of this domain is unclear but it is highly conserved in thrombomodulins from other species and would appear to be functionally important (49). C-terminal to this lectin-like domain is a region containing six epidermal growth factor-like domains (Figure 10.3). There are a number of cystine-bridges in these regions which impart structural stability to the molecule under extremes of pH and denaturants. Following the EGF-like repeats is a region of the molecule which is heterogeneous among the thrombomodulins of several species. This region contains a high proportion of serine and threonine residues which form sites for O-linked glycosylation in addition to the N-linked glycosylation sites at asparagine 115 and 420 in the extracellular domain of human thrombomodulin. C-terminal to the glycosylated domain is a putative transmembrane spanning segment which, like TF, has 23 hydrophobic residues. This region of thrombomodulin is highly conserved between species with 20 of 23 residues being identical in mouse and man. Highly conserved transmembrane domains are associated with intracellular signalling. The platelet-derived growth factor receptor has high species conservation in this region and has transmembrane signalling functions (50); in contrast the LDL receptor, which has poor conservation of this region, does not (51). The cytoplasmic tail of thrombomodulin contains several potential phosphorylation sites. Phosphorylation in cells has been shown to be associated with endocytosis and degradation of thrombomodulin (52).

The regions of the thrombomodulin molecule which are responsible for binding to thrombin and protein C been intensively studied. The three most C-terminal EGF-like domains (4, 5, and 6) contain the region responsible for thrombin binding and protein C activation. Thrombin binding has been localized to a peptide fragment generated by cyanogen bromide cleavage of rabbit thrombomodulin (53). This peptide, which consisted of the fifth and sixth EGF-like domains, bound thrombin but did not promote protein C activation. A fragment comprising the fourth, fifth and sixth EGF domains exhibited both activities (54). This region of the protein is crucial for function, since truncated recombinant thrombomodulin molecules lacking the N-terminal domain were fully functional with respect to thrombin binding and protein C activation (55).

4.2   The structure of thrombin

The zymogen for thrombin is pro-thrombin, another member of the vitamin K-dependent coagulation factor family. It circulates as a single chain glycoprotein with a relative mass of 71 kDa (56). The primary translation product has a pre-pro leader sequence from position −43 to −18 which is highly homologous to the pre-pro leader sequences of the other vitamin K-dependent γ-carboxylated proteins (Figure 10.3). This sequence has two functions: firstly the hydrophobic leader peptide targets the protein for secretion from the cell, and secondly the pro-sequence immediately C-terminal to this contains the γ-carboxylase recognition sequence which binds to a carboxylase in the liver, leading to the carboxylation of ten glutamic acid residues in the first 32 residues of the mature pro-thrombin N-terminus (57). Immediately following the Gla-domain is a short segment between residues 33–46 which has three highly conserved aromatic amino acids which organize the structure into an amphipathic helix. This region is connected by a disulfide-loop to two regions of internal homology called kringle structures. These domains of approximately 100 amino acids contain three disulfide-bonds and the folding of the kringle is defined by the close contact of sulfur atoms which form a cluster at the centre of the domain. Kringle structures are most probably involved in protein–protein interactions (58).

C-terminal to these structures is the protease domain which is released from the Gla-helix-kringle domains on activation of pro-thrombin to thrombin by the FXa-FVa complex on a phospholipid surface. Activation of pro-thrombin by FXa requires two cleavages, one at position Arg 284 releases the N-terminal heavy chain (known as fragment 1.2) and a second at position Arg 320 generates α-thrombin, the active enzyme. The enzyme therefore comprises a 36 residue A chain disulfide-linked to a 259 residue B chain (59). Thrombin is unique among the vitamin K-dependent proteases of blood coagulation in that the active enzyme does not retain the N terminal Gla-domain disulfide-liked to its C-terminal protease domain. Pro-thrombin activation leads to the release of the N-terminal portion of the molecule liberating a soluble non-surface associated enzyme. Thrombin binds to thrombomodulin through the B chain of the enzyme, since thrombin derivatives cleaved in this region do not bind the receptor efficiently (60). The sites on thrombin responsible for interactions with thrombomodulin are not clearly defined. The active site of the enzyme is not required for this binding, as thrombin with a blocked active site competes with the wild-type enzyme for thrombomodulin binding. Anti-peptide antibodies to thrombin amino acids 62–73 of the B chain inhibit the enzyme–receptor interaction (61).

4.3   The function of the thrombomodulin–thrombin complex

The concentration of thrombomodulin is highest in the micro-circulation since it is expressed on the surface of endothelial cells and it is here that the ratio of surface to volume is at its highest (62). Thrombin generated in the micro-circulation will be most readily complexed with thrombomodulin, depressing the pro-coagulant stimulus. In the micro-circulation therefore, thrombin may be regarded as an anti-coagulant. The formation of the thrombin–thrombomodulin complex has several anti-coagulant properties. The binding of thrombin to the receptor induces conformational changes in the enzyme (63) and may also sterically inhibit its action upon pro-coagulant substrates fibrinogen, FV, and FVIII (64). The preferred substrate becomes protein C which it activates through specific proteolysis (65). Protein C is another member of the vitamin K-dependent protease family which circulates as a disulfide-linked dimer and which is activated by the thrombin–thrombomodulin complex following cleavage at an arginyl peptide bond to release an activation peptide from the enzyme. The anti-coagulant effect of thrombomodulin is further enhanced by the fact that it accelerates the action of anti-thrombin III (ATIII), the serpin responsible for the covalent inactivation of several of the blood clotting proteases (66). Soluble thrombin normally binds to fibrinogen in plasma (see also Chapter 11), where it is protected from inactivation by ATIII, but thrombomodulin-complexed thrombin is readily inactivated by the serpin, in an additional anti-coagulant mechanism (67). The action of protein C is accelerated by protein S, a non-proteolytic Gla-domain containing protein cofactor (Figure 10.3) which serves to anchor the APC to the phospholipid surface, markedly reducing the Km for FV and FVIII inactivation by APC (68). This localization of the APC–protein S complex on the phospholipid surface serves to direct it to the pro-coagulant reaction complexes containing FVa and FVIIIa (Figure 10.2).

There are several levels of regulation of the pro-coagulant cascade. In the reaction complexes an enzyme combines with a cofactor on a surface and the formation of these complexes markedly alters the kinetics of substrate activation. The isolated proteases, such as FVIIa and FIXa, proteolyse their respective substrates very poorly hence the reactions are effectively limited to surfaces bearing the appropriate receptors or cofactors. Regulation of the pro-coagulant reaction complexes is also achieved through direct inactivation of these enzymes by specific serpins. Inactivation of the cofactors FV and FVIII depends on the generation of APC by thrombin–thrombomodulin complexes.

5 The regulated expression of TF

5.1 Tissue specific expression of tissue factor

Since contact of TF with blood is a major pro-coagulant stimulus, its expression in vessels must be strictly regulated to prevent activation of the cascade. TF is therefore, not normally expressed on the surface of cells within the vasculature. TF expression *in vivo* is highly cell type-specific (69). It is expressed on the surface of adventitial cells surrounding many blood vessels, on epithelial cells of the renal glomerulus, and is abundant in the outer pre-keratinized layers of the epidermis. TF is also prominent in other squamous epithelial cells and in myoepithelial layers which encapsulate many organs. The tissue distribution of TF can therefore be thought of as constituting a 'haemostatic envelope', not only around blood vessels, but encasing organ structures and the entire organism itself.

5.2   TF induction in response to inflammation and infection

TF expression by cells within the vasculature occurs in the process of inflammation and cellular immune responses (70). Two cell types within the vasculature, the monocyte and the endothelial cell, can be induced directly to express TF by a variety of agents including cytokines (71), lymphokines (72), and endotoxins (73–75) (Figure 10.4). The monocyte TF response however, is substantially augmented in the presence of T lymphocytes (76). Furthermore, in the cellular immune response, TF expression by monocytes can be induced by stimulated T helper cells. The mechanism of TF induction has been studied extensively *in vitro* using freshly isolated monocytes, monocyte cell lines (THP-1), and in primary cultures of endothelial cells.

Monocytes can be induced by endotoxins either directly, or indirectly, to express TF. Endotoxins are lipopolysaccharide (LPS) constituents of the outermost part of a Gram-negative bacterial cell membrane and are released upon bacterial lysis (77). LPS in the bloodstream rapidly binds to LPS-binding protein (LBP) (78); this complex then binds to CD14, its receptor on monocytes (79). Cellular responses to physiological concentrations of LPS are dependent on binding LBP and can be blocked by monoclonal antibodies to CD14. CD14 is a 55 kDa glycoprotein that is attached to the membrane via a phosphatidylinositiol glycan anchor (GPI). A number of GPI-linked proteins expressed on the surface of haemopoietic cells have been implicated in signal transduction (80). Exactly how GPI-linked molecules transduce activation signals is unclear. Binding of the LPS–LBP complex to CD14 results in signal transduction to the nucleus and TF gene transcription. Similarly, LPS induces TF expression on the surface of endothelial cells however, the cellular receptor for LPS on endothelial cells remains to be defined.

The induction of TF on the cell surface requires transcriptional initiation (81, 82). The initiation of transcription is a very rapid, transient response which does not require protein synthesis. TF mRNA is easily detectable in endothelial cells within 30 minutes, peaks by two hours, and has fallen to very low levels by 12 hours following stimulation with either LPS or the phorbol ester, phorbol 12-myristate 13-acetate (PMA), which is a potent activator of protein kinase C (83). Similar results have been described for TF induction in monocytes (84, 85). The isolation, characterization, and sequencing of the

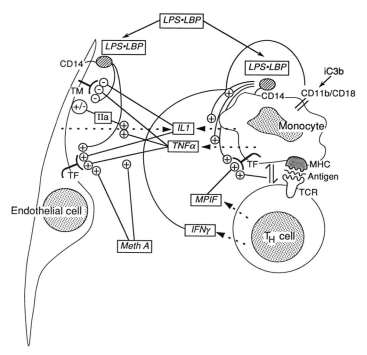

Fig. 10.4 Cellular interactions regulating coagulation in infection. The interaction of LPS with its receptor on monocytes, CD14, induces TF surface expression and synthesis and secretion of TNFα and IL-1. This response can be modulated by IFNγ or engagement of the integrin CD11b/CD18. TF expression can also be induced by T_H cells by direct cellular interaction or by the lymphokine MPIF. The interaction of LPS with its receptor on endothelial cells, which may be CD14, induces TF and represses thrombomodulin surface expression. This response can also be induced by IL-1 and TNFα. Further IL-1 is secreted by endothelial cells in response to TNFα, thrombin, and LPS. Furthermore, thrombin generated by the activation of coagulation will induce thrombomodulin gene transcription as well as thrombomodulin internalization in the absence of APC. MethA induces TF expression on endothelial cells and promotes the effect of TNFα.

TM, thrombomodulin; TF, tissue factor; LPS.LBP, lipopolysaccharide-lipopolysaccharide binding protein complex; MHC, major histocompatibility complex; TCR, T cell receptor; MPIF, monocyte pro-coagulant inducing factor; IL-1, interleukin-1; IFNγ, interferon-γ; TNFα, tumour necrosis factor-α; MethA, factor isolated from murine methylcholanthrene A-induced fibrosarcoma; +, positive stimulus inducing expression; −, negative stimulus causing down-regulation.

human TF gene has allowed studies on the control of TF gene expression to be initiated. Distinct intracellular signalling pathways, involving either protein kinase C (activated by LPS or PMA) or cyclic AMP-dependent protein kinases (activated by IL-1), appear to converge at the activation of the transcription factor NFκB (86, 87). This protein exists in the cytoplasm of unstimulated cells in an inactive state, complexed to a labile inhibitor called IκB. NFκB activation is postulated to occur through protein kinase-mediated phosphorylation of the labile IκB inhibitor, which dissociates from the NFκB complex, leaving it free to move to the nucleus (88). NFκB has also been implicated in the induction of TNFα and IL-6 by LPS in monocytes (see Chapters 3 and 4) (89, 90). LPS induction of TF in monocytes has been shown to involve a NFκB-type sequence, although other *cis*-acting sequences were found to modulate the response (91).

The increased steady state levels of TF mRNA observed upon stimulation with LPS cannot be completely accounted for by an increase in the rate of TF gene transcription. It has been shown in endothelial cells that the half-life of TF mRNA at one hour following stimulation with LPS (when levels of TF mRNA are increasing), is 12 times longer than at four hours (when levels of TF mRNA are decreasing) (83). This suggests an additional post-transcriptional control of TF mRNA stability by LPS. There are now a number of examples described in which control of cytoplasmic mRNA stability affects gene expression, however, the mechanisms which determine differential rates of mRNA degradation are poorly understood (92). This response does not require protein kinase C since depletion of protein kinase C by prolonged exposure to PMA, does not block TF induction by LPS. Similar results have now been reported in the monocyte following stimulation with LPS (28).

The effects of LPS upon monocytes, in addition to the induction of TF, include the synthesis and release of TNFα and IL-1 (93). TNFα can also induce TF expression as well as further IL-1 synthesis and secretion by endothelial cells (94). Furthermore, the IL-1 secreted by the monocyte in response to LPS, and presumably the IL-1 secreted by the endothelial cell in response to TNFα, will induce endothelial cells to express TF in an autocrine manner. Monocytes however, do not express TF in response to IL-1 or TNFα. Increased transcription of the TF gene is not a general consequence of monocyte activation since interferon-gamma (IFNγ) does not induce expression of TF. Cells exposed to IFNγ for 72 hours however, express four-fold higher levels of TNFα and IL-1 in response to LPS (95). Moreover, the expression of IL-1 is sustained over at least 16 hours instead of the more usual transient response. IFNγ may therefore serve to modulate the monocyte response, and the secreted IL-1 and TNFα may induce TF expression by the endothelium.

Monocytes can also be induced to express TF by two alternative indirect pathways which have an absolute requirement for T helper (T$_H$) cells (96). One pathway is mediated by a lymphokine, monocyte pro-coagulant inducing factor (MPIF), which is secreted by antigen-stimulated T$_H$ cells (97, 98). MPIF induces TF expression on monocytes but not on endothelial cells. The structure of MPIF remains to be established, however preliminary characterization has demonstrated that it is distinct from cyto/lymphokines described to date. A second pathway uses apparent contact collaboration between T_H cells and monocytes to induce TF expression (96, 99). The surface molecules involved in these cellular interactions remain to be defined.

Recently it has been shown that engagement of the integrin CD11b/CD18 on the surface of the monocyte results in a marked enhancement of TF expression by the monocyte in response to MPIF or LPS (100). Engagement of CD11b/CD18 alone did not elicit expression of TF. CD11b/CD18 is one of the three major integrins on the leucocyte cell surface, which functions as a receptor for iC3b, factor X, fibrinogen, and possibly LPS. Although CD11b/CD18 is not the effector molecule in the cell–cell collaboration between T_H and monocytes it may be important in enhancing the response of monocytes at sites of fibrin deposition, factor X generation, and in response to iC3b-coated micro-organisms.

5.3   TF expression in neoplasia

Neoplastic lesions have been associated with activation of the haemostatic system. Expression of pro-coagulants including TF, a factor X-activating enzyme, and expression of a surface which supports assembly of the pro-thrombinase complex constitute direct mechanisms by which malignant cells can promote fibrin formation. In addition, secretion of mediators such as IL-1 or IL-1-like molecules can promote activation of coagulation by interacting with endothelial cells, as described above. More recently a tumour-derived mediator (MethA) has been described, which induces TF expression and enhances the response of endothelial cells to TNFα (101). MethA appears to be distinct from other cytokines, such as TNFα, or IL-1, but may be related to vascular permeability factor or vascular endothelial growth factor (102, 103). MethA may be important in priming the vasculature within the tumour to respond with increased sensitivity to TNFα (see also Chapter 4). Activation of coagulation within vessels supplying the tumour will obstruct blood flow, thereby depriving the tumour of essential nutrients.

6   The expression of thrombomodulin in inflammation and infection

The unperturbed endothelium normally presents an anti-coagulant surface to flowing blood through the cell surface expression of thrombomodulin. Since TF is not expressed on the unstimulated endothelial cell surface any thrombin that is generated locally will complex with cell surface-bound thrombomodulin and activate protein C (APC), which by inactivation of factors VIIIa and Va, blocks further thrombin generation. Thrombomodulin under basal conditions has a half-life of 19 hours. However, thrombin can induce internalization of thrombin–thrombomodulin complexes with transport to the lysosomes, release and degradation of the bound thrombin, and return of thrombomodulin to the cell surface (104). Endocytosis is inhibited by protein C, but not by activated protein C, suggesting that the endocytosis will not occur until protein C activation is complete (105). Protein S, the cofactor for APC, is also synthesized by the endothelium. The complex interactions described above result in the expression of TF on the surface of either endothelial cell or monocytes in response to the various agonists (Figure 10.4). In addition, endothelium responds to TNFα, IL-1, and LPS by down-regulating cell surface expression of thrombomodulin (106–108).

Expression of thrombomodulin appears to be regulated by a variety of mechanisms: transcriptional, post-transcriptional, and internalization and degradation of the protein. The molecular mechanisms responsible for thrombomodulin down-regulation are however, controversial. Alterations in the rates of transcription and subsequent translation of thrombomodulin in response to TNFα were described by Conway and Rosenberg (109). It was therefore concluded by these authors that the down-regulation of thrombomodulin was under transcriptional control. In contrast, Scarpati and Sadler (110) reported a loss of thrombomodulin surface expression, with no change in the steady state levels of thrombomodulin mRNA in endothelial cells treated with TNFα implying a post-transcriptional mechanism of control of thrombomodulin expression in response to TNFα. A recent report however, shows a decrease in steady state levels of thrombomodulin mRNA in response to LPS, TNFα and IL-1 (111). In addition, Kapiotis *et al.* (111) demonstrate that IL-4, a product of activated T cells counteracted TNFα, IL-1, and LPS induced down-regulation of thrombomodulin in endothelial cells. IL-4 has been shown to possess anti-inflammatory activities by neutralizing LPS-induced monocyte production of IL-1, TNFα, and IL-8 (112, 113), and endothelial cell expression of the cellular adhesion molecules ICAM and ELAM (114, 115); TNFα induces a 50 per cent reduction in thrombomodulin activity at the endothelial cell surface within four hours, which is the result of endocytosis and lysosomal degradation of the receptor (116). IL-1 and LPS also cause decreased thrombomodulin activity on endothelial cell surfaces (107, 108). The mechanism of the reduction in response to these agonists is not known, but presumably involves increased endocytosis and degradation, as is seen with TNFα. The extent of this apparently unified response of the endothelium, the simultaneous and opposite regulation of TF and thrombomodulin, may however vary according to the agonist (117).

Comparison of results from the literature reporting the study of TF and thrombomodulin expression by endothelial cells is complicated by the variety of cell types, culture methods, and experimental protocols which have been used. The culture method, especially the presence or absence of heparin and growth factors (118, 119), the origin or passage number of cells (120), and their state of confluence (119, 121), can greatly influence the TF or thrombomodulin response in endothelial cells. Endothelial cell populations from different sites within the vasculature while sharing some characteristics, such as Class I major histocompatablity complex molecules may differ in other respects, such as organ-specific receptor expression (122). These organ-specific variations may reflect differences in function and result in alternative responses to various agonists (123). Despite these caveats, the induction of TF expression by both monocytes and endothelial cells, and the possible repression of thrombo-modulin expression by endothelial cells, is critical to the conversion of the vasculature from an anti-coagulant to a pro-coagulant state at sites of inflammation and infection *in vivo*. This activation of coagulation causes fibrin deposition and the resulting pathology.

7 Summary

Blood coagulation is initiated in response to vessel damage in order to preserve the integrity of the mammalian vascular system. Exposure of blood to extra-vascular tissues results in the formation of a complex between FVII and TF, which initiates the cascade of coagulation zymogen activations and leads to clot formation. The reaction complexes involved in this process form on phospholipid surfaces and comprise cofactors, enzymes, and substrates. Anti-coagulant pathways are initiated following the formation of a complex between thrombin and thrombomodulin which activates protein C.

The coagulation cascade can also be initiated by mediators of the in-flammatory response, and fibrin deposition has been noted in a variety of pathologic states including Gram-negative sepsis, glomerular nephritis, viral hepatitis, and cancer. Two proteins are pivotal in this process: TF, the cellular receptor that initiates the coagulation cascade, can be expressed on the surface of endothelial cells and monocytes in response to various inflamma-tory mediators. Thrombomodulin, the receptor responsible for the activation of the anti-coagulant protein C pathway in normal haemostasis, is down-regulated by the same inflammatory mediators under experimental conditions. The net effect of these events is to promote extra and intravascular coagula-tion, which may play a role in preventing the spread of infection throughout the tissues and vasculature.

References

1 Mann, K. G., Nesheim, M. E., Church, W., Haley, P., and Krishnaswamy, S. (1990). Surface-dependent reactions of the vitamin K-dependent enzyme com-plexes. *Blood*, **76**, 1–16.

2 Furie, B. and Furie, B. (1988). The molecular basis of blood coagulation. *Cell*, **53**, 505–18.

3 Colvin, R., Johnson, R., Mihm, M., and Dvorak H. (1973). Role of the clotting system in cell-mediated hypersensitivity. *J. Exp. Med.*, **138**, 686–9.

4 Vassalli, P. and McCluskey, R. (1971). The pathogenic role of the coagulation process in glomerular diseases of pathologic origin. *Adv. Nephrol.*, **1**, 47–63.

5 Lindquist, R., Gutterman, R., Merill, J., and Dammin, G. (1968). Human renal allografts. Interpretation of morphologic and immunohistochemical observations. *Am. J. Path.*, **53**, 851–82.

6 Levy, G. A., Leibowitz, J. L., and Edgington, T. S. (1981). Induction of monocyte pro-coagulant activity by murine hepatitis virus type 3 parallels disease susceptibility in mice. *J. Exp. Med.*, **154**, 1150–63.

7 Zwaifler, N. (1973). The immunopathology of joint inflammation in rheumatoid arthritis. *Adv. Immunol.*, **16**, 265–336.

8 Coalson, J., Benjamin, B., Archer, L., Beller, B., Gilliam, C., Taylor, F., and Hinshaw, L. (1978). Prolonged shock in the baboon subjected to infusion of *E. coli* endotoxin. *Circ. Shock*, **5**, 423–37.

9 Esmon, C., Taylor, F., and Snow, R. (1991). Inflammation and coagulation: linked processes potentially regulated through a common pathway by protein C. *Thromb. Haemostas.*, **66**, 160–5.

10 Lyberg, T. (1984). Clinical significance of increased thromboplastin activity on the monocyte surface — a brief review. *Haemostasis*, **14**, 430–9.

11 Galdal, K. (1984). Thromboplastin synthesis in endothelial cells. *Haemostasis*, **14**, 378–5.

12 Gordon, S., Franks, J., and Lewis, B. (1975). Cancer pro-coagulant A: a factor X-activating pro-coagulant from malignant tissue. *Thromb. Res.*, **6**, 127–37.

13 Nemerson, Y. (1988). Tissue factor and haemostasis. *Blood*, **71**, 1–8.

14 Davie, E. W. and Ratnoff, O. D. (1964). Waterfall sequence for intrinsic clotting. *Science*, **145**, 1310–12.

15 MacFarlane, R. (1964). Enzyme cascade in the blood clotting mechanism and its function as a biochemical amplifier. *Nature* (London), **202**, 498–9.

16 Eaton, D., Rodriguez, H., and Vehar, G. (1986). Proteolytic processing of human FVIII. Correlation of specific cleavages by thrombin, factor Xa, and activated protein C with activation and inactivation of FVIII coagulant activity. *Biochemistry*, **25**, 505–12.

17 Pieters, J., Lindhout, T., and Hemker, C. (1989). *In situ*-generated thrombin is the only enzyme that effectively activates FVIII and FV in thromboplastin activated plasma. *Blood*, **74**, 1021–4.

18 Naito, K. and Fujikawa, K. (1991). Activation of human blood coagulation factor XI independent of FXII. *J. Biol. Chem.*, **266**, 7353–58.

19 Asakai, R. and Chung, D. (1989). The molecular genetics of factor XI deficiency. In *The molecular biology of coagulation* (ed. E. G. D. Tuddenham), Baillieres Clinical Haematology, **2**, (4) 787–99. Ballière Tindall, London.

20 Dittman, W. and Majerus, P. (1990). Structure and function of thrombomodulin: a natural anti-coagulant. *Blood*, **75**, 329–36.

21 Stenflo, J. (1976). A new vitamin K-dependent protein. Purification from bovine plasma and preliminary characterization. *FEBS Lett.*, **101**, 377–81.

22 Seligsohn, U., Berger, A., Abend, M., Rubin, L., Attias, D., Zivelin, A., and Rapaport, S. (1984). Homozygous protein C deficiency manifested by massive venous thrombosis in the newborn. *N. Eng. J. Med.*, **310**, 559–62.

23 Fisher, K., Gorman, C., Vehar, G., O' Brien, D., and Lawn, R. (1987). Cloning and expression of human tissue factor cDNA. *Thromb. Res.*, **48**, 89–99.

24 Scarpati, E., Wen, D., Broze, G., Miletich, J., Flandermeyer, R., Siegal, N., and Sadler, E. (1987). Human tissue factor: cDNA sequence and chromosome location of the gene. *Biochemistry*, **26**, 5234–8.

25 Spicer, E., Horton, R., Bloem, L., Bach, R., Williams, K., GuHa, A., Kraus, J., Lin, T., Nemerson, Y., and Konigsberg, W. (1987). Isolation of cDNA clones coding for tissue factor: primary structure of the protein and cDNA. *Proc. Natl. Acad. Sci. U.S.A.*, **84**, 5148–52.

26 Morrissey, J., Fakhrai, H., and Edgington, T. (1987). Molecular cloning of the cDNA for tissue factor, the cellular receptor for the initiation of the coagulation protease cascade. *Cell*, **50**, 129–35.

27 Bach, R., Konigsberg, W., and Nemerson Y. (1988). Human tissue factor contains thiolester-linked palmitate and stearate on the cytoplasmic half-cystine. *Biochemistry*, **27**, 4227–31.

28 Edgington, T. S., Mackman, N., Brand, K., and Ruf, W. (1991). The structural biology of expression and function of tissue factor. *Thromb. Haemostas.*, **66**, 67–79.

29 Paborsky, L., Tate, K., Harris, R., Yansura, D., Band, L., McCray, G., Gorman, C., O'Brien, D., Chang, Y., Swartz, J., Fung, V., Thomas, J., and Vehar, G. (1989). Purification of recombinant human tissue factor. *Biochemistry*, **28**, 8072–7.

30 Broze, G., Leykam, J., Schwartz, B., and Miletich J. (1985). Purification of human brain tissue factor. *J. Biol. Chem.*, **260**, 10917–20.

31 Ruf, W., Rehemtulla, A., and Edgington, T. (1991). Phospholipid-independent interactions required for tissue factor receptor and cofactor function. *J. Biol. Chem.*, **266**, 2158–66.

32 Hagen, F., Gray, C., O'Hara, P., Grant, F., Saari, G., Woodbury, R., Hart, C., Insley, M., Kisiel, W., Kurachi, K., and Davie, E. (1986). Characterization of a cDNA coding for human FVII. *Proc. Natl. Acad. Sci. U.S.A.*, **83**, 2412–16.

33 Nelsestuen, G (1976). Role of gamma-carboxy glutamic acid. *J. Biol. Chem.*, **251**, 5648–56.

34 Tulinsky, A. (1991). The structures of domains of blood proteins. *Thromb. Haemostas.*, **66**, 16–31.

35 Broze, G. (1982). Binding of human factor VII and VIIa to monocytes. *J. Clin. Invest.*, **70**, 526–35.

36 Kumar, A., Blumenthal, D., and Fair, D. (1991). Identification of molecular sites on FVII which mediate its assembly and function in the extrinsic pathway activation complex. *J. Biol. Chem.*, **266**, 915–21.

37 Wildgoose, P., Kazim, A., and Kisiel, W. (1990). The importance of residues 195–206 of human blood clotting factor VII in the interaction with tissue factor. *Proc. Natl. Acad. Sci. U.S.A.*, **87**, 7290–4.

38 O'Brien, D. P., Gale, K. M., Anderson, J. S., McVey, J. H., Miller, G. J., Meade, T. W., and Tuddenham, E. G. D. (1991). Purification and characterization of FVII304-Gln: a variant molecule with reduced activity isolated from a clinically unaffected male. *Blood*, **78**, 132–40.

39 Nemerson, Y. and Gentry, R. (1986). An ordered addition essential activation model of the tissue factor pathway of coagulation. Evidence for a conformational cage. *Biochemistry*, **25**, 4020–33.

40 Zur, M., Radcliffe, R., Oberdick, J., and Nemerson, Y. (1982). The dual role of FVII in blood coagulation. Initiation and inhibition of a proteolytic system by a zymogen. *J. Biol. Chem.*, **257**, 5623–31.

41 Williams, E. and Mann, K. (1988). Zymogen/protease discrimination using fluorescent peptide fluoroprobes. *Circulation*, **78**, 512 (abstr.).

42 Wildgoose, P., Berkener, K., and Kisiel, W. (1990). Synthesis, purification, and characterization of an Arg 152 to Glu site-directed mutant of recombinant human blood clotting FVII. *Biochemistry*, **29**, 3413–20.

43 Rao, L., Rapaport, S., and Bajaj, S. (1986). Activation of human FVII in the initiation of tissue factor-dependent coagulation. *Blood*, **68**, 685–91.

44 Radcliffe, R., Bagdasarian, A., Colman, R., and Nemerson, Y. (1977). Activation of bovine FVII by Hageman factor fragments. *Blood*, **50**, 611–5.

45 Lane, D. and Caso, R. (1989). Anti-thrombin structure, genomic organization, function, and inherited deficiency. In *The molecular biology of blood coagulation* (ed. E. G. D. Tuddenham), Baillieres Clinical Haematology, **2**, (4) 962–98. Ballière Tindall, London.

46 Rao, L. and Rapaport, S. (1988). Activation of FVII bound to tissue factor. A key step in the tissue factor pathway of coagulation. *Proc. Natl. Acad. Sci. U.S.A.*, **85**, 6687–91.

47 Wen, D., Dittman, W., Ye, R., Dearen, L., Majerus, P., and Sadler, E. (1987). Human thrombomodulin. Complete cDNA sequence and chromosome location of the gene. *Biochemistry*, **26**, 4350–7.

48 Petersen, T. (1988). The amino-terminal domain of thrombomodulin and pancreatic stone protein are homologous with lectins. *FEBS Lett.*, **231**, 51–3.

49 Dittman, W. and Majerus, P. (1989). Sequence of a cDNA for mouse thrombomodulin and comparison of the predicted mouse and human amino acid sequences. *Nucleic Acids Res.*, **17**, 802.

50 Escobedo, J., Barr, P., and Williams, L. (1988). Role of tyrosine kinase and membrane spanning domains in signal transduction by the platelet-derived growth factor receptor. *Mol. Cell Biol.*, **13**, 5126–9.

51 Goldstein, J., Brown, M., Anderson, T., Russell, D., and Schneider, W. (1985). Receptor-mediated endocytosis: concepts emerging from the LDL receptor system. *Annu. Rev. Cell Biol.*, **1**, 1–6.

52 Dittman, W., Kumada, T., Sadler, J., and Majerus, P. (1988). The structure and function of mouse thrombomodulin: phorbol myristate acetate stimulates degradation and synthesis of thrombomodulin without affecting mRNA levels in haemangioma cells. *J. Biol. Chem.*, **263**, 15815–22.

53 Kurosawa, J., Stearns, D., Jackson, K., and Esmon, C. (1988). A 10 kDa cyanogen bromide fragment from the epidermal growth factor homology domain of rabbit thrombomodulin contains the primary thrombin binding site. *J. Biol. Chem.*, **263**, 5993–6.

54 Stearns, D., Kurosawa, S., and Esmon, C. (1989). Micro-thrombomodulin residues 310–486 from the epidermal growth factor precursor homology domain of thrombomodulin will accelerate protein C activation. *J. Biol. Chem.*, **264**, 3352–6.

55 Suzuki, K., Hayashi, T., Nishioka, J., Kosaka, Y., Zushi, M., Honda, G., and Yamamoto, S. (1989). A domain composed of the epidermal growth factor-like structures of human thrombomodulin is essential for thrombin-binding and protein C activation. *J. Biol. Chem.*, **264**, 4872–6.

56 Davie, E. (1987). The blood coagulation factors: their cDNAs, genes, and expression. In *Haemostasis and thrombosis* (ed. R. Colman, J. Hirsh, V. Marder, and E. Salzman), pp. 148–267. J. Lippincott Co. USA.

57   Butkowski, R., Elion, J., Downing, M., and Mann, K. (1977). Primary structure of human pro-thrombin-2 and alpha-thrombin. *J. Biol. Chem.*, **252**, 4942-7.

58   Park, C. and Tulinsky, A. (1986). Three-dimensional structure of the kringle sequence: structure of pro-thrombin fragment 1. *Biochemistry*, **25**, 3977-82.

59   Fenton, J., Fascow, M., Stackrow, M., Aronson, A., Young, A., and Finlayson, J. (1977). Human thrombins. Production, evaluation, and properties of alpha-thrombin. *J. Biol. Chem.*, **252**, 3587-98.

60   Thompson, E. and Salem, H. (1977). Modification of human thrombin: effect on thrombomodulin binding. *Thromb. Haemostas.*, **59**, 415 (abstr.).

61   Noe, G., Hofsteenge, J., Rovelli, G., and Stone, S. R. (1988). The use of sequence-specific antibodies to identify a secondary binding site in thrombin. *J. Biol. Chem.*, **263**, 11729-35.

62   Esmon, C. (1989). The roles of protein C and thrombomodulin in the regulation of blood coagulation. *J. Biol. Chem.*, **264**, 4743-6.

63   Musci, G., Berliner, L., and Esmon, C. (1988). Evidence for multiple conformational changes in the active centre of thrombin induced by complex formation with thrombomodulin. *Biochemistry*, **27**, 769-73.

64   Esmon, N., Owen, W., and Esmon, C. (1982). Isolation of a menbrane-bound cofactor for thrombin catalysed activation of protein C. *J. Biol. Chem.*, **257**, 859-64.

65   Kisiel, W. (1979). Human plasma protein C. Isolation, characterization, and mechanism of activation by alpha-thrombin. *J. Clin. Invest.*, **64**, 761-9.

66   Damus, P., Hicks, M., and Roesnberg, R. (1973). Anti-coagulant action of heparin. *Nature*, **246**, 355-7.

67   Hofsteenge, J., Taguchi, H., and Stone, S. (1986). Effect of thrombomodulin on the kinetics of the interaction of thrombin with substrates and inhibitors. *Biochem J.*, **237**, 243-51.

68   Walker, F. J. (1981). Regulation of bovine activated protein C by protein S. The role of cofactor proteins in species specificity. *Thromb. Res.*, **22**, 321-7.

69   Drake, T. A., Morrisey, J. H., and Edgington, T. S. (1989). Selective cellular expression of tissue factor in human tissues. *Am. J. Pathol.*, **134**, 1089-97.

70   Ryan, J. and Geczy, C. (1987). Coagulation and the expression of cell-mediated immunity. *Immunol. Cell Biol.*, **65**, 127-39.

71   Bevilacque, M. P., Pober, J. S., Majeau, G. R., Fiers, W., Cotran, R. S., and Gimbrone, M. A. (1986). Recombinant tumour necrosis factor induces pro-coagulant activity in cultured human vascular endothelium: characterization and comparison with the actions of interleukin-1. *Proc. Natl. Acad. Sci. U.S.A.*, **83**, 4533-7.

72   Bevilacque, M. P., Pober, J. S., Majeau, G. R., Cotran, R. S., and Gimbrone, M. A. (1984). Interleukin-1 (IL-1) induces biosynthesis and cell surface expression of pro-coagulant activity in human vascular endothelial cells. *J. Exp. Med.*, **160**, 618-23.

73   Maynard, J. R., Dreyer, B. E., Stemerman, M. B., and Pitlick, F. A. (1977). Tissue factor coagulant activity of cultured human endothelial and smooth muscle cells and fibroblasts. *Blood*, **50**, 387-96.

74 Colcucci, M., Balconi, G., Lorenzet, R., Pietra, A., Locati, D., Donati, M. B., and Semeraro, N. (1983). Cultured human endothelial cells generate tissue factor in response to endotoxin. *J. Clin. Invest.*, **71**, 1893–6.

75 Niemetz, J. and Morrison, C. (1977). Lipid A as the biologically active moiety in bacterial endotoxin (LPS)-initiated generation of pro-coagulant activity by peripheral blood leucocytes. *Blood*, **49**, 947–56.

76 Edwards, R. L. and Rickles, F. R. (1984). Macrophage pro-coagulants. *Prog. Haemostasis Thromb.*, **7**, 183–209.

77 Morrison, D. C. and Ulevitch, R. J. (1978). The effects of bacterial endotoxins on host mediation systems. *Am. J. Pathol.*, **93**, 527–617.

78 Ulevitch, R. J., Mathison, J. C., Schumann, R. R., and Tobias, P. S. (1990). A new model of macrophage stimulation by bacterial lipopolysaccharide. *J. Trauma*, **30**, 5189–92.

79 Wright, S. D., Ramos, R. A., Tobias, P. S., Ulevitch, R. J., and Mathison, J. C. (1990). CD14, a receptor for complexes of lipopolysaccharide (LPS) and LPS binding protein. *Science*, **249**, 1431–3.

80 Robinson, P. J. (1991). Phosphatidylinositol membrane anchors and T cell activation. *Immunol. Today*, **12**, 35–41.

81 Gregory, S. A., Morrissey, J. H., and Edgington, T. S. (1989). Regulation of tissue factor gene expression in the monocyte pro-coagulant response to endotoxin. *Mol. Cell Biol.*, **9**, 2752–5.

82 Conway, E. M., Bach, R., Rosenberg, R. D., and Konigsberg, W. H. (1989). Tumour necrosis factor enhances expression of tissue factor mRNA in endothelial cells. *Thromb. Res.*, **53**, 231–41.

83 Crossman, D. C., Carr, D. P., Tuddenham, E. G. D., Pearson, J. D., and McVey, J. H. (1990). The regulation of tissue factor mRNA in human endothelial cells in response to endotoxin or phorbol ester. *J. Biol. Chem.*, **265**, 9782–7.

84 Mackman, N., Morrissey, J. H., Fowler, B., and Edgington, T. S. (1989). Complete sequence of the human tissue factor gene, a highly regulated cellular receptor that initiates the coagulation protease cascade. *Biochemistry*, **28**, 1755–62.

85 Mackman, N., Fowler, B., Edgington, T. S., and Morrissey, J. H. (1990). Functional analysis of the human tissue factor promoter and induction by serum. *Proc. Natl. Acad. Sci. U.S.A.*, **87**, 2254–8.

86 Shirakawa, F. and Mizel, S. B. (1989). *In vitro* activation and nuclear translocation of NFκB catalysed by cyclic AMP-dependent protein kinase and protein kinase C. *Mol. Cell Biol.*, **9**, 2424–30.

87 Shirakawa, F., Chedid, M., Suttles, J., Pollok, B. A., and Mizel, S. B. (1989). Interleukin-1 and cyclic AMP induce κ immunoglobulin light chain expression via activation of an NFκB-like DNA binding protein. *Mol. Cell Biol.*, **9**, 959–64.

88 Ghosh, S. and Baltimore, D. (1990). Activation *in vitro* of NFκB by phosphorylation of its inhibitor IκB. *Nature*, **394**, 678–83.

89 Shakhov, A. N., Collart, M. A., Vassalli, P., Nedospasov, S. A., and Jongeneel, C. V. (1990). κB-type enhancers are involved in lipopolysaccharide-mediated transcriptional activation of the tumour necrosis factor-α gene in primary macrophages. *J. Exp. Med.*, **171**, 35–47.

90 Libermann, T. A. and Baltimore, D. (1990). Activation of interleukin-6 gene expression through the NFκB transcription factor. *Mol. Cell Biol.*, **10**, 2327–34.

91 Mackman, N., Brand, K., and Edgington, T. S. (1991). Regulation of the human tissue factor gene in THP-1 monocyte cells exposed to bacterial lipopolysaccharide. *Thromb. Haemostas.*, **65**, 701 (abstr.).

92 Cleveland, D. W. (1989). Gene regulation through messenger RNA stability. *Curr. Opinion Cell Biol.*, **1**, 1148–53.

93 Kornbluth, R. S. and Edgington, T. S. (1986). Tumour necrosis factor production by human monocytes is a regulated event: induction of IFNγ mediated cellular cytotoxicity by endotoxin. *J. Immunol.*, **137**, 2585–91.

94 Nawroth, P. P., Bank, I., Handley, D., Cassimeres, J., Chess, I. L., and Stern, D. (1986). Tumour necrosis factor/cachectin interacts with endothelial cell receptors to induce release of interleukin-1. *J. Exp. Med.*, **163**, 1363–75.

95 Uncla, C., Roux-Lombard, P., Fey, S., Dayer, J-M., and Mach, B. (1990). Interferon-γ drastically modifies the regulation of interleukin-1 genes by endotoxin in U937 cells. *J. Clin. Invest.*, **85**, 185–91.

96 Gregory, S. A. and Edgington, T. S. (1985). Tissue factor induction in human monocytes. *J. Clin. Invest.*, **76**, 2440–5.

97 Gregory, S. A., Kornbluth, R. S., Helin, H., Remold, H. G., and Edgington, T. S. (1986). Monocyte pro-coagulant inducing factor: a lymphokine involved in the T cell instructed monocyte pro-coagulant response to antigen. *J. Immunol.*, **137**, 3231–9.

98 Ryan, J. and Geczy, C. L. (1986). Characterization and purification of mouse macrophage pro-coagulant inducing factor. *J. Immunol.*, **137**, 2864–70.

99 Fan, S-T. and Edgington, T. S. (1988). Clonal analysis of mechanisms of murine T helper cell collaboration with effector cells of macrophage lineage. *J. Immunol.*, **141**, 1819–27.

100 Fan, S-T. and Edgington, T. S. (1991). Coupling of the adhesive receptor CD11b/CD18 to functional enhancement of effector macrophage tissue factor response. *J. Clin. Invest.*, **87**, 50–57.

101 Clauss, M., Murray, J. C., Viannu, M., de Waal, R., Thurston, G., Nawroth, P., Gerlach, H., Gerlach, M., Bach, R., Familletti, P. C., and Stern, D. (1990). A polypeptide factor produced by fibrosarcoma cells that induces endothelial tissue factor and enhances the pro-coagulant response to tumour necrosis factor/cachectin. *J. Biol. Chem.*, **265**, 7078–83.

102 Keck, P. J., Hauser, S. D., Krivir, G., Sanzo, K., Warren, T., Feder, J., and Connolly, D. T. (1989). Vascular permeability factor, an endothelial cell mitogen related to PDGF. *Science*, **246**, 1309–12.

103 Leung, D. W., Cachianes, G., Kuang, W-J., Goeddel, D. V., and Ferrara, N. (1989). Vascular endothelial growth factor is a secreted angiogenic mitogen. *Science*, **246**, 1306–9.

104 Muruyama, I. and Majerus, P. W. (1985). The turnover of thrombin–thrombomodulin complex in cultured human umbilical vein endothelial cells and A549 lung cancer cells. Endocytosis and degradation of thrombin. *J. Biol. Chem.*, **260**, 5432–8.

105 Murayama, I. and Majerus, P. W. (1987). Protein C inhibits endocytosis of thrombin–thrombomodulin complexed in A549 lung cancer cells and human vein endothelial cells. *Blood*, **69**, 1481–4.

106 Nawroth, P. P. and Stern, D. M. (1986). Modulation of endothelial cell haemostatic properties by tumour necrosis factor. *J. Exp. Med.*, **163**, 740–5.

107   Nawroth, P. P., Handley, D. A., Esmon, C. T., and Stern, D. M. (1986). Interleukin-1 induces endothelial cell pro-coagulant while suppressing cell surface anti-coagulant activity. *Proc. Natl. Acad. Sci. U.S.A.*, **83**, 3460–4.

108   Moore, K. L., Andreoli, S. P., Esmon, N. L., Esmon, C. T., and Bang, N. U. (1987). Endotoxin enhances tissue factor and suppresses thrombomodulin expression of human vascular endothelium *in vitro*. *J. Clin Invest.*, **79**, 124–30.

109   Conway, E. M. and Rosenberg, R. D. (1988). Tumour necrosis factor suppresses transcription of the thrombomodulin gene in endothelial cells. *Mol. Cell Biol.*, **8**, 5588–92.

110   Scarpati, E. M. and Sadler, J. E. (1989). Regulation of endothelial cell coagulant properties: Modulation of tissue factor, plasminogen activator inhibitors, and thrombomodulin by phorbol 12-myristate 13-acetate and tumour necrosis factor. *J. Biol. Chem.*, **264**, 20705–13.

111   Kapiotis, S., Besemer, J., Bevec, D., Valent, P., Bettenheim, P., Lechner, K., and Speiser, W. (1991). Interleukin-4 counteracts pyrogen-induced downregulation of thrombomodulin in cultured human vascular endothelial cells. *Blood*, **78**, 410–5.

112   Hart, P. H., Vetti, G. F., Burgess, D. R., Whitly, G. A., Piccoli, D. S., and Hamilton, J. A. (1989). Potential anti-inflammatory effects of interleukin-4: suppression of human monocyte tumour necrosis factor-α, interleukin-1, and prostaglandin E$_2$. *Proc. Natl. Acad. Sci. U.S.A.*, **86**, 3803–7.

113   Standiford, T. J., Strieter, R. M., Chensue, S. W., Westwick, J., Kasahara, K., and Kunkel, S. L. (1990). IL-4 inhibits the expression of IL-8 from stimulated human monocytes. *J. Immunol.*, **145**, 1435–9.

114   Thornhill, M. H. and Haskard, D. O. (1990). IL-4 regulates endothelial cell activation by IL-1, tumour necrosis factor, or IFNγ. *J. Immunol.*, **145**, 865–72.

115   Thornhill, M. H. Kyan-Aung, U., and Haskard, D. O. (1990). IL-4 increases human endothelial cell adhesiveness for T cells but not for neutrophils. *J. Immunol.*, **144**, 3060–5.

116   Moore, K. L., Esmon, C. T., and Esmon, N. L. (1989). Tumour necrosis factor leads to internalization and degradation of thrombomodulin from the surface of bovine aortic endothelial cells in culture. *Blood*, **73**, 159–65.

117   Archipoff, G., Beretz, A., Freyssinet, J-M., Klein-Soyer, C., Brisson, C., and Cazenave, J-P. (1991). Heterologous regulation of constitutive thrombomodulin or inducible tissue factor activities on the surface of human saphenous vein endothelial cells in culture following stimulation by interleukin-1, tumour necrosis factor, thrombin, or phorbol ester. *Biochem. J.*, **273**, 679–84.

118   Almus, F. E., Rao, L. V. M., and Rapaport, S. I. (1988). Decreased inducibility of tissue factor activity on human umbilical vein endothelial cells cultured with endothelial cell growth factor and heparin. *Thromb. Res.*, **50**, 339–44.

119   Andoh, K., Petterson, K. S., Filion-Myklebust, C., and Prydz, H. (1990). Observations on the cell biology of tissue factor in endothelial cells. *Thromb. Haemostas.*, **63**, 298–302.

120   Dichek, D. and Quertermous, T. (1989). Variability in messenger RNA levels in human umbilical vein endothelial cells of different lineage and time of culture. *In vitro Cell Dev.*, **25**, 289–92.

121   Gerlach, H., Lieberman, H., Bach, R., Godman, G., Brett, J., and Stern, D. (1989). Enhanced responsiveness of endothelium in the growing/motile state to tumour necrosis factor/cachectin. *J. Exp. Med.*, **170**, 913–31.

122 Huber, S. A., Hausch, C., and Lodge, P. A. (1990). Functional diversity in vascular endothelial cells: role in coxsackievirus tropism. *J. Virol.*, **64**, 4516–22.
123 Meyrick, B., Christman, B., and Jesmok, G. (1991). Effects of recombinant tumour necrosis factor-α on cultured pulmonary artery and lung microvascular endothelial monolayers. *Am. J. Pathol.*, **138**, 93–101.

11 Platelet adhesion molecules in natural immunity

K. T. PREISSNER AND P. G. DE GROOT

1 Introduction

Many biological systems depend on the adherence of cells to the extracellular matrix, and this phenomenon is crucial for the maintenance of tissue integrity, cellular movement, or extracellular recognition processes. In particular, defence mechanisms of the organism such as wound healing, tissue repair, the humoral/cellular immune system, and the haemostasis system require different types of adhesive cells such as epithelial cells, keratinocytes, B, T lymphocytes, monocytes/macrophages, or platelets and endothelial cells, respectively, which all bear variable subtypes of adhesion receptors of the integrin and non-integrin type. The respective adhesive ligands for these receptors are either available as humoral factors in the circulating blood, in other body fluids, or in intracellular storage pools in circulating platelets, or they are found in association with extracellular matrices or basal membranes (Figure 11.1). The most abundant members of this group of proteins include fibrinogen, fibronectin, vitronectin, and von Willebrand factor and current knowledge about the role of these glycoproteins in natural defence mechanisms will be summarized in this chapter.

2 Platelet adhesion molecules

Upon vessel wall injury, initial adhesion of platelets to the exposed sub-endothelium and subsequent platelet aggregation are dependent on adhesive glycoproteins, present in the subendothelial cell matrix as well as stored inside platelets and secreted during this initial phase of haemostatic plug formation. In addition to their potent attachment promoting activity, pre-dominantly residing in an Arg-Gly-Asp (RGD)-containing epitope (1) and being one of the recognition sites for platelet membrane integrin receptors, these proteins express multiple functions and thus may interact with other ligands such as heparan sulfate, collagens, or mediators of humoral defence mechanisms. The circulating forms of these adhesive proteins may differ from those in the subendothelium and α-granules of platelets. This can be due to alternative splicing forms as for fibronectin, differences in the state of poly-merization as for von Willebrand factor, different conformational forms

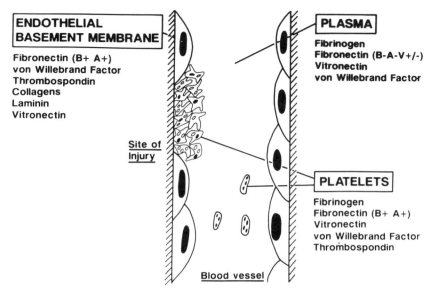

Fig. 11.1 The presence and availability of adhesive glycoproteins which contribute to cell-matrix interaction. Adhesive proteins present in plasma, platelet α-granules, or the endothelial basement membrane contribute to the integrity of the endothelial cell layer, or initial platelet adhesion and aggregation at the site of injury. Due to alternatively spliced segments designated A, B, and V, the available fibronectins at different sites may vary.

as for vitronectin, or the transition into a self-aggregating molecule as for fibrinogen. The partitioning of these proteins between humoral and cell surface or matrix phases together with inducible receptor sites on platelets or inflammatory cells indicates that these molecules and responding cells occur in a 'pre-activated' state under quiescent conditions but may become 'activated' into a functionally relevant form once natural defence mechanisms are initiated. Thus, these platelet adhesion molecules provide versatile molecular linkers mediating adhesive processes and responsive reactions of humoral defence mechanisms at localized sites.

In order to appreciate their multiple functions, the biochemical properties, site(s) of biosynthesis, and distribution of these molecules will be considered with emphasis on the human proteins (Table 11.1).

2.1   Fibrinogen

Fibrinogen is a major plasma glycoprotein which constitutes the macromolecular substrate for thrombin in the blood clotting cascade (see Chapter 10). Although the conformation of the molecule appears to be rather rigid based on models, deduced from electron microscopy (2), a considerable flexibility

Table 11.1 Properties of platelet adhesion molecules

Parameter	Fibrinogen	Fibronectin	von Willebrand factor	Vitronectin
Molecular weight	3.4×10^5	4.5×10^5	$0.44–20 \times 10^6$	0.8×10^5
Chains	2×3	2	subunit (0.22×10^6)	1
Carbohydrate, % (w/w)	3	5 – 10	19	10 – 15
Alternative spliced forms	no	yes	no	no
Plasma concentration (mg/ml)	2 – 4	0.2 – 0.4	0.015	0.2 – 0.4

of fibrinogen is appreciated using hydrodynamic or conformation-specific antibody approaches (3). The primary structure of fibrinogen has been elucidated by protein (4, 5) and cDNA (6) sequencing. Fibrinogen is composed of two identical sets of three polypeptide chains, Aα, Bβ, and γ, which are disulfide-bridged and organized in an anti-parallel fashion such that all amino-termini of the individual chains are arranged in the inner domain of the mature protein, whereas the carboxy-termini represent both outer domains of the symmetrical trinodular molecule. Upon selective and specific proteolytic attack by α-thrombin, two pairs of fibrino-peptides A and B (representing 3 per cent of the total mass of the protein) are sequentially released, and the occurrence of these peptides in the circulation is an indicator for thrombin activity *in vivo*. Covalent stabilization of the fibrin clot which forms is mediated by transglutaminase/factor XIIIa-dependent cross-linking between α and γ chains. Together with invading cells and aggregating platelets, the fibrin clot constitutes the predominant network for sealing the wound site and thereby protecting this area against infiltration by infectious micro-organisms.

Interaction of fibrin(ogen) with collagen, fibronectin, components of the fibrinolytic system, or binding to a variety of eukaryotic cells as well as to bacteria underlines the multi-functional role of the protein in natural defence mechanisms. In particular, at the same time the fibrin clot is being organized, it may already serve as a cofactor surface for tissue plasminogen activator-dependent plasminogen activation, ultimately leading to clot lysis. Also, binding of α_2-plasmin inhibitor to fibrin accounts for effective control of plasmin formation at that site. Early and late degradation products derived from plasmin proteolysis of fibrin(ogen) have been well characterized (7), and elevated levels of these fragments in the circulation are indicators for acquired disorders of the blood coagulation system.

Cell surface receptors for fibrinogen that belong to the family of integrins (see Section 3.1) have been identified on mammalian cells of which the platelet integrin α_{IIb}-β_3 (GP IIb/IIIa) is a major representative (8). Integrin α_M-β_2 (CR3) on phagocytes may recognize the ligand as well (9). While the platelet integrin appears to be responsible for fibrinogen binding to activated platelets and platelet–platelet aggregation, CR3 may be involved in the phagocytotic clearance of fibrin(ogen) associated clot or cell fragments. The recognition of two RGD containing sites as well as an additional site at the distal end of the γ chain of fibrinogen by these integrins (10, 11) indicates that fibrinogen may serve as a bridging component between surface receptors on different cells or other extracellular sites once they become exposed.

The liver parenchymal cells are the main source for secreted fibrinogen while megakaryocytes and circulating platelets contain an intracellular pool of fibrinogen also, although platelet- and plasma-fibrinogens are identical (12). Biosynthetic processing of the three individual polypeptide chains of fibrinogen in a cell-free system is accomplished by separate translation of three distinct mRNAs (13). As an acute phase response, plasma fibrinogen levels will also rise as a consequence of an increase in mRNA synthesis, probably due to glucocorticoid responsive elements in the fibrinogen gene (14) (see Chapter 1). Hereditary disorders with variable inheritance pattern of fibrinogen synthesis such as congenital afibrinogenaemia, hypofibrinogenaemia, or dysfibrinogenaemia have been described in many instances and are well defined. In affected patients, a wide variety of phenotypic abnormalities, involving the majority of known functional properties of fibrinogen, have been analysed on the molecular level (15) particularly by analysis of the respective DNA structures.

2.2   Fibronectin

Fibronectin is an ubiquitious adhesive protein and essential for the adhesion of almost all types of cells. Fibronectin is abundant in the circulation and at various extracellular sites. The characteristic form of the molecule in solution is a dimer generated by disulfide-bridging at the carboxy-terminus of two similar subunits, each with molecular weight of about 220 kDa [for reviews see (16, 17)]. Visualization by electron microscopy reveals that the molecule is a strand of independent, globular domains connected by short, flexible segments (18). In addition to approximately 30 intrachain disulfide-bonds, two free sulfhydryl groups per subunit are involved in the formation of high molecular weight polymers of fibronectin which are predominantly found in extracellular tissues (19). The heterogeneity observed in fibronectin molecules isolated from plasma or tissue is due to variation in both the amino acid sequence and post-translational modifications. Although only one gene has been identified, the primary transcript of the gene can be processed by alternative splicing resulting in variation of the domain structure such that segments at three positions (A, B, V) can either be spliced out or be included during RNA processing. Variations in the carbohydrate content/structure, phosphorylation, sulfation, and acetylation are responsible for additional heterogeneities.

The primary structure of human fibronectin was elucidated first by protein sequencing and by analysing cDNA and genomic clones (20). The major part of fibronectin is built up out of three types of homologous repeats, including 12 type I repeats, 2 type II repeats, and 17 type III repeats. The splice variations (A+/−, B+/−) relate to type III-8 and III-13 repeats, both encoded by exactly one exon each but which are not found in plasma fibronectin and the corresponding mRNA derived from the liver (21). Fibronectin synthesized by fibroblasts in culture contains about 25 per cent type III-8 repeats (22) as does platelet-derived fibronectin (23). Another variation of fibronectin mRNA corresponds to a type III connecting strand (V segment) which contains additional cell attachment site(s) (24). Different cDNA forms of fibronectin, both containing or lacking this segment have been isolated from liver and different cells in culture (25), and the V segment has been implicated in attachment, spreading, and movement of cells.

The sensitivity of fibronectin towards proteolytic degradation has been used to dissect the molecule into different independent domains in order to study their structure/function relationship. The 30 kDa amino-terminal fragment contains the major acceptor site for factor XIIIa-mediated cross-linking and also bears the binding sites for heparin, fibrin, and *Staphylococcus aureus* (26–28). The well known property of fibronectin to bind to collagen or gelatin and to complement C1q is contained within the adjacent 40 kDa fragment (29), while the central portion of the molecule has no well defined binding functions. The versatile integrin recognition sequence RGD was first recognized in the type III-11 repeat of fibronectin (30) and has been found in a large number of adhesive and non-adhesive proteins since then. Additional heparin-binding and fibrin-binding domains are located towards the carboxy-terminal portion of the fibronectin molecule. Together with the RGD containing cell attachment site the heparin-binding domain is crucial for the establishment of stable focal adhesions as has been demonstrated in fragment complementation assays (31). Synthesis and deposition of fibronectin into the growing extracellular matrix of adhesive cells occurs by an active process (32), and the accumulation of fibronectin into an insoluble form is potentiated by disulfide-bridge formation as well as covalent cross-linking by transglutaminase/factor XIIIa (33). Although no appreciable binding of plasma fibronectin to unstimulated platelets occurs, binding to the $\alpha_{IIb}\text{-}\beta_3$ integrin on platelets is induced by platelet activation or by supplying fibronectin on a surface (34). Moreover, fibronectin appears to be essential for platelet adhesion at all shear rates tested (35), and the molecule also contributes to proper thrombus formation (36). The level of fibronectin synthesis in various cell types *in vitro* or *in vivo*, relevant for cell differentiation and development, differs greatly depending on the stimulus used; yet, no inherent deficiency of fibronectin has been described in humans so far. However, based on animal studies, it had been proposed that acquired fibronectin deficiencies may predispose the organism for multi-organ failure and weaken the immune response (37).

2.3   Vitronectin

Human vitronectin is found as a single chain polypeptide with a molecular weight of 78 kDa in the circulation and may be associated with different extracellular sites. Liver cells predominantly synthesize vitronectin (38), and there is no indication for alternative splicing mechanisms during processing (39). Only a limited number of cell types such as mesothelial cells, monocytes/macrophages, megakaryocytes, and some transformed cell lines produce this adhesive protein, whereas fibroblastic cells as well as vascular endothelial cells or other non-hepatic cells do not produce vitronectin.

Several immunofluorescent and histochemical studies suggest the deposition of vitronectin in a fibrillar pattern in loose connective tissue (40), in association with dermal elastic fibres in skin (41), as well as with renal tissue (42), and the media of the vascular wall (43–45). Moreover, the accumulation of terminal complement complexes (C5b–9 and/or SC5b–9) along elastic fibres later in life, the association of vitronectin with keratin bodies during keratino-cyte programmed cell death (apoptosis) (46), and co-localization of vitronectin with deposits of the terminal complement complex in kidney tissue from patients with glomerulonephritis (42, 47) suggest a role for vitronectin in preventing tissue damage in proximity to local complement activation. The deposits of vitronectin in fibrotic and necrotic regions of arteriosclerotic blood vessels (43, 45, 48) point to a possible but yet uncharacterized role of vitronectin in the pathogenesis of arteriosclerotic lesions. It remains to be established whether these pathological sites throughout the organism are the cause or the consequence for subsequent vitronectin accumulation. Available data, however, demonstrate that appreciable amounts of vitronectin may become deposited at sites distant from actual biosynthesis of the protein. Although the mechanism of deposition of exogenous vitronectin alone or in association with other proteins into different tissues remains unclear at present, it may occur in a similar fashion as described for fibronectin. The interaction of vitronectin with glycosaminoglycans (49) or different types of native collagens (50), and cross-linking of vitronectin by transglutaminase/factor XIIIa (51) are reactions that are likely to occur at extracellular matrix sites *in vivo* as well.

The molecular structure of vitronectin has mostly been elucidated by se-quencing human and rabbit cDNA's (48, 52, 53) which share appreciable high homology, also seen for the cDNA derived amino acid sequence from mouse (54; H. J. Ehrlich and K. T. Preissner, unpublished data). Localization of binding sites, which include (from the amino- to the carboxy-terminus) those for integrins, collagens, heparin, complement components, and perforin, plasminogen and plasminogen activator inhibitor-1, was mostly established by *in vitro* binding experiments. Vitronectin forms stable ternary complexes with thrombin–serine protease inhibitor complexes, and binary complexes with plasminogen activator inhibitors and may thereby control the distribution of anti-proteolytic activity in the pericellular micro-environment (55). Vitronectin functions as an inhibitor of cytolytic reactions of the terminal complement pathway as well as of perforin in cytolytic T cells (see Section 11.5 and Chapter 9).

Stabilized by internal heteropolar interactions, the predominant form of vitronectin in plasma appears to exhibit a folded conformation. Hydro-dynamic data have suggested a conformational lability/flexibility of vitro-nectin (56, 57) reflected by a transition of vitronectin from this folded into an extended form. This process may be provoked by different ligands or surface coating and denaturation, and concomitant to unfolding, binding sites for heparin, thrombin–anti-thrombin III complex, or complement C5b–7 become exposed. The RGD-dependent attachment site of vitronectin appears to be unaffected by these transitions. It is worthwhile noting that distant sequence homology exists between vitronectin and the haem-binding plasma protein haemopexin (39) whose ligand-binding properties strongly depend on conformational flexibility of the protein as well (58). Detailed description of structure–function relationships of vitronectin are found in recently published reviews (59, 60).

A complete genetic deficiency of vitronectin has not been described; acquired deficiencies with up to 50 per cent reduction of vitronectin plasma levels have been diagnosed in several patients suffering from disseminated intra-vascular coagulation and degenerative liver diseases (61, 62).

2.4   Von Willebrand factor

Von Willebrand factor is an exception in the family of adhesive proteins, because it mainly contributes to haemostatic plug formation and its function is limited to the maintenance of intact blood vessels. Von Willebrand factor is only produced by endothelial cells (63) and megakaryocytes (64). It is synthesized as a precursor protein with a short signal peptide followed by an unusually long pro-peptide, about 25 per cent of the total protein [for review see (65)]. While processed in the endoplasmic reticulum, the protein dimerizes by disulfide-bond formation between the carboxy-terminal ends of two chains. During passage through Golgi compartments, multimerization of dimers occurs by subsequent disulfide-bridging between the amino-termini; the presence of the pro-peptide is essential for this process after which it is cleaved off. Highly multimerized von Willebrand factor is stored in the α-granules of platelets or in endothelial cell-specific Weibel–Palade bodies (66, 67) and may become deposited into the subendothelium. Part of the synthetic route in endothelial cells is designated as constitutive pathway (68, 69) and involves secretion of multimers of von Willebrand factor into the circulation where they function as a transport and stabilizing protein for coagulation factor VIII.

Von Willebrand factor is strongly involved in the attachment of endo-thelial cells to basement membranes (70), and plasma–, endothelial cell–, and platelet–von Willebrand factor contribute to the adhesion of platelets to an injured vessel wall (71). Both adhesive processes are unique since the high shear stresses of blood flow require a stronger interaction between the cells and the adhesive ligand as compared to static conditions. Consequently, multi-merization of von Willebrand factor (72) offers the possibility for multiple interactions between the adhesive protein and cell surface receptors. Two types of receptors recognize distinct parts of the von Willebrand factor mole-cule. The RGD recognition site located towards the carboxy-terminus of the protein (69) interacts with integrin α_{IIb}-β_3 on platelets, whereas a unique binding site for another platelet surface glycoprotein complex, GP Ib/IX, encompasses two short sequences in the middle portion of von Willebrand factor which are held in close proximity by disulfide-bonds (73).

Although different proteins related to the natural immune system, including β_2-type integrins (e.g. those of the LFA-1 family with CD18 as β chain) or complement factors C2 and B, share appreciable structural homology in a domain common to von Willebrand factor (74), the contribution of von Willebrand factor in immune defence has not been recognized so far.

2.5   Other adhesive proteins

A number of additional adhesive proteins not present in plasma contribute to platelet–vessel wall interaction (75), or participate in the establishment of intact basement membranes to which cells involved in the immune defence mechanisms may adhere. Subendothelium and connective tissue structures contain at least seven different types of collagens (76), and the importance of collagens for optimal platelet adhesion *in vivo* is demonstrated by the bleeding tendency of patients with congenital disorders of collagen metabolism known as osteogenesis imperfecta or Ehlers–Danlos syndrome (77) (Table 11.3).

Laminin is an ubiquitous basement membrane component of 800 kDa and has a unique cross shaped structure consisting of one long arm and three short arms (78). The interactions of laminin with collagen type IV and heparan sulfate proteoglycans form the basis for the structural part of different basement membranes and its functional role during cell differentiation and development. Platelet adherence to laminin occurs in a metal ion-dependent manner via α_6-β_1 integrin (VLA-6) (79).

Thrombospondin is synthesized by endothelial, smooth muscle, or other cells (80) and is secreted upon platelet activation as a disulfide-linked homotrimer with an overall molecular weight of 510 kDa (81). Rotary shadowing images revealed a bola-like structure with amino-terminal globular domains that bind to heparin (82). Due to the interaction of thrombospondin with collagen type V, fibronectin, and fibrinogen, the adhesive protein not only participates in platelet aggregation but also plays a role in the structural organization of the subendothelial cell matrix. Under static conditions thrombospondin may bind to the α_{IIb}-β_3 or α_2-β_1 integrin receptors on the platelet surface, whereas under flow conditions the receptor is unknown (83).

3   Role of adhesive proteins in haemostatic plug formation and wound healing

As a defence mechanism, haemostatic plug formation refers to a sequence of events culminating in spontaneous arrest of bleeding from disrupted blood vessels. Fibrinogen and von Willebrand factor contribute to platelet adhesion and aggregation by forming molecular bridges between adjacent platelets, but also thrombospondin and fibronectin play a role in strengthening this process, whereas vitronectin is believed to govern organization of the thrombus by attracting and stabilizing plasminogen activator inhibitor-1 to this site. Immediately following injury, wound healing is initiated to replace the formation of a temporary haemostatic plug. This process starts with the induction of adhesive receptors in adjacent cells to enable them to migrate into the wound area via locally deposited fibrin and fibronectin.

3.1   Integrins: cell surface receptors for adhesive proteins

The cell attachment activity of platelet adhesion molecules often resides in the versatile RGD epitope (1, 30) and is shared by different collagens and laminin, as well as by other plasma proteins such as complement component C3 and (pro)thrombin. In focal adhesions, tight interactions between extracellular matrix components and the cytoskeleton inside a particular adherent cell are formed by 'integral' cell contacts through transmembranous moieties such as integrins (84, 85) and non-integrin-type receptors. Other cytoskeleton-associated proteins provide a further linkage between the cytoplasmic tail of these receptors and the end of the microfilamental stress fibre bundles inside the cell (86). Due to clustering of integrins in focal adhesions, the cumulative effect of the low affinity of individual receptor–ligand interaction may be increased considerably. Most cell types express receptors of the integrin-type and they are composed of non-related α and β subunits, which share about 50 per cent structural homology within the different classes and whose non-covalent association and ligand binding is promoted by divalent cations. The compositional diversity within the integrin gene family is reflected by the variable subunit composition of each receptor, i.e. the ability of a given β subunit to associate with multiple α subunits and of a few α subunits to assemble with more than one β subunit (87). Consequently, integrins may be divided into certain subfamilies of β_1-type (very late antigens), β_2-type (leucocyte cell adhesion molecules), or β_3-type (cytoadhesins) (88), but also a α_v-type subfamily exists (89). The resulting heterodimers not only exhibit variable ligand recognition but also bind with different affinity and to distinct sites within a common ligand (90, 91) and may be expressed at variable combinations in different cell types. Thus, the stereochemistry of the RGD flanking region in a given ligand (92) as well as the availability of integrins determines the multiplicity of ligand recognition which is not simply a reflection of cell type specific differences. Examples of integrins involved in the natural immune system with regard to the present context are listed in Table 11.2.

In addition to the RGD containing epitope, other sites on adhesive ligands such as the C-terminal fibrinogen γ chain peptide HHLGGAKQAGDV as well as epitopes in fibronectin with the minimal sequence REDV or LDV have been characterized as adhesive motifs that constitute alternative binding sites for integrins (93) and may thereby contribute to the specificity and selectivity of ligand recognition (94). Fibronectin, thrombospondin and von Willebrand factor each possess domains distinct from these sites which are recognized by non-

Table 11.2 Selection of integrins that recognize humoral factors involved in immune defence

Integrin	Ligands	Tissue distribution
α_L-β_2 (LFA-1)	ICAM-1, ICAM-2	Leucocytes
α_M-β_2 (MAC-1, CR3)	iC3b*, fibrinogen, factor X, ICAM-1, lipopolysaccharide	Phagocytes
α_X-β_2 (p150,95, CR4)	iC3b	Phagocytes
α_{IIb}-β_3 (GP IIb/IIIa)	Fibronectin, fibrinogen, vitronectin, von Willebrand factor	Megakaryocytes, platelets
α_v-β_3 (VNR)	Vitronectin, fibrinogen, von Willebrand factor, thrombospondin	Endothelial cells, osteosarcoma cells, mesothelial cells, melanoma cells
α_v-β_5	Vitronectin	Monocytes/macrophages, osteosarcoma cells

The nomenclature of integrins is such that: α denotes the type of α chain; β denotes the type of β chain; β_1 is equivalent to CD29; β_2 is equivalent to CD18; and β_3 is equivalent to CD61. See Section 11.3.1

*iC3b is a degradation product of complement component C3 (see Figures 5.3 and 7.6).

integrin cell surface receptors such as proteoglycans or GP Ib/IX complex, but which also contribute to adhesive function.

Although the factors determining the relative abundance of different adhesion protein-specific integrins in tissues are unknown at present, *in vitro* data have led to an understanding of biosynthetic processing and distinct ligand-binding properties of these receptors. The biosynthesis of both β_3-type integrins is similar and involves separate mRNA synthesis for α and β subunits and subsequent trans-Golgi processing (95, 96). Furthermore, the assembly of newly synthesized α chain(s) with a pre-existing pool of β subunits is believed to be a pre-requisite for expression of distinct heterodimeric complexes on the cell surface (97).

Both integrin subunits appear to participate in ligand binding, involving not only highly conserved Ca^{2+} binding sites on the α chain but also additional highly homologous regions within the β chains of different integrins. These conclusions are based on biochemical evidence (98, 99) and on genetic analysis of functionally defective receptors (100). Moreover, binding of the adhesive ligand to the receptor(s) may alter its shape and conformation of the ligand, resulting in exposure of ligand-induced binding sites on the receptor and receptor-induced binding sites on the ligand, respectively (101).

The β_2-type subfamily of integrins whose expression is restricted to different leucocytes and haematopoetic stem cells (102, 103) plays an important role in the functions of these types of cells with regard to cell activation and differentiation in the immune system (104). Due to the expression of a limited number of β_2-type integrins on the cell surface and their storage in intracellular pools (105, 106) a rapid acquisition and up-regulation of these integrins upon cell stimulation is attained such that leucocytes are converted from circulating into adherent tissue cells upon induction. This process is distinct from 'activation' of cell surface expressed α_{IIb}-β_3 integrin from a cryptic form into a functionally active form upon platelet stimulation. Moreover, concomitant up-regulation and recruitment of respective ligands such as ICAM-1 on endothelial cells results in, for example, increased leucocyte adherence via α_L-β_2 and α_M-β_2 to endothelium and subsequent extravasation. Cell surface expressed ICAM-1 and other members of the immunoglobulin superfamily (107) thereby act as 'counter receptors' generating potent cell–cell contacts relevant during inflammatory reactions (103). Integrins α_M-β_2 and α_X-β_2 (also designated as complement receptors CR3 and CR4) may recognize complement component iC3b and fibrinogen in a RGD-dependent manner or iC3b and fibrinogen γ chain peptide, respectively (11, 108). Since iC3b may be the preferred ligand for α_X-β_2 integrin as well, the latter two receptors appear to be mainly involved in the recognition of iC3b bearing particles and subsequent phagocytosis of these opsonized particles. Different examples for variable integrin–ligand interactions are schematically depicted in Figure 11.2. The participation of another family of cell surface receptors, designated 'selectins' (109, 110) that mediate leucocyte–endothelial interaction is beginning to

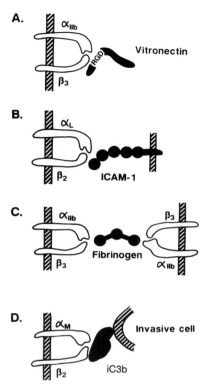

Fig. 11.2 Examples for principle integrin–ligand interactions. **(A)** Recognition of vitronectin by a β_3-type integrin in a typical RGD-dependent manner. Other related adhesion proteins present in an extracellular matrix network are recognized according-ly. **(B)** Interaction of a β_2-type integrin with an insoluble ligand present on the cell surface of another cell. Binding of β_2-type integrins to counter receptor molecules such as ICAM-1, abundantly present, e.g. after induction of endothelial cells, results in close cell–cell contacts, necessary for leucocyte adhesion to the vessel wall during inflammation. **(C)** Multiple binding of fibrinogen to more than one integrin. Due to the presence of more than one RGD-dependent attachment site as well as additional recognition domains in the γ chain, fibrinogen (and also von Willebrand factor) may function as bridging molecules during platelet aggregation and thereby mediate cell–cell contacts. **(D)** Recognition of an opsonized invasive cell by a β_2-type integrin. Through recognition of the iC3b fragment of complement component C3 which has been bound covalently to invasive cells or other micro-organisms during complement activation, iC3b bearing particles may be recognized by phagocytes and thereby mediate the initial events for subsequent ingestion.

emerge, and the expression of the p-selectin (GMP-140 or CD62), specific for leucocytes, on activated platelets and endothelial cells points to a direct role of platelets in the events of inflammation and wound repair.

3.2   Non-integrin receptors

Differential interaction of platelet adhesion molecules with cell surfaces also involves different cell surface-associated proteoglycans. These complex macro-molecules are present in adhesion plaques as well and thereby facilitate cell attachment and spreading events, whereas soluble proteoglycans may have an opposing effect by regulating cell adhesion processes (111). In particular, thrombospondin interaction with various cell types predominantly depends on the presence of the heparin-binding domain of this adhesive protein and complementary proteoglycan cell surface binding sites (112). Also, in addition to the RGD containing cell attachment domain, the heparin binding or other domain(s) in fibronectin and von Willebrand factor are crucial for the establishment of stable focal adhesions and may account for differences in the response of adherent cells exposed to the particular adhesive ligand (113).

Among the platelet adhesion molecules, only vitronectin is found associated within a ternary complex together with thrombin–anti-thrombin III, being the ultimate reaction product of the enzyme in plasma following blood clotting (114–117) (see Chapter 10). Owing to a conformational transition of vitronectin concomitant to ternary complex formation (118), the exposure of the heparin-binding domain of vitronectin converts these products into potent heparin scavengers. Specific proteoglycan-dependent binding of ternary complexes to endothelial cell monolayers with an affinity similar to the vitronectin–heparin interaction has been observed (119), indicating a possible role for the vessel wall in the clearance of these high molecular weight complexes. The RGD-dependent cell attachment activity within this complex (120) as well as additional active site-independent mitogenic properties of thrombin (121) may very well act in concert to promote cell adhesion/invasion and support natural defence mechanisms at sites of vessel wall injury where these products are most likely to be concentrated.

3.3   Events in haemostatic plug formation and wound healing

The onset of bleeding is immediately followed by accumulation of platelets on the connective tissue at the wound edge. Histological observations with biopsies from human skin wounds showed that the earliest event is the adhesion of single platelets to collagen-like fibres (122). In this phase, the functional activity of von Willebrand factor depends on its interaction with various types of collagen (type I, III, VI) (123, 124) and is mediated by interaction with GP Ib/IX to form a molecular bridge between platelets and the injured vessel wall (75). Subsequent platelet spreading on the subendothelium requires integrin α_2-β_1–collagen as well as α_{IIb}-β_3–fibronectin/von Willebrand factor interaction (125). Due to its higher local concentration *in vivo*, fibronectin seems to be more important for the latter process, but von Willebrand factor rather than fibrinogen appears to be the predominant adhesive ligand contributing to platelet–platelet interaction during the formation of a primary haemostatic plug at high shear rates (126). Although initially platelets are loosely packed and rebleeding may occur, early fibrin formation in the periphery of the plug and later on within the thrombus as well as concomitant platelet degranulation and retraction result in further sealing of the wound area. The haemostatic plugs of arterioles are in general larger than those of venules and bleeding in capillaries is stopped by contraction and contact formation of vessel edges. Fibronectin and von Willebrand factor are also incorporated into the growing network of thick fibrin strands and become covalently cross-linked by activated factor XIII. Due to high concentration of platelet secretion products as well as other inflammatory mediators, pronounced infiltration of monocytes and granulocytes occurs inside and around the plug, and also in the vessel near the wound to manage the immune response and subsequent phagocytotic processes.

Fibrin and fibronectin deposits not only form the essential network of the haemostatic plug, but this provisional wound matrix induces integrin-mediated attachment and migration of epidermal cells (keratinocytes) into the wound area, the formation of granulation tissue beneath the epidermal layer, and subsequent neo-vascularization (127, 128), the formation of granulation tissue beneath the epidermal layer and migration of epidermal cells (keratinocytes) into the wound area. Also, invasion of neutrophils and macrophages into this area appears to be mediated by fibronectin (129) and thrombospondin (130). Additional fibronectin may be produced by migrating fibroblasts, and TGFβ released from platelet α-granules might even induce fibronectin synthesis (131) to amplify the adhesion processes, and at later stages of granulation collagens also appear. An important process in the ultimate stage of wound healing which can be detected about two days after injury involves proliferation of endothelial cells (132). Moreover, basic fibroblast growth factor, heparin, but also laminin may induce endothelial cell growth at these sites.

Effective control of plasminogen activators during early haemostatic plug formation is attained through endothelial cell-derived plasminogen activator inhibitor type-1 (PAI-1) (133) which is found deposited in its active form within the subendothelium (134). PAI-1 also acts to inhibit secretion during platelet aggregation. However, PAI-1 requires vitronectin as a binding and stabilizing protein which not only increases the *in vitro* half-life of the inhibitor (135, 136) but, more importantly, retains and stabilizes PAI-1 in the subendothelium *in vitro* (137–139) (Figure 11.3). In addition, vitronectin–PAI-1 complexes are also secreted during platelet activation and aggregation (140). As a functional consequence, the concentration of vitronectin–PAI-1 complexes in a haemostatic plug may control the lag phase before plasminogen activators overcome the inhibitory potential to invoke fibrinolysis. By serving as a specific cofactor for PAI-1, vitronectin changes the specificity of the

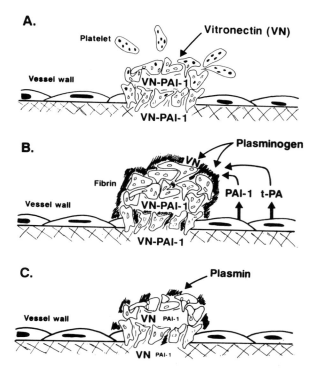

Fig. 11.3 Schematic illustration for contribution of vitronectin (VN)–plasminogen activator inhibitor-1 (PAI-1) complexes to stabilization of the haemostatic plug. Active PAI-1, stabilized by platelet- as well as matrix-associated vitronectin prevents the onset of the fibrinolytic system during the early phase of thrombin formation (A). The forming fibrin network (B) provides a template to which fibrinolytic components may bind and where plasminogen activation starts. Due to neutralization of vitronectin bound PAI-1 by plasminogen activators and by thrombin the balance of the haemostatic system is gradually shifted towards clot lysis (C).

inhibitor such that thrombin also becomes neutralized (141), particularly at the subendothelium (142). Vitronectin–PAI-1-rich adhesion sites may be protected against proteolysis as well (143), such that vitronectin functions as a unique matrix-associated regulator of pericellular proteolysis.

3.4   Dysfunction of adhesive proteins or receptors

The most severe disease in which platelet adhesion is abnormal is von Willebrand's disease, which represents about 30–40 per cent of all bleeding disorders. This genetic disorder, transmitted in an autosomal manner is characterized by the partial absence (type I), the total absence (type III), or an abnormality (type II) of von Willebrand factor. The severest forms of the disease present major bleeding episodes early in life (144). Patients with congential afibrinogenaemia may exhibit haemorrhagic diseases of variable severity, and clinical manifestations of dysfibrinogenaemias include delayed wound healing and wound dehiscence (15), but no direct effect on natural immune defence has been reported. Defects in platelet adhesion can also be due to deficiencies of platelet membrane receptors such as integrin α_{IIb}-β_3 or GP Ib/IX. These inherited disorders are very rare and the clinical symptoms are in general more severe (145). Other congenital disorders of adhesive proteins and receptors which may result in bleeding complications are mentioned in Table 11.3 and are extensively described by Lowe (77).

The physiological importance of the group of integrins expressed on leucocytes is demonstrated by the fact that a congenital deficiency or absence of the common β_2 subunit (146) constitutes the primary defect in 'Leucocyte Adhesion Deficiency', which is associated with abnormal wound healing, recurrent infections, and abnormalities of leucocyte functions *in vitro*.

4   Role of adhesive proteins in humoral immune defence

Following invasion of the blood circulation system by infectious micro-organisms, the humoral factors of the immune system and the complement cascade together with polymorphonuclear leucocytes and monocytes/marcophages, designated as phagocytes, contribute to effective lysis and subsequent phagocytosis of the invading bacteria, viruses, or other micro-particles. Although through covalent deposition of C3b during complement activation, which is converted to iC3b, effective recognition and subsequent sequestration of micro-organisms by phagocytes is attained, the immune response needs to be restricted to the foreign particles and not affect the host cells. Platelet adhesive proteins participate in both clearance and control processes. In the initial adhesive phase which is the critical step in the phagocytic process, specific particle-associated opsonins (e.g. C1q and C3b, see Chapters 5–7) as well as fibronectin or vitronectin as non-specific opsonins may promote the attachment between phagocyte and foreign particle. Moreover, as an inhibitor of the membrane damaging effect of the terminal cytolytic complement pathway, vitronectin is part of the protecting machinery limiting autologous cell lysis.

4.1   Role of adhesive proteins in phagocytosis

Phagocytosis refers to the final events leading to sequestration of sensitized foreign particles by phagocytes of the host attracted to the site of inflammation (147) and is also involved in clearance of immune complexes and initiation of tissue repair. Migration of the phagocyte to the site of microbial infiltration is provoked by reaction products of complement activation such as anaphylatoxins (Chapter 8) or other inflammatory inducers such as leuko-

Table 11.3 Genetic disorders associated with adhesion molecules

Disorders	Defect	Clinical symptoms
Afibrinogenaemia	Fibrinogen absence	Bleeding, delayed wound healing
Dysfibrinogenaemia	Dysfunctional fibrinogen	Thrombus or bleeding
von Willebrand's disease	von Willebrand factor:	
type I	partial absence	Variable
type II	abnormal	Variable
type III	total absence	Severe bleeding
Osteogenesis imperfecta	Collagen type I	Purpura, hemoptysis, intracranial bleeding
Ehler–Danlos syndrome IV	Collagen type III	Easy bruising, hemoptysis, bleeding from tract and after surgery
Marfan's syndrome	Collagen crosslinking	Spontaneous bruising and operative bleeding
Bernard–Soulier syndrome	Glycoprotein Ib/IX	Mild to severe bleeding
Glanzmann's thrombasthenia	α_{IIb}-β_3 integrin (GP IIb/IIIa)	Mild to severe bleeding
Glycoprotein IIa deficiency	α_2-β_1 integrin (VLA-2)	Mild bleeding
Leucocyte adhesion deficiency	β_2 integrins	Impaired leucocyte function, abnormal wound healing

triene B_4 (see Chapters 12 and 13). Phagocytes in turn are induced to produce components which contribute to the panoply of inflammatory mediators. Although fibronectin does not promote the early phase migration of neutrophils *per se*, peripheral blood monocytes respond to fibronectin with increased motility (148). Activated neutrophils (149) and macrophages (150) themselves produce additional fibronectin which thereby leads to chemoattraction of monocytes and fibroblasts to the inflammatory area. Thus, due to the neutrophil influx into the inflammatory site, neutrophil-derived enzymes may generate fibronectin adhesion fragments which in turn are responsible for the later phase monocyte migration (151). Similarly, vitronectin has been reported to stimulate haptotaxis* and migration of cells *in vitro* (152). Neutrophil migration in response to fibronectin and vitronectin involves integrins (Table 11.2) and is controlled by calcium ions (153). As in wound healing, fibronectin-mediated macrophage adhesion may lead to production of growth factors which act as stimuli for further cell activation processes resulting in positive feed back regulation (154).

Following this critical primary adhesive step in recognition, the subsequent phase is characterized by the action of particle-associated opsonins, mainly IgG and iC3b, which bind to specific receptors (Fc receptors, β_2 integrins) on the phagocyte surface. In particular, neutrophils lacking β_2 integrins fail to amplify ingestion of opsonized particles in response to inflammatory mediators, but possess the mechanism of β_2 integrin-independent phagocytosis (155).

While plasma components such as the acute phase reactants, C-reactive protein, or serum amyloid P component have been implicated in facilitating phagocytosis (156) (see Chapter 1) fibronectin and vitronectin alone are not efficient promotors. However, together with fibrin and/or collagen the association of fibronectin with monocytes is enhanced (157), and also phagocyte ingestion of gelatin-coated particles is promoted by fibronectin (158). Similar effects in augmenting the function of β_2 integrins on monocytes are provoked by vitronectin (159). Thus, attachment of macrophages to fibronectin or vitronectin through respective β_1 or β_5 integrins (89, 160) brings about enhancement of the phagocytic process by activation of Fc and complement receptors (161, 162). Clustering of integrins (163), G protein mediated signalling, as well as integrin phosphorylation-dephosphorylation events (164) are involved to optimize or to modulate the phagocyte response.

Integrin α_M-β_2 is also involved in binding of coagulation factor X to ADP treated monocytes (165) and subsequent conversion to factor Xa. Additional factor V/Va related cell surface sites, designated 'effector cell protease receptors', may induce pro-thrombinase activity (166) independent of other coagulation factors and offer an alternate route for fibrin formation. α_M-β_2 may recognize other related serine proteases such as granzymes (167) which are possibly relevant in natural killer and cytolytic T cell-mediated target cell lysis

---

* Movement in response to contact.

indicating that pericellular proteolysis in these inflammatory areas may be of significance also for phagocytosis. Moreover, phagocyte (macrophage) recognition of cells (both neutrophils and lymphocytes) that have undergone apoptosis (168) involves the direct role of the macrophage α_V-β_3 integrin (VNR), rather than other vitronectin recognizing receptors on these cells (169). Both, vitronectin and fibronectin inhibited this process, indicating that integrin occupancy by adhesive protein ligands may control macrophage recognition and clearance of apoptotic cells in order to limit tissue injury at sites of inflammation.

4.2   Role of platelet adhesive proteins in bacterial adhesion

Bacterial adherence to host cells is likely to be a pre-requisite both for the activation of the host's immune system as well as for colonization by certain micro-organisms and the initial process of infectious diseases. Among other plasma proteins, specific and independent binding of fibrinogen, fibronectin, and vitronectin to strains of staphylococci, streptococci, and Gram-negative bacteria has been described (170–172). The predominant staphylococcal binding site of fibronectin lies in the amino-terminal domain (173), while two streptococcal binding sites for vitronectin, one being heparin-dependent the other being RGD-dependent could be identified (174). Neither adhesive protein binds to group B streptococci. Since Gram-negative bacteria adhere less well to fibronectin-coated surfaces or to endothelial cells than do staphylococci or streptococci (175), fibronectin-coating may thereby protect these cells against invasion by Gram-negative bacteria. The fibronectin receptor on *Staphylococcus aureus* has been cloned and sequenced (176) and represents a heavily glycosylated polypeptide of 110 kDa, while *Pneumocystis carinii* utilize a membrane glycoprotein of 120 kDa for fibronectin-mediated attachment to alveolar epithelial cells (177). Certain strains of *Escherichia coli* provide coiled surface structures, composed of subunits designated curlin (178) that mediate fibronectin binding during, for example, wound colonization. The adherence of streptococci to the luminal side of cultured endothelial cells (179) or to epithelial cells (180) was mediated by fibronectin-independent but vitronectin-specific interactions. The respective bacterial binding site(s) for vitronectin remain to be characterized.

Adhesion of infectious micro-organisms (*Bordetella pertussis*) to host cells may also be directly mediated through recognition of RGD containing bacterial adhesins by the α_M-β_2 integrin on macrophages (181). The invasion-mediated pathway for the entry of *Yersinia pseudotuberculosis* into non-phagocytic mammalian cells necessary for bacterial replication may be initiated by multiple β_1-type integrins, although the bacterial adhesion molecule (designated invasin) does not contain a RGD motif (182). A possible infection in these instances, however, may be prevented due to the occupation of integrins which are involved by platelet adhesion molecules of the host.

While intravascular release of tissue fibronectin and possibly other adhesive proteins may occur at sites of vascular injury where inflammatory responses are provoked (183), these areas are also most commonly infected by strains of staphylococci. Thus, it remains to be established in individual situations whether occupation of certain binding sites in platelet adhesive molecules by bacterial receptors results in recognition and subsequent attack of the micro-organisms by the immune system, involving complement and adhesive protein supported phagocytosis, or whether the pathogenesis predominates, following interaction between platelet adhesive molecules and bacteria.

5   Vitronectin as cytolysis inhibitor

The humoral immune response is supported by the complement system, whose activation via proteolytic cascade mechanisms may be initiated by antibody opsonized invasive cells or micro-organisms which become ultimately damaged or lysed (184) (summarized in Chapter 5). The transition of hydrophilic terminal complement components C5b, C6, C7, and C8 into amphiphilic complexes within the membrane of the attacked cells and subsequent poly-merization of component C9 results in formation of the lytic complement pore (185) (see Chapter 9). Since vitronectin (186, 187) and lipoproteins (188, 189) inhibit this process, these components are denoted as membrane attack complex inhibitors and are believed to play a specific role in protecting the host organism against innocent bystander cell lysis. In particular, *in vitro* data suggest that vitronectin (complement 'S protein') occupies the metastable membrane binding 'site' (190) of the nascent precursor complex C5b–7 such that the formed water soluble SC5b–7 macromolecule is unable to insert into cell membranes (Figure 11.4). Although the SC5b–7 complex may take up C8 and C9 molecules to form the SC5b–8 and SC5b–9 complexes, respectively (191), the latter one is non-lytic. It can be isolated from complement activated serum (192) and, compatible with these findings, exhibits a wedge-shaped ultras-tructural morphology unlike the characteristic circular complement lesion (193). Conversely, a hydrophilic–amphiphilic transition occurs if the vitronectin component is dissociated from the SC5b–8 or SC5b–9 complexes by limited proteolysis (194, 195) or detergent treatment (196). Furthermore, C9 poly-merization itself is inhibited by vitronectin in a concentration-dependent manner in solution (185) such that ongoing cell-associated pore formation is limited in the presence of the inhibitor (Figure 11.4), and even fully assembled membrane attack complexes are associated with non-stoichiometric amounts of vitronectin (197). This process may be particular important at those loca-tions which are rich in vitronectin, (i.e. the vessel wall), with the implication that these sites are protected against autologous complement attack. Vitro-nectin also participates in the control of cell killing by blocking perforin pore formation (198), the lytic principle characteristic for cytolytic T lymphocytes.

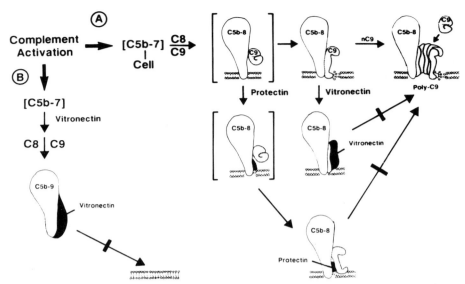

Fig. 11.4 Schematic representation of the function of complement inhibitors. Following complement activation in the presence of invading cells (A), precursor complexes (C5b-7) become bound and insert into the cell membrane providing the recognition site for C9 molecules to bind. After substantial conformational change from a hydrophilic into an amphilic C9 molecule further binding sites for additional C9 molecules are exposed which lead to the assembly of the complement pore containing a poly-C9 torus. Since the assembly of the complement pore would be harmful on autologous cells, protectin or vitronectin may limit 'innocent bystander cell lysis' by either not allowing a functional pore to assemble or by blocking polymerization into poly-C9, respectively. Alternatively (B), insertion of precursor complexes of the lytic membrane attack complex are recognized by soluble vitronectin, such that macromolecular complexes containing the terminal complement components as well as vitronectin are formed, which are lytically inactive. Other alternatives in restriction of homologous cell lysis are also available which are mentioned in the text. The illustrated morphology of the macromolecular complexes is derived from electron microscopical analysis (185, 193); see also Chapter 9.

Initial observations already indicated that several anionic as well as cationic molecules may inhibit C9 activity (199). The molecular mechanism by which vitronectin interferes with both lytic mechanisms involves the heparin-binding domain of the molecule (198) which is unique among the other platelet adhesion molecules since it contains heavily clustered basic amino acid residues. Upon unfolding of vitronectin, this domain may occupy and thereby block complementary negatively charged domain(s) on the C9 or perforin molecules, necessary for assembly of the lytic pores. Likewise, binding of vitronectin to cysteine-rich, acidic 'C9-type' repeats in C6, C7, and C8 (200) relevant for assembly of the lytic complex may strengthen vitronectin's inhibitory action. Moreover, association of vitronectin within the SC5b-9 complex does not affect the RGD-dependent cell attachment activity of the adhesive protein (54), indicating that the macromolecular SC5b–9 complex may induce integrin-dependent cell invasion at sites of inflammation and phagocytosis where these molecules are likely to be accumulated.

Interaction of the hydrophobic binding site of the nascent C5b–7 with lipo-proteins appears to be sufficient for preventing it from insertion into cell membranes (189), yet no complementary hydrophobic binding site has been characterized in the vitronectin molecule. Interestingly however, another plasma protein of 80 kDa and denoted as SP40–40/clusterin has been found asso-ciated with the SC5b–9 complex as well (201). Structural analysis of clusterin revealed putative hydrophobic binding domains (202), which may associate with high density lipoprotein particles and may thereby constitute the active inhibi-tor of the cytolytic complex, previously associated with lipoproteins themselves (203). Although no structural similarity between clusterin and vitronectin was noted, both proteins may thereby limit autologous cytolysis by complementary mechanisms. Also, the co-localization of clusterin with vitronectin in diseased renal tissue (204) suggests a concerted action of both molecules for the regu-lation of terminal complement attack phase during inflammatory processes.

5.1 Other complement regulatory proteins equivalent to vitronectin

Autologous or homologous complement-mediated cell lysis is prevented by membrane-associated 'homologous restriction factors' present on various blood cells and the vascular endothelium. The major proteins involved are homo-logous restriction factor (HRF) (205) also denoted as C8/C9 binding protein of 60 kDa (206) and membrane attack complex inhibition factor, denoted as MACIP, MIRL, or protectin of 20 kDa (207–209). Both limit lytic pore forma-tion by either mutually interacting with precursor complexes of the membrane attack complex or by not allowing proper pore formation, respectively (210, 211) (Figure 11.4) (see Table 5.2). Like decay accelerating factor which represents another regulator protein in the initial phase of complement activation, both HRF or protectin are associated with cell membranes via a glycosyl-phospha-tidylinositol moiety (212). Due to inadequate anchorage in the membrane, patients suffering from paroxysmal nocturnal haemoglobinuria lack these regu-latory proteins (Table 5.3) (208, 213), but the fatal outcome of this acquired haemolytic anaemia may be significantly reduced by vitronectin, present in the circulation. *In vitro* experiments indicated a complementary action of vitronectin as inhibitor of autologous lysis (214), whereas antibodies against vitronectin enhanced haemolysis of paroxysmal noctural haemoglobinuria cells.

The most prominent route by which nucleated cells involved in inflam-mation escape damage by non-lethal doses of the membrane attack complex of complement is by shedding pore-containing vesicles (215). In the case of platelets and endothelial cells these micro-particles contain pro-thrombinase

activity (216, 217) representing a further molecular link between the coagulation and humoral immune systems. However, the processes of homologous
restriction serve to minimize these inflammation potentiating effects of the
lytic complement complex.

6   Summary

The platelet adhesion proteins fibrinogen, fibronectin, von Willebrand factor,
and vitronectin express multiple functions in defence mechanisms of the
organism mainly devoted to haemostatic plug formation, wound repair, and
inflammation or protective mechanisms. Most of these processes are governed
by the interchangeable roles of these proteins: to be present either as humoral
factors in the blood circulation, contained in platelet α-granules or associated
as insoluble network with extracellular matrices. Due to the presence of
complementary receptors (integrins) on almost all cell types that are involved
in the immune system, multiple recognition reactions of platelet adhesion
molecules may occur. Mostly at sites of vascular injury a controlled sequence
of adhesion events may lead to proper platelet aggregation and wound healing,
as well as to a regulated influx of neutrophils and subsequently monocytes
into the inflammatory area. Ingestion of invasive material by phagocytes may
also be augmented by adhesive proteins, however, the particular beneficial
action with respect to bacterial adhesion to host cells has to be clarified in
individual situations. In particular, vitronectin has been implicated in many
physiological and pathophysiological situations due to its protective function
against autologous cell lysis and ensuing localized proteolysis.

Congenital or acquired deficiencies, described for von Willebrand factor
and fibrinogen, are associated with bleeding and wound healing complications
in patients. Further approaches such as molecular genetics are required to
understand the spectrum of multiple functional properties of fibronectin and
vitronectin throughout the organism.

As the most abundant humoral ligands for integrin receptors, platelet
adhesion molecule play an important multi-functional role by providing
molecular bridges between different activation and defence mechanisms.

Acknowledgement

We gratefully acknowledge the skillful secretarial assistance of Angelika
Püschel.

References

1 Ruoslahti, E. and Pierschbacher, M. D. (1986). Arg-Gly-Asp: a versatile cell
   recognition signal. *Cell*, **44**, 517–8.

2   Hall, C. E. and Slayter, H. S. (1959). The fibrinogen molecule: its size, shape, and mode of polymerization. *J. Biophys. Biochem. Cytol.*, **5**, 11–5.

3   Plow, E. F. and Edgington, T. S. (1982). Surface markers of fibrinogen and its physiologic derivatives revealed by antibody probes. *Sem. Thromb. Hemostas.*, **8**, 36–56.

4   Henschen, A., Lottspeich, F., Töpfer-Petersen, E., and Warbinek, R. (1979). Primary structure of fibrinogen. *Thromb. Haemostas.*, **41**, 662–70.

5   Doolittle, R. F., Watt, K. W. K., Cottrell, B. A., and *et al.* (1979). The amino acid sequence of the α chain of human fibrinogen. *Nature*, **280**, 464–8.

6   Chung, D. W., Chan, W.-Y., and Davie, E. W. (1983). Characterization of a complementary deoxyribonucleic acid coding for the γ chain of human fibrinogen. *Biochemistry*, **22**, 3250–6.

7   Francis, C. W. and Marder, V. J. (1982). A molecular model of plasmic degradation of cross-linked fibrin. *Sem. Thromb. Hemostas.*, **8**, 25–35.

8   Marguerie, G. A., Plow, E. F., and Edgington, T. S. (1979). Human platelets possess an inducible and saturable receptor specific for fibrinogen. *J. Biol. Chem.*, **254**, 5357–63.

9   Trezzini, C., Jungi, T. W., Kuhnert, P., and Peterhans, E. (1988). Fibrinogen association with human monocytes: evidence for constitutive expression of fibrinogen receptors and for involvement of Mac-1 (CD18, CR3) in the binding. *Biochem. Biophys. Res. Commun.*, **156**, 477–84.

10   Kloczewiak, M., Timmons, S., Lukas, T. J., and Hawiger, J. (1984). Platelet receptor recognition site on human fibrinogen. Synthesis and structure–function relationship of peptides corresponding to the carboxy-terminal segment of the gamma chain. *Biochemistry*, **23**, 1767–74.

11   Wright, S. D., Weitz, J. I., Huang, A. J., *et al.* (1988). Complement receptor type three (CD11b/CD18) of human polymorphonuclear leucocytes recognizes fibrinogen. *Proc. Natl. Acad. Sci. U.S.A.*, **85**, 7734–8.

12   Doolittle, R. F., Takagi, T., and Cottrell, B. A. (1974). Platelet and plasma fibrinogens are identical gene products. *Science*, **185**, 368–70.

13   Chung, D. W., MacGillivray, R. T. A., and Davie, E. W. (1980). The biosynthesis of bovine fibrinogen, pro-thrombin, and albumin in a cell-free system. *Ann. N. Y. Acad. Sci.*, **408**, 330–43.

14   Fowlkes, D. M., Mullis, N. T., Comeau, G. M., and Crabtree, G. R. (1984). Potential basis for regulation of the co-ordinately expressed fibrinogen genes: homology in 5′-flanking regions. *Proc. Natl. Acad. Sci. U.S.A.*, **81**, 2313–16.

15   Lane, D. A. and Southan, G. (1987). Inherited abnormalities of fibrinogen synthesis and structure. In *Haemostasis and thrombosis* (ed. A. L. Bloom and D. P. Thomas), pp. 442–51. Churchill Livingstone, Edinburgh.

16   Hynes, R. O. (1989). *Fibronectins* (ed. A. Rich). Springer-Verlag New York.

17   Petersen, T. E., Skorstengaard, K., and Vibe-Pedersen, K. (1989). Primary structure of fibronectin. In *Fibronectin* (ed. D. F. Mosher), pp. 1–24. Academic Press, San Diego.

18   Odermatt, E. and Engel, J. (1989). Physical properties of fibronectin. In *Fibronectin* (ed. D. F. Mosher), pp. 25–45. Academic Press, San Diego.

19   Wagner, D. D. and Hynes, R. O. (1979). Domain structure of fibronectin and its relation to function. *J. Biol. Chem.*, **254**, 6746–54.

20   Kornblihtt, A. R., Vibe-Pedersen, K., and Baralle, M. (1983). Isolation and characterization of cDNA clones from human and bovine fibronectins. *Proc. Natl. Acad. Sci. U.S.A.*, **80**, 3218–22.

21 Schwarzbauer, J. E., Tamkun, J. W., Lemischka, l. R., and Hynes, R. O. (1983). Three different fibronectin mRNA arise by alternative splicing within the coding region. *Cell*, **35**, 421–31.

22 Kornblihtt, A. R., Vibe-Petersen, K., and Baralle, M. (1984). Human fibronectin: molecular cloning evidence for two mRNA species different by an internal segment coding for a structural domain. *EMBO J.*, **3**, 221–6.

23 Paul, J. I., Schwarzbauer, J. E., Tamkun, J. W., and Hynes, R. O. (1986). Cell-type specific fibronectin subunits generated by alternative splicing. *J. Biol. Chem.*, **261**, 12258–65.

24 Bernard, M. P., Kolbe, M., Weil, D., and Chu, M. L. (1985). Human cellular fibronectin: comparison of the C-terminal portion with rat identifies primary structural domains separated by hypervariable regions. *Biochemistry*, **24**, 2698–704.

25 Humphries, M. J., Akiyama, S. K., Komoriya, A., Olden, K., and Yamada, K. M. (1986). Identification of an alternatively spliced site in human plasma fibronectin that mediates cell type-specific adhesion. *J. Cell Biol.*, **103**, 2637–47.

26 McDonagh, R. P., McDonagh, J., Petersen, T. E., Thogersen, H. C., Skorstengaard, K., Sottrup-Jensen, L., Magnusson, S., Dell, A., and Morris, H. R. (1981). Amino acid sequence of the factor XIIIa acceptor site in bovine plasma fibronectin. *FEBS Lett.*, **127**, 174–8.

27 Hörmann, H. and Seidl, M. (1980). Affinity chromatography on immobilized fibrin monomer III, the fibrin affinity centre of fibronectin. *Hoppe-Seyler's Z. Physiol. Chem.*, **361**, 1449–52.

28 Mosher, D. F. and Proctor, R. A. (1980). Binding and factor XIIIa-mediated cross-linking of a 27-kilodalton fragment of fibronectin to *Staphylococcus aureus*. *Science*, **209**, 927–9.

29 McDonald, J. A. and Kelley, D. G. (1980). Degradation of fibronectin by human leucocyte elastase. Release of biological active fragments. *J. Biol. Chem.*, **255**, 8848–58.

30 Pierschbacher, M. D. and Ruoslahti, E. (1984). Cell attachment activity of fibronectin can be duplicated by small synthetic fragments of the molecule. *Nature*, **309**, 30–3.

31 Obara, M., Kang, M. S., and Yamada, K. M. (1988). Site-directed mutagenesis of the cell-bindung domain of human fibronectin: separable, synergistic sites mediate adhesive function. *Cell*, **53**, 649–57.

32 McKeown-Longo, P. J. and Mosher, D. F. (1985). Interaction of the 70 000 mol-wt amino-terminal fragment of fibronectin with the matrix-assembly receptor of fibroblasts. *J. Cell Biol.*, **100**, 364–74.

33 Barry E. L. R. and Mosher D. F. (1989). Factor XIIIa-mediated cross-linking of fibronectin in fibroblast cell layers. *J. Biol. Chem.*, **264**, 4179–85.

34 Plow, E. F. and Ginsberg, M. H. (1981). Specific and saturable binding of plasma fibronectin to thrombin-stimulated human platelets. *J. Biol. Chem.*, **256**, 9477–82.

35 Houdijk, W. P. M. and Sixma, J. J. (1985). Fibronectin in artery subendothelium is important for platelet adhesion. *Blood*, **65**, 598–604.

36 Bastida, E. B., Escolar, G., Ordinas, O., and Sixma, J. J. (1987). Fibronectin is required for platelet adhesion and for thrombus formation on subendothelium and on collagen surfaces. *Blood*, **70**, 1437–42.

37 Saba, T. M. (1989). Kinetics of plasma fibronectin: relationship to phagocytic function and lung vascular integrity. In *Fibronectin* (ed. D. F. Mosher), pp. 395–439. Academic Press, San Diego.

38 Barnes, D. W. and Reing, J. (1985). Human spreading factor: synthesis and response by HepG2 hepatoma cells in culture. *J. Cell. Physiol.*, **125**, 207–14.

39 Jenne, D. and Stanley. K. K. (1987). Nucleotide sequence and organization of the human S protein gene: repeating peptide motifs in the 'pexin' family and a model for their evolution. *Biochemistry*, **26**, 6735–742.

40 Hayman, E. G., Pierschbacher, M. D., Ohgren, Y., and Ruoslahti, E. (1983). Serum spreading factor (vitronectin) is present at the cell surface and in tissues. *Proc. Natl. Acad. Sci. U.S.A.*, **80**, 4003–7.

41 Dahlbäck, K., Löfberg, H., and Dahlbäck, B. (1986). Localization of vitronectin (S protein of complement) in normal human skin. *Acta Derm. Venereol.*, **66**, 461–7.

42 Falk, R. J., Podack, E., Dalmasso, A. P., and Jennette, J. C. (1987). Localization of S protein and its relationship to the membrane attack complex of complement in renal tissue. *Am. J. Pathol.*, **127**, 182–90.

43 Niculescu, F., Rus, H. G., and Vlaicu, R. (1987). Immunohistochemical localization of C5b–9, S protein, C3d, and apolipoprotein B in human arterial tissues with atherosclerosis. *Atherosclerosis*, **65**, 1–11.

44 Reilly, J. T. and Nash, J. R. G. (1988). Vitronectin (serum spreading factor): its localization in normal and fibrotic tissue. *J. Clin. Pathol.*, **41**, 1269–72.

45 Guettier, C., Hinglais, N., Bruneval, P., Kazatchkine, M., Bariety, J., and Camilleri, J.-P. (1989). Immunohistochemical localization of S protein/vitronectin in human atherosclerotic versus arteriosclerotic arteries. *Virchows Arch. A Pathol. Anat.*, **414**, 309–13.

46 Dahlbäck, K., Löfberg, H., Alumets, J., and Dahlbäck, B. (1989). Immunohistochemical demonstration of age-related deposition of vitronectin (S protein of complement) and terminal complement complex on dermal elastic fibres. *J. Invest. Dermatol.*, **92**, 727–33.

47 Bariety, J., Hinglais, N., Bhakdi, S., Mandet, C., Rouchon, M., and Kazatchkine, M. D. (1989). Immunohistochemical study of complement S protein (vitronectin) in normal and diseased human kidneys: relationship to neoantigens of the C5b–9 terminal complex. *J. Clin. Exp. Immunol.*, **75**, 76–81.

48 Sato, R., Komine, Y., Imanaka, T., and Takano, T. J. (1990). Monoclonal antibody EMR 1a/212D recognizing site of deposition of extracellular lipid in atherosclerosis. Isolation and characterization of a cDNA clone for the antigen. *J. Biol. Chem.*, **265**, 21232–6.

49 Lane, D. A., Flynn, A. M., Pejler, G., Lindahl, U., Choay, J., and Preissner, K. T. (1987). Structural requirements for the neutralization of heparin-like saccharides by complement S protein/vitronectin. *J. Biol. Chem.*, **262**, 16343–9.

50 Gebb, C., Hayman, E. G., Engvall, E., and Ruoslahti, E. (1986). Interaction of vitronectin with collagen. *J. Biol. Chem.*, **261**, 16698–703.

51 Sane, D. C., Moser, T. L., Parker, C. J., Seiffert, D., Loskutoff, D. J., and Greenberg, C. S. (1990). Highly sulfated glycosaminoglycans augment the cross-linking of vitronectin by guinea pig liver transglutaminase. Functional studies of the cross-linked vitronectin multimers. *J. Biol. Chem.*, **265**, 3543–48.

52 Suzuki, S., Oldberg, A., Hayman, E. G., Pierschbacher, M. D., and Ruoslahti, E. (1985). Complete amino acid sequence of human vitronectin deduced from cDNA. Similarity of cell attachment sites in vitronectin and fibronectin. *EMBO J.*, **4**, 2519–24.

53 Jenne, D. and Stanley, K. K. (1985). Molecular cloning of S protein, a link between complement, coagulation, and cell-substrate adhesion. *EMBO J.*, **4**, 3153–7.

54 Seiffert, D., Keeton, M., Eguchi, Y., Sawdey, M., and Loskutoff, D. J. (1991). Detection of vitronectin mRNA in tissues and cells of the mouse. *Proc. Natl. Acad. Sci. U.S.A.*, **88**, 9402–6.

55 Preissner, K. T. and Jenne, D. (1991). Structure of vitronectin and its biological role in haemostasis. *Thromb. Haemostas.*, **66**, 123–30.

56 Preissner, K. T. and Müller-Berghaus, G. (1987). Neutralization and binding of heparin by S protein/vitronectin in the inhibition of factor Xa by anti-thrombin III. Involvement of an inducible heparin binding domain of S protein/vitronectin. *J. Biol. Chem.*, **262**, 12247–53.

57 Tomasini, B. R., Mosher, D. F., Owen, M. C., and Fenton, J. W. (1989). Conformational lability of vitronectin: induction of an antigenic change by alpha-thrombin–serpin complexes and by proteolytically modified thrombin. *Biochemistry*, **28**, 832–42.

58 Smith, A., Tatum, F. M., Muster, P., Burch, M. K., and Morgan, T. (1988). Importance of ligand-induced conformational changes in haemopexin for receptor-mediated haem transport. *J. Biol. Chem.*, **263**, 5224–9.

59 Tomasini, B. R. and Mosher, D. F. (1990). Vitronectin. *Prog. Haemost. Thromb.*, **10**, 269–305.

60 Preissner, K. T. (1991). Structure and biological role of vitronectin. Annu. Rev. Cell Biol., **7**, 275–310.

61 Conlan, M. G., Tomasini, B. R., Schultz, R. L., and Mosher, D. F. (1988). Plasma vitronectin polymorphism in normal subjects and patients with disseminated intravascular coagulation. *Blood*, **72**, 185–90.

62 Kemkes-Matthes, B., Preissner, K. T., Langenscheidt, F., Matthes, K. J., and Müller-Berghaus, G. (1987). S protein/vitronectin in chronic liver diseases: correlations with serum cholinesterase, coagulation factor X, and complement component C3. *Eur. J. Haematol.*, **39**, 161–5.

63 Jaffe, E. A., Hoyer, L. W., and Nachman, R. L. (1973). Synthesis of anti-haemophilic factor antigen by cultured human endothelial cells. *J. Clin. Invest.*, **52**, 2757–64.

64 Nachman, R., Levine, R., and Jaffe, E. A. (1977). Synthesis of factor VIII antigen by cultured guinea pig megakaryocytes. *J. Clin. Invest.*, **60**, 914–21.

65 Wagner, D. D. (1990). Cell biology of von Willebrand factor. *Annu. Rev. Cell Biol.*, **6**, 217–46.

66 Zucker, M. B., Broekman, M. J., and Kaplan, K. L. (1979). Factor VIII-related antigen in human blood platelets. *J. Lab. Clin. Med.*, **94**, 675–82.

67 Wagner, D. D., Olmsted, J. B., and Marder, V. J. (1982). Immunolocalization of von Willebrand protein in Weibel-Palade bodies of human endothelial cells. *J. Cell Biol.*, **95**, 355–60.

68 Loesberg, C., Gonsalves, M. D., Zandbergen, J., Willems, C., van Aken, W. G., Stel, H. V., van Mourik, J. A., and de Groot, P. G. (1983). The effect of calcium on the secretion of factor VIII-related antigen by cultured endothelial cells. *Biochim. Biophys. Acta*, **763**, 160–8.

69 Girma, J. P., Meyer, D., Verweij, C. L., Pannekoek, H., and Sixma, J. J. (1987). Structure-function relationship of human von Willebrand factor. *Blood*, **70**, 605–11.

70 Dejana, E., Lampugnani, M. G., Giorgi, M., Gaboli, M., Federici, A. B., Ruggeri, Z. M., and Marchisio, P. C. (1989). Von Willbrand factor promotes endothelial cell adhesion via an Arg-Gly-Asp-dependent mechanism. *J. Cell Biol.*, **109**, 367–75.

71 Tschopp, T. B., Weiss, H. J., and Baumgartner, H. R. (1974). Decreased adhesion of platelets to subendothelium in von Willebrand's disease. *J. Lab. Clin. Med.*, **83**, 296–300.

72 Ruggeri, Z. M. and Zimmerman, T. S. (1980). Variant von Willebrand disease: characterization of two subtypes by analysis of multimeric composition of factor VIII/von Willebrand factor in plasma and platelets. *J. Clin. Invest.*, **65**, 1318–25.

73 Mohri, H., Fujimura, Y., Shima, M., Yoshioka, A., Houghten, R. A., Ruggeri, Z. M., and Zimmerman, T. S. (1988). Structure of the von Willebrand factor domain interacting with glycoprotein lb. *J. Biol. Chem.*, **263**, 17901–4.

74 Colombatti, A. and Bonaldo, P. (1991). The superfamily of proteins with von Willebrand factor type A-like domains: one theme common to components of extracellular matrix, haemostasis, cellular adhesion, and defence mechanisms. *Blood*, **77**, 2305–15.

75 de Groot, P. G. and Sixma, J. J. (1990). Platelet-adhesion. *Br. J. Haematol.*, **75**, 308–12.

76 Mayne, R. (1986). Collagenous proteins of blood vessels. *Arteriosclerosis*, **6**, 585–93.

77 Lowe, G. D. O. (1991). Vascular disease and vasculitis. In *Disorders of haemostasis* (ed. O. D. Ratnoff and C. D. Forbes), pp. 532–49. W. B. Saunders Company, Philadelphia.

78 Beck K., Hunter I., and Engel J. (1990). Structure and function of laminin—anatomy of a multidomain glycoprotein. *FASEB J.*, **4**, 148–60.

79 Sonnenberg, A., Modderman, P. W., and Hogervorst, F. (1988). Laminin receptor on platelets is the integrin VLA-6. *Nature*, **366**, 487–9.

80 Mosher, D. F. (1990). Physiology of thrombospondin. *Annu. Rev. Med.*, **41**, 85–97.

81 Lawler, J. W., Slayter, H. S., and Coligan, J. A. (1978). Isolation and characterization of a high molecular weight glycoprotein from human blood platelets. *J. Biol. Chem.*, **253**, 8609–16.

82 Coligan, J. E. and Slayter, H. S. (1984). Structure of thrombospondin. *J. Biol. Chem.*, **259**, 3944–8.

83 Tuszynski, G. P. and Kowalska, M. A. (1991). Thrombospondin-induced adhesion of human platelets. *J. Clin. Invest.*, **87**, 1387–94.

84 Hynes, R. O. (1987). Integrins: a family of cell surface receptors. *Cell*, **48**, 549–54.

85 Ruoslahti, E. and Pierschbacher, M. D. (1987). New perspectives in cell adhesion: RGD and integrins. *Science*, **238**, 491–7.

86 Burridge, K., Fath, K., Kelly, T., Nuckolls, G., and Turner, C. (1988). Focal adhesions: transmembrane junctions between the extracellular matrix and the cytoskeleton. *Annu. Rev. Cell Biol.*, **4**, 487–525.

87 Ruoslahti, E. (1991). Integrins. *J. Clin. Invest.*, **87**, 1–5.

88 Ginsberg, M. H., Loftus, J. C., and Plow, E. F. (1988). Cytoadhesins, integrins, and platelets. *Thromb. Haemostas.*, **59**, 1–6.

89   Krissansen, G. W., Elliott, M. J., Lucas, C. M., Stomski, F. C., Berndt, M. C., Cheresh, D. A., Lopez, A. F., and Burns, G. F. (1990). Identification of a novel integrin β subunit expressed on cultured monocytes (marcophages). Evidence that one alpha subunit can associate with multiple β subunits. *J. Biol. Chem.*, **265**, 823–30.

90   Cheresh, D. A., Berliner, S. A., Vicente, V., and Ruggeri, Z. M. (1989). Recognition of distinct adhesive sites on fibrinogen by related integrins on platelets and endothelial cells. *Cell*, **58**, 945–53.

91   Smith, J. W., Ruggeri, Z. M., Kunicki, T. J., and Cheresh, D. A. (1990). Interaction of integrins α_v–β_3 and glycoprotein IIb-IIIa with fibrinogen. Differential peptide recognition accounts for distinct binding sites. *J. Biol. Chem.*, **265**, 12267–71.

92   Pierschbacher, M. D. and Ruoslahti, E. (1987). Influence of stereochemistry of the sequence Arg-Gly-Asp-Xaa on binding specificity in cell adhesion. *J. Biol. Chem.*, **262**, 17294–8.

93   Humphries, M. J. (1990). The molecular basis and specificity of integrin–ligand interactions. *J. Cell Sci.*, **97**, 585–92.

94   Yamada, K. M. (1991). Adhesive recognition sequences. *J. Biol. Chem.*, **266**, 12809–12.

95   Duperray, A., Berthier, R., Chagnon, E., Ryckewaert, J.-J., Ginsberg, M., Plow, E., and Marguerie, G. (1987). Biosynthesis and processing of platelet GPIIb-IIIa in human megakaryocytes. *J. Cell Biol.*, **104**, 1665–73.

96   Polack, B., Duperray, A., Troesch, A., Berthier, R., and Marguerie, G. (1989). Biogenesis of the vitronectin receptor in human endothelial cell: evidence that the vitronectin receptor and GPIIb-IIIa are synthesized by a common mechanism. *Blood*, **73**, 1519–24.

97   Cheresh, D. A. and Spiro, R. C. (1987). Biosynthetic and functional properties of an Arg-Gly-Asp-directed receptor involved in human melanoma cell attachment to vitronectin, fibrinogen, and von Willebrand factor. *J. Biol. Chem.*, **262**, 17703–11.

98   D'Souza, S. E., Ginsberg, M. H., Lam, S. C.-T., and Plow, E. F. (1988). Chemical cross-linking of arginyl-glycyl-aspartic acid peptides to an adhesion receptor on platelets. *J. Biol. Chem.*, **263**, 3943–51.

99   Smith, J. W. and Cheresh, D. A. (1988). The arg-gly-asp binding domain of the vitronectin receptor. Photoaffinity cross-linking implicates amino acid residues 61–203 of the β subunit. *J. Biol. Chem.*, **263**, 18726–31.

100   Loftus, J. C., Otoole, T. E., Plow, E. F., Glass, A., Frelinger, A. L., and Ginsberg, M. H. (1990). A β_3 integrin mutation abolishes ligand-binding and alters divalent cation-dependent conformation. *Science*, **249**, 915–18.

101   Frelinger III, A. L., Lam, S. C.-T., Plow, E. F., Smith, M. A., Loftus, J. C., and Ginsberg, M. H. (1988). Occupancy of an adhesive glycoprotein receptor modulates expression of an antigenic site involved in cell adhesion. *J. Biol. Chem.*, **263**, 12397–402.

102   Yong, K. and Khwaja, A. (1990). Leucocyte cellular adhesion molecules. *Blood Rev.*, **4**, 211–25.

103   Springer, T. A. (1990). Adhesion receptors of the immune system. *Nature*, **346**, 425–34.

104   Kishimoto, T. K., Larson, R. S., Corbi, A. L., Dustin, M. L., Staunton, D. E., and Springer, T. A. (1989). The leucocyte integrins: LFA-1, Mac-1, and p150,95. *Adv. Immunol.*, **46**, 149–82.

105 Todd III, R. F., Arnaout, M. A., Rosin, R. E., Crowley, C. A., Peters, W. A., and Babior, B. M. (1984). Subcellular localization of the large subunit of Mo1 (Mo1 alpha; formerly gp110), a surface glycoprotein associated with neutrophil adhesion. *J. Clin. Invest.*, **74**, 1280–90.

106 Miller, L. J., Bainton, D. F., Borregaard, N., and Springer, T. A. (1987). Stimulated mobilization of monocyte Mac-1 and p150,95 adhesion proteins from an intracellular vesicular compartment to the cell surface. *J. Clin. Invest.*, **80**, 535–44.

107 Diamond, M. S., Staunton, D. E., de Fougerolles, A. R., Stacker, S. A., Garcia-Aguilar, J., Hibbs, M. L., and Springer, T. A. (1990). ICAM-1 (CD54): a counter-receptor for Mac-1 (CD11b/CD18). *J. Cell Biol.*, **111**, 3129–39.

108 Wright, S. D., Reddy, P. A., Jong, M. T. C., and Erickson, B. W. (1987). iC3b receptor (complement receptor type 3) recognizes a region of complement protein C3 containing the sequence arg-gly-asp. *Proc. Natl. Acad. Sci. U.S.A*, **84**, 1965–8.

109 Bevilacqua, M., Butcher, E., Furie, B., Furie, B., Gallatin, M., Gimbrone, M., *et al.* (1991). Selectins: a family of adhesion receptors. *Cell*, **67**, 233.

110 Johnston, G. I., Cook, R. G., and McEver, R. P. (1989). Cloning of GMP-140, a granule membrane protein of platelets and endothelium: sequence similarity to proteins involved in cell adhesion and inflammation. *Cell*, **56**, 1033–44.

111 Ruoslahti, E. (1988). Fibronectin and its receptors. *Annu. Rev. Biochem.*, **57**, 375–413.

112 Murphy-Ullrich, J. E. and Mosher, D. F. (1987). Interactions of thrombospondin with endothelial cells: receptor-mediated binding and degradation. *J. Cell Biol.*, **105**, 1603–11.

113 Woods, A. and Couchman, J. R. (1988). Focal adhesions and cell-matrix interactions. *Collagen Rel. Res.*, **8**, 155–182.

114 Podack, E. R. and Müller-Eberhard, H. J. (1979). Isolation of human S protein, an inhibitor of the membrane attack complex of complement. *J. Biol. Chem.*, **254**, 9908–14.

115 Ill, C. R. and Ruoslahti, E. (1985). Association of thrombin–anti-thrombin III complex with vitronectin in serum. *J. Biol. Chem.*, **260**, 15610–15.

116 Jenne, D., Hugo, F., and Bhakdi, S. (1985). Interaction of complement S protein with thrombin–anti-thrombin complexes: a role for the S protein in haemostasis. *Thromb. Res.*, **38**, 401–12.

117 Preissner, K. T., Zwicker, L., and Müller-Berghaus, G. (1987). Formation, characterization, and detection of a ternary complex between S protein, thrombin, and anti-thrombin III in serum. *Biochem. J.*, **243**, 105–11.

118 Tomasini, B. and Mosher, D. F. (1988). Conformational states of vitronectin: preferential expression of an antigenic epitope when vitronectin is covalently and non-covalently complexed with thrombin–anti-thrombin III or treated with urea. *Blood*, **72**, 903–12.

119 de Boer, H. C., Preissner, K. T., Bouma, B. N., and de Groot, P. G. (1992). Binding of vitronectin–thrombin–anti-thrombin III complex to human endothelial cells is mediated by the heparin binding site of vitronectin. *J. Biol. Chem.*, **267**, 2264–8.

120 Preissner, K. T., Anders, E., Grulich-Henn, J., and Müller-Berghaus, G. (1988). Attachment of cultured human endothelial cells is promoted by specific association with S protein (vitronectin) as well as with the ternary S protein–thrombin–anti-thrombin III complex. *Blood*, **71**, 1581–9.

121 Bar-Shavit, R. and Wilner, G. D. (1986). Mediation of cellular events by thrombin. *Int. Rev. Exp. Path.*, **29**, 213–41.

122 Sixma, J. J. and Wester, J. (1977). The haemostatic plug. *Sem. Thromb. Haemostas.*, **14**, 265–99.

123 Baumgartner, H. R., Tschopp, T. B., and Weiss, H. J. (1977). Platelet interaction with collagen fibrils in flowing blood. II. Impairment adhesion aggregation in bleeding disorders. A comparison with subendothelium. *Thromb. Haemostas.*, **37**, 17–28.

124 de Groot, P. G., Ottenhof-Rovers, M., van Mourik, J. A., and Sixma, J. J. (1988). Evidence that the primary binding site of von Willebrand factor that mediates platelet adhesion to subendothelium is not collagen. *J. Clin. Invest.*, **82**, 65–73.

125 Weiss, H. J., Turitto, V. T., and Baumgartner, H. R. (1986). Platelet adhesion and thrombus formation on subendothelium in platelets deficient in glycoprotein GPIIb-IIIa and storage organelles. *Blood*, **67**, 322–31.

126 Weiss, H. J., Hawiger, J., Ruggeri, Z. M., Turitto, V. T., Thiagarajan, P., and Hoffmann, T. (1989). Fibrinogen-independent platelet adhesion and thrombus formation on subendothelium mediated by glycoprotein IIb-IIIa complex at high shear rate. *J. Clin. Invest.*, **83**, 288–97.

127 Colvin, R. B. (1989). Fibronectin in wound healing. In *Fibronectins* (ed. D. F. Mosher), pp. 213–54. Academic Press, San Diego.

128 Clark, R. A. F. (1990). Fibronectin matrix deposition and fibronectin receptor expression in healing and normal skin. *Invest. Dermatol.*, **6**, 128S–34S.

129 Knox, P., Crooks, S., and Rimmer, C. S. (1986). Role of fibronectin in the migration of fibroblasts into plasma clots. *Thromb. Haemostas*, **102**, 2318–23.

130 Mansfield, P. J., Boxer, L. A., and Suchard, S. J. (1990). Thrombospondin stimulates motility of human neutrophils. *J. Cell Biol.*, **111**, 3077–86.

131 Madri, J. A., Pratt, B. M., and Tucker, A. M. (1988). Phenotypic modulation of endothelial cells by transforming growth factor-β depends upon the composition and organization of the extracellular matrix. *J. Cell Biol.*, **106**, 1375–84.

132 Clark, R. A., DellaPelle, P., Manseau, E., Lanigan, J. M., Dvorak, H. F., and Colvin, R. B. (1982). Blood vessel fibronectin increases in conjuction with endothelial cell proliferation and capillary ingrowth during wound healing. *Invest. Dermatol.*, **79**, 269–76.

133 Loskutoff, D. J., Sawdey, M., and Mimuro, J. (1989). Type-1 plasminogen activator inhibitor. *Prog. Haemost. Thromb.*, **9**, 87–115.

134 Levin, E. G. and Santell, L. (1987). Association of a plasminogen activator inhibitor (PAI-1) with the growth substratum and membrane of human endothelial cells. *J. Cell Biol.*, **105**, 2543–9.

135 Wiman, B., Almquist, A., Sigurdardottir, O., and Lindahl, T. (1988). Plasminogen activator inhibitor-1 (PAI) is bound to vitronectin in plasma. *FEBS Lett.*, **242**, 125–8.

136 Declerck, P. J., De Mol, M., Alessi, M.-C., Baudner, S., Paques, E.-P., Preissner, K. T., Müller-Berghaus, G., and Collen, D. (1988). Purification and characterization of a plasminogen activator inhibitor-1 binding protein from human plasma. Identification as a multimeric form of S protein (vitronectin). *J. Biol. Chem.*, **263**, 15454–61.

137 Mimuro, J. and Loskutoff, D. J. (1989). Purification of a protein from bovine plasma that binds to type-1 plasminogen activator inhibitor and prevents its

interaction with extracellular matrix—evidence that the protein is vitronectin. *J. Biol. Chem.*, **264**, 936–9.

138 Preissner, K. T., Grulich-Henn, J., Ehrlich, H. J., Declerck, P., Justus, C., Collen, D., Pannekoek, H., and Müller-Berghaus, G. (1990). Structural requirements for the extracellular interaction of plasminogen activator inhibitor-1 with endothelial cell matrix-associated vitronectin. *J. Biol. Chem.*, **265**, 18490–8.

139 Seiffert, D., Wagner, N. N., and Loskutoff, D. J. (1990). Serum-derived vitronectin influences the pericellular distribution of type-1 plasminogen activator inhibitor. *J. Cell Biol.*, **111**, 1283–91.

140 Preissner, K. T., Holzhüter, S., Justus, C., and Müller-Berghaus, G. (1989). Identification and partial characterization of platelet vitronectin: evidence for complex formation with platelet-derived plasminogen activator inhibitor-1. *Blood,* **74**, 1989–96.

141 Ehrlich, H. J., Klein Gebbink, R., Keijer, J., Linders, M., Preissner, K. T., and Pannekoek, H. (1990). Alteration of serpin specificity by a protein cofactor. Vitronectin endows plasminogen activator inhibitor-1 with thrombin inhibitory properties. *J. Biol. Chem.*, **265**, 13029–35.

142 Ehrlich, H. J., Klein Gebbink, R., Preissner, K. T., Keijer, J., Esmon, N. L., Mertens, K., and Pannekoek, H. (1991). Thrombin neutralizes plasminogen activator inhibitor-1 (PAI-1) that is complexed with vitronectin in the endothelial-cell matrix. *J. Cell Biol.*, **115**, 1773–81.

143 Ciambrone, G. J. and McKeown-Longo, P. J. (1990). Plasminogen activator inhibitor type-1 stabilizes vitronectin-dependent adhesions in HT-1080 cells. *J. Cell Biol.*, **111**, 2183–95.

144 Ruggeri, Z. M. (1987). Classification of von Willebrand disease. In *Thrombosis and Haemostasis* (ed. M. Verstraete, J. Vermeylen, R. Lijnen, and J. Arnout), pp. 419–45. Leuven University Press, Leuven.

145 Marcus, A. J. (1991). Platelets and their disorders. In *Disorders of haemostasis* (ed. O. D. Ratnoff and C. D. Forbes), pp. 75–140. W. B. Saunders Company, Philadelphia.

146 Kishimoto, T. K., Hollander, N., Roberts, T. M., Anderson, D. C., and Springer, T. A. (1987). Heterogeneous mutations in the β subunit common to the LFA-1, Mac-1, and p150,95 glycoproteins cause leucocyte adhesion deficiency. *Cell*, **50**, 193–202.

147 Absolom, D. R. (1986). Opsonins and dysopsonins: an overview. *Meth. in Enzymol.*, **132**, 281–318.

148 Norris, D. A., Clark, R. A., Swigart, L. M., Huff, J. C., Westen, W. L., and Howell, S. E. (1982). Fibronectin fragment(s) are chemotactic for human peripheral blood monocytes. *J. Immunol.*, **129**, 1612–18.

149 LaFleur, M., Beaulieu, A. D., Kreis, C., and Poubell, P. (1987). Fibronectin gene expression in polymorphonuclear leucocytes. Accumulation of mRNA in inflammatory cells. *J. Biol. Chem.*, **262**, 2111–5.

150 Tskukamoto, Y., Helsel, W. E., and Wahl, S. M. (1981). Macrophage production of fibronectin, a chemoattractant for fibroblasts. *J. Immunol.*, **127**, 673–8.

151 Doherty, D. E., Henson, P. M., and Clark, R. A. F. (1990). Fibronectin fragments containing the RGDS cell-binding domain mediate monocyte migration into the rabbit lung. *J. Clin. Invest.*, **86**, 1065–75.

152 Basara, M. L., McCarthy, J. B., Barnes, D. W., and Furcht, L. T. (1985). Stimulation of haptotaxis and migration of tumour cells by serum spreading factor. *Cancer Res.*, **45**, 2487–94.

153 Marks, P. W., Hendey, B., and Maxfield, F. R. (1991). Attachment to fibronectin or vitronectin makes human neutrophil migration sensitive to alterations in cytosolic free calcium concentration. *J. Cell Biol.*, **112**, 149–58.

154 Thorens, B., Mermod, J. J., and Vassalli, P. (1987). Phagocytosis and inflammatory stimuli induce GM-CSF mRNA in macrophages through post-transcriptional regulation. *Cell*, **48**, 671–9.

155 Gresham, H. D., Graham, l. L., Anderson, D. C., and Brown, E. J. (1991). Leucocyte adhesion-deficient neutrophils fail to amplify phagocytic function in response to stimulation. Evidence for CD11b/CD18-dependent and independent mechanisms of phagocytosis. *J. Clin. Invest.*, **88**, 588–97.

156 Schultz, D. R. and Arnold, P. I. (1990). Properties of four actue phase proteins: C-reactive protein, serum amyloid A protein, α-acid glycoprotein, and fibrinogen. *Sem. Arthr. Rheum.*, **20**, 129–47.

157 Hörmann, H., Richter, H., and Jelinic, V. (1987). The role of fibronectin fragments and cell-attached transamidase on the binding of soluble fibrin to macrophages. *Thromb. Res.*, **46**, 39–50.

158 van de Water, L., Schroeder, S., Crenshaw, E. B., and Hynes, R. O. (1981). Phagocytosis of gelatin-latex particles by a murine macrophage line is dependent on fibronectin and heparin. *J. Cell Biol.*, **90**, 32–9.

159 Parker, C. J., Frame, R. N., and Elstad, M. R. (1988). Vitronectin (S protein) augments the functional activity of monocyte receptors for IgG and complement C3b. *Blood*, **71**, 86–93.

160 Vogel B. E., Tarone G., Giancotti F. G., Gailit J., and Ruoslahti E. (1990). A novel fibronectin receptor with an unexpected subunit composition. *J. Biol. Chem.*, **265**, 5934–7.

161 Wright, S. D., Craigmyle, L. S., and Silverstein, S. C. (1983). Fibronectin and serum amyloid P component stimulate C3b and C3bi-mediated phagocytosis in cultured human monocytes. *J. Exp. Med.*, **158**, 1338–43.

162 Proctor, R. A. (1987). Fibronectin: an enhancer of phagocyte function. *Rev. Infect. Dis.*, **9** (Suppl. 4), S412–19.

163 Detmers, P. A., Wright, S. D., Olsen, E., Kimball, B., and Cohn, Z. A. (1987). Aggregation of complement receptors on human neutrophils in the absence of ligand. *J. Cell Biol.*, **105**, 1137–45.

164 Chatila, T. A., Geha, R. S., and Arnaout, M. A. (1989). Constitutive and stimulus-induced phosphorylation of CD11/CD18 leucocyte adhesion molecules. *J. Cell Biol.*, **109**, 3435–44.

165 Altieri, D. C. and Edgington, T. S. (1988). The saturable high affinity association of factor X to ADP-stimulated monocytes defines a novel function of the Mac-1 receptor. *J. Biol. Chem.*, **263**, 7007–15.

166 Altieri, D. C. and Edgington, T. S. (1989). Sequential receptor cascade for coagulation proteins on monocytes. Constitutive biosynthesis and functional pro-thrombinase activity of a membrane form of factor V/Va. *J. Biol. Chem.*, **264**, 2969–72.

167 Masson, D. and Tschopp, J. (1987). A family of serine esterases in lytic granules of cytolytic T lymphocytes. *Cell*, **49**, 679–85.

168 Wyllie, A. H. (1987). Apoptosis: cell death in tissue regulation. *J. Pathol.*, **153**, 313–16.

169 Savill, J., Dransfield, I., Hogg, N., and Haslett, C. (1990). Vitronectin receptor-mediated phagocytosis of cells undergoing apoptosis. *Nature*, **343**, 180–3.

170 Fuquay, J. I., Loo, D. T., and Barnes, D. W. (1986). Binding of *Staphylococcus aureus* by human serum spreading factor in an *in vitro* assay. *Infect. Immun.*, **52**, 714–17.

171 Chhatwal, G. S. and Blobel, H. (1986). Binding of host plasma proteins to streptococci and their possible role in streptococcal pathogenicity. *IRCS Med. Sci.*, **14**, 1–3.

172 Proctor, R. A. (1990). Fibronectin–staphylococcal interactions in endovascular infections. *Zbl. Bakt.*, **274**, 342–9.

173 Kuusela, P., Vartio, T., Vuento, M., and Myhre, E. B. (1984). Binding sites for streptococci and staphylococci in fibronectin. *Infect. Immun.*, **45**, 433–6.

174 Chhatwal, G. S., Preissner, K. T., Müller-Berghaus, G., and Blobel, H. (1987). Specific binding of the human S protein (vitronectin) to streptococci, *Staphylococcus aureus*, and *Escherichia coli*. *Infect. Immun.*, **55**, 1878–83.

175 Vercellotti, G. M., Lussenhop, D., Peterson, P. K., Furcht, L. T., McCarthy, J. B., Jacob, H. S., and Moldow, C. F. (1984). Bacterial adherence to fibronectin and endothelial cells: a possible mechanism for bacterial tissue tropism. *J. Lab. Clin. Med.*, **103**, 34–43.

176 Signäs, C., Raucci, G., Jonsson, K., Lindgren, P. E., Anantharamaiah, G. M., Höök, M., and Lindberg, M. (1989). Nucleotide sequence of the gene for a fibronectin-binding protein from *Staphylococcus aureus* and its use in the synthesis of biologically active peptides. *Proc. Natl. Acad. Sci. U.S.A.*, **86**, 699–703.

177 Pottratz, S. T., Paulsrud, J., Smith, J. S., and Martin II, W. J. (1991). *Pneumocystis carinii* attachment to cultured lung cells by pneumocystis gp120, a fibronectin binding protein. *J. Clin. Invest.*, **88**, 403–7.

178 Olsén, A., Jonsson, A., and Normark, S. (1989). Fibronectin binding mediated by a novel class of surface organelles on *Escherichia coli*. *Nature*, **338**, 652–4.

179 Valentin-Weigand, P., Grulich-Henn, J., Chhatwal, G. S., Müller-Berghaus, G., Blobel, H., and Preissner, K. T. (1988). Mediation of adherence of streptococci to human endothelial cells by complement S protein (vitronectin). *Infect. Immun.*, **56**, 2851–5.

180 Filippsen, L. F., Valentin-Weigand, P., Blobel, H., Preissner, K. T., and Chhatwal, G. S. (1990). Role of complement S protein (vitronectin) in adherence of *Streptococcus dysgalactiae* to bovine epithelial cells. *Am. J. Vet. Res.*, **51**, 861–5.

181 Relman, D., Tuomanen, E., Falkow, S., Golenbock, D. T., Saukkonen, K., and Wright, S. D. (1990). Recognition of a bacterial adhesin by an integrin: macrophase CR3 (alphaMβ2, CD11b/CD18) binds filamentous haemagglutinin of *Bordetella pertussis*. *Cell*, **61**, 1375–82.

182 Isberg, R. R. and Leong, J. M. (1990). Multiple β1 chain integrins are receptors for invasin, a protein that promotes bacterial penetration into mammalian cells. *Cell*, **60**, 861–71.

183 Peters, J. H., Ginsberg, M. H., Bohl, B. P., Sklar, L. A., and Cochrane, C. G. (1986). Intravascular release of intact cellular fibronectin during oxidant-induced injury of the *in vitro* perfused rabbit lung. *J. Clin. Invest.*, **78**, 1596–603.

184 Müller-Eberhard, H. J. (1988). Molecular organization and function of the complement system. *Annu. Rev. Biochem.*, **57**, 321–47.

185 Podack, E. R. and Tschopp, J. (1984). Membrane attack by complement. *Mol. Immunol.*, **21**, 589–603.

186   Kolb, W. P. and Müller-Eberhard, H. J. (1975). The membrane attack mechanism of complement. Isolation and subunit composition of the C5b–9 complex. *J. Exp. Med.*, **141**, 724–35.

187   McLeod, B., Baker, P., and Gewurz, H. (1975). Studies on the inhibition of C56-initiated lysis (reactive lysis). III. Characterization of the inhibitory activity C567-Inh and its mode of action. *Immunology*, **28**, 133–49.

188   Lint, T. F., Behrends, C. L., and Gewurz, H. (1977). Serum lipoproteins and C567-Inh activity. *J. Immunol.*, **119**, 883–8.

189   Podack, E. R. and Müller-Eberhard, H. J. (1978). Binding of deoxycholate, phosphatidylcholine vesicles, lipoprotein, and of the S protein to complexes of terminal complement components. *J. Immunol.*, **121**, 1025–30.

190   Preissner, K. T., Podack, E. R., and Müller-Eberhard, H. J. (1985). The membrane attack complex of complement: relation of C7 to the metastable membrane binding site of the intermediate complex C5b–7. *J. Immunol.*, **135**, 445–51.

191   Bhakdi, S. and Tranum-Jensen, J. (1983). Molecular composition of the terminal membrane and fluid-phase C5b–9 complexes of rabbit complement. *Biochem. J.*, **209**, 753–61.

192   Ware, C. F., Wetsel, R. A., and Kolb, W. P. (1981). Physicochemical characterization of fluid-phase (SC5b–9) and membrane derived (MC5b–9) attack complexes of human complement purified by immunoadsorbent affinity chromatography or selective detergent extraction. *Mol. Immunol.*, **18**, 521–31.

193   Preissner, K. T., Podack, E. R., and Müller-Eberhard, H. J. (1989). SC5b–7, SC5b–8, and SC5b–9 complexes of complement: ultrastructure and localization of the S protein (vitronectin) within the macromolecules. *Eur. J. Immunol.*, **19**, 69–75.

194   Bhakdi, S., Bhakdi-Lehnen, B., and Tranum-Jensen, J. (1979). Proteolytic transformation of SC5b–9 into an amphiphilic macromolecule resembling the C5b–9 membrane attack complex of complement. *Immunology*, **37**, 901–12.

195   Bhakdi, S. and Tranum-Jensen, J. (1982). Hydrophilic–amphiphilic transition of the terminal SC5b–8 complement complex through tryptic modification: biochemical and ultrastructural studies. *Mol. Immunol.*, **19**, 1167–77.

196   Podack, E. R. and Müller-Eberhard, H. J. (1980). SC5b–9 complex of complement: formation of the dimeric membrane attack complex by removal of S protein. *J. Immunol.*, **124**, 1779–83.

197   Bhakdi, S., Käflein, R., Halstensen, T. S., Hugo, F., Preissner, K. T., and Mollnes, T. E. (1988). Complement S protein (vitronectin) is associated with cytolytic membrane-bound C5b–9 complexes. *Clin. Exp. Immunol.*, **74**, 459–64.

198   Tschopp, J., Masson, D., Schäfer, S., Peitsch, M., and Preissner, K. T. (1988). The heparin binding domain of S protein/vitronectin binds to complement components C7, C8, C9, and perforin from cytolytic T cells and inhibits their lytic activities. *Biochemistry*, **27**, 4103–9.

199   Baker, P. J., Lint, T. F., McLeod, B., Behrends, C. L., and Gewurz, H. (1975). Studies on the inhibition of C56-induced lysis (reactive lysis). VI. Modulation of C56-induced lysis by polyanions and polycations. *J. Immunol.*, **114**, 554–8.

200   Tschopp, J. and Mollnes, T. E. (1986). Antigenic cross-reactivity of the β subunit of complement component C8 with the cysteine-rich domain shared by complement component C9 and low density lipoprotein receptor. *Proc. Natl. Acad. Sci. U.S.A.*, **83**, 4223–7.

201 Murphy, B. F., Kirszbaum, L., Walker, I. D., and d'Apice, A. J. F. (1988). SP40–40, a newly identified normal human serum protein found in the SC5b–9 complex of complement and in the immune deposits in glomerulonephritis. *J. Clin. Invest.*, **81**, 1858–64.

202 Jenne, D. E. and Tschopp, J. (1989). Molecular structure and functional characterization of a human complement cytolysis inhibitor found in blood and seminal plasma: identity to sulfated glycoprotein-2, a constituent of rat testis fluid. *Proc. Natl. Acad. Sci. U.S.A.*, **86**, 7123–7.

203 Jenne, D. E., Lowin, B., Peitsch, M. C., Böttcher, A., Schmitz, G., and Tschopp, J. (1991). Clusterin (complement lysis inhibitor) forms a high density lipoprotein complex with apolipoprotein AI in human plasma. *J. Biol. Chem.*, **266**, 11030–6.

204 Murphy, B. F., Davies, D. J., Morrow, W., and d'Apice, A. J. F. (1989). Localization of terminal complement components, S protein, and SP40–40 in renal biopsies. *Pathology*, **21**, 275–8.

205 Zalman, L. S., Wood, L. M., and Müller-Eberhard, H. J. (1986). Isolation of a human erythrocyte membrane protein capable of inhibiting expression of homologous complement transmembrane channels. *Proc. Natl. Acad. Sci. U.S.A.*, **83**, 6975–9.

206 Schönermark, S., Rauterberg, E. W., Shin, M. L., Loke, S., Roelcke, D., and Hänsch, G. M. (1986). Homologous species restriction in lysis of human erythrocytes: a membrane-derived protein with C8-binding capacity functions as an inhibitor. *J. Immunol.*, **136**, 1772–6.

207 Sugita, Y., Nakano, Y., and Tomita, M. (1988). Isolation from human erythrocytes of a new membrane protein which inhibits the formation of complement transmembrane channels. *J. Biochem.*, **104**, 633–7.

208 Holguin, M. H., Frederick, L. R., Bernshaw, N. J., Wilcox, L. A., and Parker, C. J. (1989). Isolation and characterization of a membrane protein from normal human erythrocytes that inhibits reactive lysis of the erythrocytes of paroxysmal nocturnal haemoglobinuria. *J. Clin Invest.*, **84**, 7–17.

209 Davies, A., Simmons, D. L., Hale, G., Harrison, R. A., Tighe, H., Lachmann, P. J., and Waldmann, H. (1989). CD59, an LY-6-like protein expressed in human lymphoid cells, regulates the action of the complement membrane attack complex on homologous cells. *J. Exp. Med.*, **170**, 637–54.

210 Rollins, S. A. and Sims, P. J. (1990). The complement-inhibitory activity of CD59 resides in its capacity to block incorporation of C9 into membrane C5b–9. *J. Immunol.*, **144**, 3478–83.

211 Meri, S., Morgan, B. P., Davies, A., Daniels, R. H., Olavesen, M. G., Waldmann, H., and Lachmann, P. J. (1990). Human protein (CD59), an 18 000–20 000 MW complement lysis restricting factor, inhibits C5b–8 catalysed insertion of C9 into lipid bilayers. *Immunology*, **71**, 1–9.

212 Rosse W. F. (1990). Phosphatidylinositol-linked proteins and paroxysmal nocturnal haemoglobinuria. *Blood*, **75**, 1595–601.

213 Hänsch, G. M., Schönermark, S., and Roelcke, D. (1987). Paroxysmal nocturnal haemoglobinuria type III. Lack of an erythrocyte membrane protein restricting the lysis by C5b–9. *J. Clin. Invest.*, **80**, 7–12.

214 Salama, A., Preissner, K. T., Goettsche, B., Müller-Berghaus, G., and Mueller-Eckhardt, C. (1988). Complement inhibitor S protein is associated with membranes of red blood cells from patients with paroxysmal nocturnal haemoglobinuria. *Br. J. Haematol.*, **68**, 41–5.

215 Morgan, B. P. (1989). Complement membrane attack on nucleated cell: resistance, recovery, and non-lethal effects. *Biochem.*, **264**, 1–14.

216 Sims, P. J., Wiedmer, T., Esmon, C. T., Weiss, H. J., and Shattil, S. J. (1989). Assembly of the platelet pro-throminase complex is linked to vesiculation of the platelet plasma membrane. *J. Biol. Chem.*, **264**, 17049–57.

217 Hamilton, K. K., Hattori, R., Esmon, C. T., and Sims, P. J. (1990). Complement proteins C5b–9 induce vesiculation of the endothelial plasma membrane and expose catalytic surface for assembly of the pro-thrombinase enzyme complex. *J. Biol. Chem.*, **265**, 3809–14.

12 Eicosanoids in defence

J. STANKOVA AND M. ROLA-PLESZCZYNSKI

1 Introduction

Specific immune responses in the host are most often preceded or accompanied by non-specific inflammation. Such inflammation may be triggered by numerous substances, including infectious agents, toxic material, foreign particles, or cells. It may and often does significantly affect the natural defence mechanisms of the host, as well as its more sophisticated specific immune responses.

With the identification of many molecular and cellular components of the inflammatory response, investigators have initiated studies of the interactions that link inflammation and immunity. In particular, soluble mediators of inflammation, produced by phagocytes, endothelial cells, platelets, and many other cell types, have been studied in regard to their possible modulation of lymphocyte, monocyte/macrophage, and neutrophil functions. In this chapter, we will focus on eicosanoids, derived from the oxidative metabolism of arachidonic acid. Whenever possible, we will include comparisons of their actions with those of another lipid mediator, PAF, described in greater detail in the following chapter.

1.1 Eicosanoids: production and biological activities

Following membrane perturbations and activation of phospholipase A_2 (PLA_2), arachidonic acid is released from membrane phospholipids. When the latter consist of arachidonoyl-phosphatidylcholine, arachidonic acid and lyso-PAF, the precursor of PAF, are produced simultaneously. Arachidonic acid undergoes oxygenation either by cyclo-oxygenase, which results in the formation of the various prostaglandins (PG), or by one of several lipoxygenases. Leukotrienes (LT) (1) are derived from the action of 5-lipoxygenase (5-LO), which becomes activated, after translocation to the membrane, by the 5-LO activating protein (FLAP) (2). The initial 5-LO metabolite of arachidonic acid is 5-hydroperoxyeicosatetraenoic (5-HPETE) acid, followed by LTA_4. LTB_4, which is an enzymically produced, hydrolytic product of LTA_4 differs from the other leukotrienes LTC_4, LTD_4 and LTE_4 in that it has no peptidic component. LTB_4 is a more stable molecule than the peptido-leukotrienes, but can be rapidly degraded through omega-oxidation by polymorphonuclear leucocytes (PMN) to the relatively less active metabolites, $20-OH-LTB_4$ and $20-COOH-LTB_4$ (3). The combined activities of

5-LO and 15-LO can give rise to a family of trihydroxytetraene compounds called lipoxins (4) (Figure 12.1).

While sharing some of the myotropic properties of the other leukotrienes, LTB_4 has been found to exert very strong leucocytotropic activities. It is one of the most powerful chemokinetic (5) and chemotactic (6) agents, and it can induce neutrophil aggregation (5), degranulation (7), hexose uptake (8), and enhanced binding to endothelial cells (9). It can also induce cation fluxes (10), augment cytoplasmic calcium concentrations from intracellular pools (11, 12), and activate phosphatidylinositol hydrolysis (13, 14). LTB_4 can also synergize with prostaglandins E_1 and E_2 in causing macromolecule leakage in the skin, through increased vascular permeability (15), and when injected into guinea pig skin, it induces leucocytoclastic vasculitis (16). Two sets of plasma membrane receptors for LTB_4 have been described on human neutrophils (17). The high affinity receptor set mediates aggregation, chemokinesis, and increased adherence to surfaces, while the low affinity receptor set mediates degranulation and increased oxidative metabolism. In contrast to human cells, rat leucocytes lack the lower affinity receptor (18). Signal transduction via high affinity receptors appears to involve a guanine nucleotide regulatory protein (19). In contrast, little is known at present about potential LTB_4 receptors on lymphocytes, although a fraction of $CD4^+$ and $CD8^+$ T cells bind LTB_4 (20).

LTB_4 is rapidly synthesized by phagocytic cells, principally neutrophils (1) and alveolar macrophages (21), upon challenge with a variety of stimuli such as microbial pathogens (22), toxins, aggregated immunoglobulin (23), particulate material (24), or ionophores, especially when exogenous arachido-

PHOSPHOLIPID METABOLITES

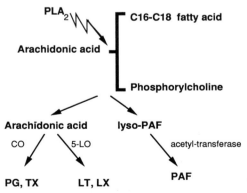

Fig. 12.1 Metabolic pathways which convert membrane phospholipids to arachidonic acid and its metabolites, on the one hand, and to PAF on the other. PLA_2, phospholipase A_2; CO, cyclo-oxygenase; 5-LO, 5-lipoxygenase; PG, prostaglandins; TX, thromboxane A_2; LT, leukotrienes; LX, lipoxins; PAF, platelet activating factor.

nic acid is available (Figure 12.2). Its synthesis can also be induced by platelet-derived 12-HPETE (25) or PAF-acether (26, 27). Certain cell types, which lack 5-LO activity, can still produce LTB_4 from LTA_4 received from other cells. This transcellular biosynthetic pathway appears to be operative in red blood cells and endothelial cells which contain LTA_4 hydrolase but no 5-LO (28, 29). Similarly, human T cells and B cells, as well as some lymphocytic cell lines have been shown to convert LTA_4 to LTB_4, while failing to produce LTB_4 following stimulation with ionophore alone (30).

Effective cell separation techniques suggest that LTB_4 is not a product of lymphocytes (31–33), in spite of several earlier reports to the contrary. Under a variety of situations, LTB_4 seems to be found in lymphocyte cultures only in the presence of contaminating monocytes (32). That the gene(s) involved in LT synthesis may be derepressed is suggested however by the observed production of LTC_4 by a human hybridoma formed by fusing $CD8^+$ T cells with CEM-6 lymphoma ($CD4^+$) cells (34). With the use of 5-LO and FLAP cDNA probes, T cells were found not to express either gene product under normal conditions (35).

LTB_4 has been detected in significant concentrations in inflammatory synovial exudates (36), psoriatic skin lesions (37), peritonitis (38), and inflammatory bowel disease (39).

Cytotoxic cells and their various effector mechanisms are thought to play an important role in host defences against a whole array of foreign invaders, including parasites, viruses, neoplastic and grafted cells. Many effector cell types (T cells, NK cells and other natural cytotoxic lymphocytes, macrophages, polymorphonuclear leucocytes) participate in these functions and, while many of the effector mechanisms appear distinct, they are still largely undefined.

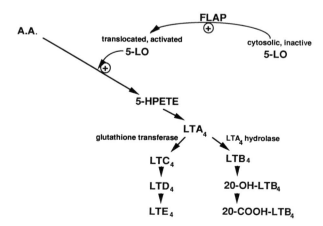

Fig. 12.2 Metabolic pathways leading from arachidonic acid to the formation of leukotrienes. A.A., arachidonic acid; FLAP, five-lipoxygenase activating protein; 5-LO, 5-lipoxygenase; LT, leukotriene.

2   Lymphocyte-mediated natural defences

Non-MHC restricted lymphocyte-mediated natural defences involve both NK cells and natural cytotoxic (NC) lymphocytes, as well as some cytotoxic T cells. NK cell cytotoxicity is measured over four hours using classically the human erythroleukaemia K562 cell line or the murine YAC-1 cell line as targets. NK cytotoxicity involves effector-target cell contact and soluble factors such as proteases, pore-forming protein, and NK cytotoxic factor(s). In contrast, NC activity is measured using solid tumour targets, usually over 18 hours and $TNF\alpha$ production is measured (40). Several lines of evidence indicate that NK cell activation involves membrane phospholipid metabolism and we and others have described the modulation of NK cell functions by arachidonic acid metabolites.

2.1   Modulation by leukotrienes

Among its various effects on lymphocytes, LTB_4 was shown to modulate the activity of both NK and NC cells. NC activity was measured using MA-160 target cells infected with herpes simplex virus type 1. At concentrations of $10^{-12}-10^{-8}$ M, LTB_4 and, to a lesser extent, LTA_4, markedly augmented NK and NC activities (41, 42). The relatively non-specific lipoxygenase inhibitor nordihydroguaiaretic acid (NDGA) inhibited NC activity and this inhibition could be effectively reversed by LTB_4, indicating that, under these conditions, exogenous lipoxygenase products could overcome lipoxygenase inhibition (43). Other laboratories have also shown that lipoxygenase inhibitors could reversibly block NK activity (44–46). However, while human NK cells pre-treated with interferons or poly I:C are partially resistant to suppression by lipoxygenase inhibitors (46), lymphokine (IL-2) activated killer (LAK) cells can be reversibly inhibited by those drugs (47). LTB_4 acted on effector NK or NC lymphocytes rather than on their target cells, as demonstrated by pre-incubation experiments (48). LTB_4 was also shown to increase both the binding of effector lymphocytes to their target cells and the rate of target cell killing. These effects were rapid, within 30 minutes for binding and two hours for lysis of target cells. No IL-2 or $IFN\gamma$ was detectable in these cultures (48).

In contrast to LTB_4, lipoxins which can antagonize several activities of LT (49), have been shown to inhibit NK cell activity by affecting a post-binding event in effector–target cell interactions, possibly the generation of a lytic signal (50).

2.2   Modulation by prostaglandins and thromboxane A_2

Both PGE_2 and PGI_2 are known to inhibit mitogen-induced lymphocyte proliferation (51), cytokine production (52–54), and NK cell activity (55–57). The latter appears to be due to a decrease of NK target cell binding linked with induction of cAMP by PG. We have also shown them to inhibit NC cell function (58). Interestingly, while inhibitors of CO often enhance NK and NC cell activities, inhibition of the thromboxane (TX) A_2 pathway by specific inhibitors, such as dazoxiben or OKY-1581, significantly inhibited NC and NK cell functions (68). This appeared to be due to reorientation of cyclic endoperoxide metabolism toward the more inhibitory mediators PGE_2 and PGI_2 (59). On the other hand, U44069, a TXA_2 analogue, was also inhibitory by itself at high concentrations, while it caused a modest enhancement of NC activity at concentrations below 10^{-8} M. As with PGE_2, these effects may be related to differential involvement of cyclic nucleotides.

2.3   Modulation by PAF

Preliminary data from several laboratories suggest that PAF may play a role during certain cytotoxic activities, in as much as PAF receptor antagonists inhibit them. Thus the antagonist BN 52021 can inhibit rat splenic lympho-cyte-mediated lysis of Langerhan islet cells (60). In other non-lymphocyte systems, keratinocyte killing of *Candida albicans* (61) and eosinophil-mediated cytotoxicity against *Schistosoma mansoni* (62) were also found to be blocked by the PAF antagonist.

When human monocyte-depleted lymphocytes were cultured with the NK-sensitive K562 target cells in the presence of graded concentrations of PAF, we found NK activity to be significantly enhanced (32 to 110 per cent) at all effector:target cell ratios, but predominantly at lower ratios (63, 64). Peak activity was found at PAF concentrations of 10^{-13} to 10^{-11} M, and this was not blocked by the PAF antagonist BN 52021. In contrast, PAF concentra-tions of 10^{-7} or greater were often associated with inhibition of NK activity, with reversal using PAF antagonists. While optimal enhancement was observed when PAF was added at the initiation of the cytotoxicity co-culture, or within the first 30 minutes, significant enhancement was also seen when PAF was added as late as one hour into the culture. Lymphocytes could also be pre-incubated for one to 18 hours with PAF, followed by washing to avoid inter-action of PAF with target cells, and significant enhancement of NK activity still ensued. Both binding of lymphocytes to K562 cells and post-binding single cell lytic efficiency were augmented by PAF (64). Mandi *et al.* (65) reported a marked inhibition of both rat and human NK cell function by BN 52021.

Although impossible to verify at the present time, the above findings could be explained by the presence of two PAF receptors on NK cells, one with a lower affinity, which would be linked with inhibition of cell function, and another with high affinity, linked with augmentation of cell function. The recent cloning of a guinea pig PAF receptor may help shed some light on the potential existence of more than one PAF receptor (66).

Recently, we studied the modulation of lung NK cell activity by PAF and the mechanisms involved in this regulation. Rat lung large granular lymphocytes (LGL) showed an enhanced NK cell activity when cultured with PAF (67): peak effect was observed at 10^{-9} M PAF. Both short-term (one hour) and longer-term (18 hours) pre-incubation of LGL with PAF resulted in augmented NK activity. The 18 hour pre-treatment involved protein synthesis since cycloheximide could inhibit the PAF-induced effect. The mechanisms of activation also appeared to involve protein kinase C, 5-LO, and extracellular Ca^{2+}, as suggested by inhibition of the PAF-induced effect with PKC and 5-LO inhibitors, and Ca^{2+} channel blockers, respectively (67).

In several transplantation models, PAF appears to act as a pro-rejection mediator (68). BN 52021 increases cardiac allograft survival in rats, acting synergistically with azathioprine and cyclosporine A (69). Analogous findings are also reported with skin, liver, and kidney grafts. The mechanism(s) and cells involved in these phenomena in relation to PAF are essentially unknown at this time.

3   Monocyte/macrophage-mediated effects

When appropriately stimulated, monocytes and macrophages can produce a variety of cytokines (discussed below in this chapter) as well as inhibiting tumour cell growth or destroying susceptible target cells (70).

3.1   Modulation by leukotrienes and prostaglandins

The potential regulatory role of endogenous and exogenous LT on mono-cyte/macrophage functions has come under study, in view of the findings that LT are synthesized and released by these cells following immunological and non-immunological stimuli (as indicated earlier in this chapter). For instance, as assessed by use of lipoxygenase inhibitors, activation of macro-phage phagocytic capacity by endotoxins seems to be dependent on lipoxygenase metabolites of arachidonic acid (71). LTs have also been shown to induce the release of PGs and lysosomal enzymes by macrophages (72–74).

When mouse resident peritoneal macrophages were co-cultured with MOPC-315 myeloma cells for 42 hours, the cytostatic activity of the former was measured by the inhibition of [^{3}H] thymidine uptake by the latter during the last 18 hours of the co-culture (75). In this system, LTD_4 at concentrations of 10^{-6} and 10^{-7} M caused a modest augmentation of macrophage cytostatic activity. Indomethacin alone also induced an enhanced cytostatic activity and both LTD_4 and indomethacin were additive in causing a marked (>80 per cent) inhibition of tumour cell proliferation (75, 76).

Human peripheral blood monocytes can lyse several types of tumour target cells, as indicated by the release of ^{51}Cr from the targets following an 18–24 hour co-culture. When they were incubated with increasing concentrations of LTB_4 during an 18 hour micro-cytotoxicity assay, we observed a very significant augmentation of monocyte-mediated cytotoxicity against K562 target cells (77). The strongest augmentation of cytotoxicity was seen at concentrations of 10^{-12} to 10^{-8} M. In contrast, a 10^{-6} M concentration of LTB$_4$ inhibited cytotoxic activity, without evidence of toxicity, as determined by trypan blue exclusion. Superimposable findings were observed when we used P815 mastocytoma cells as targets for monocyte cytotoxicity (77).

Since binding of effector cells to target cells is the initial step in cell-mediated cytotoxicity, we measured effector–target conjugate formation in the presence or absence of LTB$_4$ to determine whether this initial step was affected by LTB$_4$. Our results showed that LTB$_4$ (10^{-8} M) doubled the binding of human monocytes to K562 target cells (77). Following the initial binding of effector cells to target cells, the lytic signal transmitted to the target cell may be composed of cytotoxic factor(s), to be found in culture supernatants. When monocytes were incubated (18 hours) in the presence of increasing concentrations of LTB$_4$ (10^{-14} to 10^{-8} M), we observed an augmentation in the rate of killing of K562 target cells by the culture supernatants (77). LTB$_4$, by itself, had no effect on K562 cell viability.

Inhibitors of cyclo-oxygenase (indomethacin, 10^{-6} M) and lipoxygenase (NDGA and BW755C, 10^{-5} M) induced a modest enhancement and a marked inhibition, respectively, in monocyte-mediated cytotoxicity. Exogenous LTB$_4$ could restore by 75–110 per cent the activity inhibited by NDGA (77). These findings corroborate those of others (78, 79) indicating that PGs, possibly through activation of adenylate cyclase, inhibit cytotoxic functions of mononuclear phagocytes, as they do that of NK cells. In contrast, both endogenous and exogenous LT have a positive effect on cytotoxic functions.

3.2 Modulation by PAF

Although several studies are in progress to assess the effects of PAF in monocyte/macrophage-mediated cytotoxicity, relatively little is known at the present time. Valone *et al.* (80) reported enhanced human monocyte-mediated cytotoxicity in response to PAF. In contrast, Bonavida *et al.* (81) suggested that the presence of TNF inhibitors may be responsible for lack of cytotoxicity in the face of enhanced TNF production by human monocytes in response to PAF. In our hands, PAF treated rat alveolar macrophages show augmented killing of P815 (TNF-resistant) target cells and WEHI-164 (TNF-sensitive) targets (see Chapter 4).

4 Cytokine-mediated natural defences

Host defence mechanisms involve not only cells such as lymphocytes, macrophages, and other leucocytes, as well as parenchymal cells, but also a whole array of soluble cell products. The interactions of eicosanoids with other humoral factors in defence is only beginning to be unravelled.

4.1   Modulation of TNF production by leukotrienes

Tumour necrosis factor alpha (TNF) is a potent mediator of cytotoxic activity exerted by monocytes and macrophages (see Chapter 4), and possibly natural cytotoxic (NC) lymphocytes. LTB_4 markedly enhances cytotoxicity mediated by NC cells and monocyte-mediated cytotoxicity is also augmented by LTB_4 (see above sections). To further define the underlying mechanism(s), we studied the effect of LTB_4 on TNF production by human monocytes, as measured by lysis of L929 target cells (77). Addition of 10^{-14}–10^{-8} M LTB_4 to monocyte cultures enhanced TNF activity in the supernatant after 24 hours by an average of 50 per cent with maximal enhancement at 10^{-10}–10^{-8} M LTB_4. Higher concentrations of LTB_4 were inhibitory. Kinetic studies indicated a maximal effect during the first eight hours of incubation. Addition of indomethacin to the cultures augmented TNF production, while addition of the lipoxygenase inhibitor NDGA diminished TNF production (82). These data suggest that LTB_4 may affect the cytotoxic activity of human monocytes, at least in part, by augmenting their production of the cytolytic cytokine TNF.

Alveolar macrophages can play a crucial role in the host natural defence. When exposed to asbestos fibres or silica particles, alveolar macrophage produce large amounts of TNF (24). They also produce LTB_4 and their pre-treatment with 5-LO inhibitors stops both LTB_4 and TNF production. These findings suggest that 5-LO metabolites, including LTB_4, may play a major role as 'second messengers' in TNF production by alveolar macrophage.

Endogenous lipoxygenase metabolites may also be involved in enhanced TNF production and TNFα gene expression following other stimuli, such as PAF (83), LPS (84), phorbol esters, or TNF itself (85–87). Under the latter conditions, inhibition of PLA_2 by bromophenacyl bromide or quinacrine, or of lipoxygenases by ketoconazole or NDGA results in inhibition of TNF mRNA accumulation and TNF gene transcription (85-87). Furthermore, exogenous LTB_4 can increase TNF mRNA (86). In contrast, inhibition of 5-LO activation using MK-886, which binds the five-lipoxygenase-activating protein (FLAP), does not affect TNFα production in response to phorbol ester, concanavalin A, LPS, or zymosan (88). Interestingly, the dual CO/5-LO inhibitor, tebufelone, at 20–25 μM, inhibits TNF mRNA accumulation while enhancing TNF protein production (89).

4.2   Modulation of TNF production by PG

In comparison to 5-LO metabolites, CO metabolites such as PGE_2 have been shown to inhibit TNF production at high concentrations (90), presumably by augmenting cAMP levels in the cells. Low concentrations of PGE_2, however, appear to stimulate guanylate cyclase and result in augmented TNF production (91, 92). TNF mRNA accumulation can also be inhibited by PGE_2 (93), an effect associated with decreased TNF transcription (85) (Figure 12.3).

4.3   Modulation of TNF and NK cell cytotoxic factor production by PAF

Following the observations that PAF could modulate NK cell activity, additional studies were undertaken to assess whether this effect was associated with the production of cytotoxic cytokines. To do so, LGL, which contain most of NK and NC activity, were incubated with various target cell lines, in the presence or absence of PAF. Supernatants were collected and assayed for cytotoxicity in a 20 hour ^{51}Cr release assay against WEHI 164 and U937 target cells which are sensitive to cytotoxic cytokines. The results showed that LGL, incubated with target cells in the presence of PAF, released significantly increased amounts of cytotoxic factors (94). The maximal release was obtained after 8 to 10 hours of incubation. Mannose-6-phosphate, which inhibits NK cell cytotoxic factor, was not able to block supernatant cytotoxicity against U937 target cells, while anti-TNF antibody completely abolished supernatant activity. These findings suggest that picomolar concentrations of PAF enhance the release of cytotoxic factor(s), mainly TNF, by LGL following interaction with target cells.

The concomitant addition of PAF and muramyl dipeptide to rat alveolar macrophage cultures markedly enhanced TNF production in a concentration-dependent fashion with peak effect at 10^{-10} M PAF (83, 94). This enhancement occurred when muramyl dipeptide and PAF were present together at

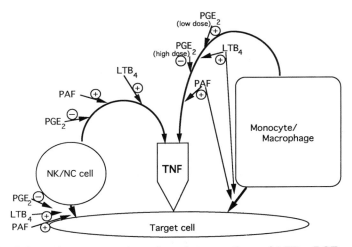

Fig. 12.3   Schematic representation of regulatory actions of LTB_4, PGE_2, and PAF in natural defence mechanisms.

the initiation of the 24 hour culture. Stimulation of TNF production by PAF was blocked by specific PAF receptor antagonists, BN 52020, BN 52021, and WEB 2086. Additionally, the stereoisomer of PAF, [S]PAF, and the biologically inactive precursor/metabolite of PAF, lyso-PAF, used at 10^{-10}–10^{-12} M failed to induce significant enhancement in TNF production. In parallel, addition of PAF to alveolar macrophage triggered LTB_4 release in a concentration-dependent manner. Inhibition of 5-LO by NDGA or AA-861 blocked the PAF-induced augmentation of both TNF and LTB_4 production. These findings suggest that PAF stimulates TNF production in alveolar macrophage by interaction with a specific putative receptor and by subsequent induction of endogenous leukotriene production.

Human monocytes or macrophages can also be stimulated by PAF to produce augmented quantities of TNF (80, 94–96). TNF production is enhanced at two concentration ranges of PAF, 10^{-15}–10^{-13} M and 10^{-9}–10^{-7} M in LPS or MDP treated monocytes. WEB 2086 blocks both effects, while pertussis toxin partially inhibits the effect of higher PAF concentrations, suggesting a mediation through a N_i type guanine nucleotide (G_i) regulatory protein. Because denser, less differentiated monocytes respond to PAF with a single, higher concentration peak, we studied the human pro-myelocytic HL-60 cell line, during differentiation towards the macrophage lineage with $1,25(OH)_2$ vitamin D_3. While undifferentiated HL-60 cells failed to respond to PAF in terms of TNF production, partially differentiated cells responded only to the nanomolar concentrations of PAF, while fully differentiated cells responded to both concentration ranges (96). A similar bimodal effect of PAF was observed in human monocytes when IL-1 production was measured (97). Evidence has also been obtained which suggests the existence of two types of PAF receptors on guinea pig eosinophils (98).

PAF, or IL-1, can prime monocytes to respond to LPS with enhanced production of TNF during a subsequent culture with IL-1 or PAF, respectively (99, 100). These findings suggest again that a cascade of inflammatory signals may have much greater effects than simultaneous or individual activities. Analogous findings have been reported in PMN primed with PAF, TNF, or endotoxin (101–103).

5   Conclusions

The ability of lipoxygenase products, mainly leukotriene B_4, to participate in inflammatory and immunoregulatory processes, and to modulate cytokine production has been previously documented (104). Exogenous and endogenous LTB_4 was found to enhance IL-2, IL-6, and IFNγ production in lymphocytes, in addition to the cytokines described in this chapter and their potential participation in defence may contribute to the global network linking mediators of inflammation with mediators of more specific immune responses.

Acknowledgement

The authors' work was supported by a grant from the National Cancer Institute of Canada.

References

1 Borgeat, P. and Samuelsson, B. (1979). Transformation of arachidonic acid by rabbit polymorphonuclear leucocytes: formation of a novel dihydro-eicosatetraenoic acid. *J. Biol. Chem.*, **254**, 2643–6.

2 Miller, D. K., Gillard, J. W., Vickers, P. J., Sadowski, S., Léveillé, C., Mancini, J. A., Charleson, P., Dixon, R. A. F., Ford-Hutchinson, A. W., Fortin, R., Gauthier, J. Y., Rodkey J., Rosen, R., Rouzer, C., Sigal, I. S., Strader, C. D., and Evans, J. F. (1990). Identification and isolation of a membrane protein necessary for leukotriene production. *Nature*, **343**, 278–81.

3 Shak, S. and Goldstein I. M. (1984). Omega-oxidation is the major pathway for the catabolism of leukotriene B$_4$ in human polymorphonuclear leucocytes. *J. Biol. Chem.*, **259**, 10181–7.

4 Serhan, C. N., Hamberg, M., and Samuelsson, B. (1984). Lipoxin: novel series of biologically active compounds formed from arachidonic acid in human leucocytes. *Proc. Nat. Acad. Sci. U.S.A.*, **81**, 5335–9.

5 Ford-Hutchinson, A. W., Bray, M. A., Doig, M. V., Shipley, M. E., and Smith, M. J. H. (1980). Leukotriene B, a potent chemokinetic and aggregating substance released from polymorphonuclear leucocytes. *Nature*, **286**, 264–5.

6 Palmblad, J., Malmsten, C. L., Uden, A. M., Radmar, K. O., Engstedt, L., and Samuelsson, B. (1981). Leukotriene B$_4$ is a potent stereospecific stimulator of neutrophil chemotaxis and adherence. *Blood*, **58**, 658–65.

7 Showell, H. J., Naccache, P. H., Borgeat, P., Picard, S., Valerand, P., Becker, E. L., and Sha'afi, R. I. (1982). Characterization of the secretory activity of LTB$_4$ toward rabbit neutrophils. *J. Immunol.*, **128**, 811–16.

8 Bass, D. A., Thomas, M. J., Goetzl, E. J., DeChatelet, E. R., and McCall, C. E. (1981). Lipoxygenase-derived products of arachidonic acid mediate stimulation of hexose uptake in human polymorphonuclear leucocytes. *Biochem. Biophys. Res. Commun.*, **100**, 1–6.

9 Bray, M. A., Ford-Hutchinson, A. W., and Smith, M. J. H. (1981). Leukotriene B$_4$: an inflammatory mediator *in vivo*. *Prostaglandins*, **22**, 213–19.

10 Molski, T. F. P., Naccache, P. H., Borgeat, P., and Sha'afi, R. I. (1981). Similarities in the mechanisms by which formylmethionyl-leucyl-phenylalanine, arachidonic acid, and leukotriene B$_4$ increase calcium and sodium influxes in rabbit neutrophils. *Biochem. Biophys. Res. Commun.*, **103**, 227–34.

11 Lew, D. P., Dayer, J.-M., Wollheim, C. B., and Pozzan, T. (1984). Effect of leukotriene B$_4$ and arachidonic acid on cytosolic-free calcium in human neutrophils. *FEBS Lett.*, **166**, 44–7.

12 Goldman, D. W., Gifford, L. A., Olson, D. M., and Goetzl, E. J. (1985). Transduction by leukotriene B$_4$ receptors of increases in cytosolic calcium in human polymorphonuclear leucocytes. *J. Immunol.*, **135**, 525–29.

13 Andersson, T., Schlegel, W., Monod, A., Krause, K-H., Stendahl, O., and Lew, D. P. (1986). Leukotriene B_4 stimulation of phagocytes results in the formation of inositol-1, 4, 5-triphosphate. *Biochem. J.*, **240**, 333–8.

14 Mong, S., Chi-Rosso, G., Miller, J., Hoffman, K., Raggaitis, K. A., Bender, P., and Crooke, S. T. (1986). Leukotriene B_4 induces formation of inositol phosphates in rat peritoneal polymorphonuclear leucocytes. *Mol. Pharmacol.*, **30**, 235–9.

15 Bray, M. A., Cunningham, F. M., Ford-Hutchinson, A. W., and Smith, M. J. H. (1981). Leukotriene B_4: a mediator of vascular permeability. *Br. J. Pharmacol.*, **72**, 483–7.

16 Ruzicka, T. and Burg, G. (1987). Effects of chronic intracutaneous administration of arachidonic acid and its metabolites. Induction of leucocytoclastic vasculitis by leukotriene B_4 and 12-hydroxyeicosatetraenoic acid and its prevention by prostaglandin E_2. *J. Invest. Dermatol.*, **88**, 120–6.

17 Watson, S. P. and Abbott, A. (1992). Tips receptor nomenclature supplement. *Trends Pharmacol. Sci.*, **13**, 519.

18 Kreisle, R. A., Parker, C. W., Griffin, G. L., Senior, R. M., and Stenson, W. F. (1986). Studies of leukotriene B_4-specific binding and function in rat polymorphonuclear leucocytes: absence of a chemotactic response. *J. Immunol.*, **134**, 3356–9.

19 Goldman, D. W., Chang, F.-H., Gifford, L. A., Goetzl, E. J., and Bowne, H. R. (1985). Pertussis toxin inhibition of chemotactic factor-induced calcium mobilization and function in human polymorphonuclear leucocytes. *J. Exp. Med.*, **162**, 145–51.

20 Payan, D. G., Missirian-Bastian, A., and Goetzl, E. J. (1984). Human T lymphocyte subset specificity of the regulatory effects of leukotriene B_4. *Proc. Natl. Acad. Sci. U.S.A.*, **81**, 3501–4.

21 Fels, A. O., Pawlowski, N. A., Cramer, E. B., King, T. K., Cohen, A. Z., and Scott, W. A. (1982). Human alveolar macrophages produce leukotriene B_4. *Proc. Natl. Acad. Sci. U.S.A.*, **79**, 7866–70.

22 Hewricks, P. A. J., VanDertol, M. E., Engels, F., Nijkamp, F. P., and Verhoef, J. (1986). Human polymorphonuclear leucocytes release leukotriene B_4 during phagocytosis of *Staphylococus aureus*. *Inflammation*, **10**, 37–42.

23 Ferreri, N. R., Howland, W. C., and Spiegelberg, H. L. (1986). Release of leukotrienes C_4 and B_4 and prostaglandin E_2 from human monocytes stimulated with aggregated IgG, IgA, and IgE. *J. Immunol.*, **136**, 4188–92.

24 Dubois, C., Bissonnette, E., and Rola-Pleszczynski, M. (1989). Asbestos fibres and silica particles stimulate rat alveolar macrophages to release TNF; autoregulatory role of leukotriene B_4. *Am. Rev. Resp. Dis.*, **139**, 1257–64.

25 Maclouf, J., Fruteau de Laclos, B., and Borgeat, P. (1982). Stimulation of leukotriene biosynthesis in human blood leucocytes by platelet- derived 12-hydroperoxy-icosatetraenoic acid. *Proc. Natl. Acad. Sci. U.S.A.*, **79**, 6042–8.

26 Chilton, F. H., O'Flaherty, J. T., Walsh, C. E., Thomas, M. J., Wykle, R. L., DeChatelet, L. R., and Waite, B. M. (1982). Stimulation of the lipoxygenase pathway in polymorphonuclear leucocytes by 1-0-alkyl-2-0-acetyl-*SN*-glycero-3-phosphocholine. *J. Biol. Chem.*, **257**, 5402–6.

27 Lin, A. H., Morton, D. R., and Gorman, R. R. (1982). Acetyl glyceryl ether phosphorylcholine stimulates leukotriene B_4 synthesis in human polymorphonuclear leucocytes. *J. Clin. Invest.*, **70**, 1058–63.

28 McGee, J. E. and Fitzpatrick, F. A. (1986). Erythrocyte neutrophil interactions: formation of leukotriene B_4 by transcellular biosynthesis. *Proc. Natl. Acad. Sci. U.S.A.*, **83**, 1349–53.

29 Renkonen, R. and Ustinov, J. (1990). Interferon-gamma augments hydrolysis of LTA_4 to LTB_4 by endothelial cells. *Prostaglandins*, **39**, 205–11.

30 Odlander, B., Jakobsson, P.-J., Rosen, A., and Claesson, H.-E. (1988). Human B and T lymphocytes convert leukotriene A_4 into leukotriene B_4 *Biochem. Biophys. Res. Commun.*, **153**, 203–8.

31 Goldyne, M. E., Burrish, G. F., Poubelle, P., and Borgeat, P. (1984). Arachidonic acid metabolism among human mononuclear leucocytes. Lipoxygenase related pathways. *J. Biol. Chem.*, **259**, 8815–21.

32 Poubelle, P., Borgeat, P., and Rola-Pleszczynski, M. (1987). Assessment of leukotriene B_4 synthesis in human lymphocytes using high performance liquid chromatography and radioimmunoassay methods. *J. Immunol.*, **139**, 1273–7.

33 Goldyne, M. E. and Rea, L. (1987). Stimulated T cell and natural killer (NK) cell lines fail to synthesize leukotriene B_4. *Prostaglandins*, **34**, 783–90.

34 Ambrus, J. L., Jurgensen, C. H., Witzel, N. L., Lewis, R. A., Butler, J. L., and Fauci, A. S. (1988). Leukotriene C_4 produced by a human T–T hybridoma suppresses Ig production by human lymphocytes. *J. Immunol.*, **140**, 2382–6.

35 Vickers, P. J., Miller, D. K., Coppolino, M. G., Mancini, J. A., Reid, G. K., and Evans, J. F. (1991). The cellular specificity of 5-lipoxygenase-activating protein (FLAP) expression. In *Prostaglandins, leukotrienes, lipoxins, and PAF* (ed. J. M. Bailey), pp. 267–75. Plenum Press, New York.

36 Davidson, E. M., Rae, S. A., and Smith, M. J. H. (1982). Leukotriene B_4 in synovial fluid. *J. Pharm. Pharmacol.*, **34**, 410–17.

37 Brain, S. D., Camp, R. D. R., Dowd, P. M., Black, A. K., Woolard, P. M., Mallet, A. I., and Greaves, M. W. (1982). Psoriasis and leukotriene B_4. *Lancet*, **2**, 762–63.

38 Kikawa, Y., Shigematsu, Y., and Sudo, M. (1986). Leukotriene B_4 and 20-OH-LTB_4 in purulent peritoneal, exudates demonstrated by GC-MS. *Prostagl. Leukotr. Med.*, **23**, 85–9.

39 Sharon, P. and Stenson, W. F. (1983). Production of leukotrienes by colonic mucosa from patients with inflammatory bowel disease. *Gastroenterol.*, **84**, 1306–16.

40 Ortaldo, J. R., Mason, L. H., Mathieson, B. J., Liang, S.-M., Flick, D. A., and Herberman, R. B. (1986). Mediation of mouse natural cytotoxic activity by tumour necrosis factor. *Nature*, **321**, 700–2.

41 Rola-Pleszczynski, M., Gagnon, L., and Sirois, P. (1983). Leukotriene B_4 augments human natural cytotoxic cell activity. *Biochem. Biophys. Res. Commun.*, **113**, 531–7.

42 Rola-Pleszczynski, M., Gagnon, L., Rudzinska, P., Borgeat, P., and Sirois, P. (1984). Human natural cytotoxic cell activity: enhancement by leukotrienes (LT) A_4, B_4 and D_4 but not by stereoisomers of LTB_4 or HETEs. *Prostaglandins Leukotrienes Med.*, **13**, 113–116.

43 Rola-Pleszczynski, M., Gagnon, L., and Sirois, P. (1984). Natural cytotoxic cell activity enhanced by leukotriene B_4 modulation by cyclo-oxygenase and lipoxygenase inhibitors. In *Icosanoids and cancer* (ed. H. Thaler-Dao), pp. 235–42. Raven Press, New York.

44 Seaman, W. E. (1983). Human natural killer cell activity is reversibly inhibited by antagonists of lipoxygenation. *J. Immunol.*, **131**, 2953–8.

45   Bray, R. A. and Brahmi, Z. (1986). Role of lipoxygenation in human natural killer cell activation. *J. Immunol.*, **136**, 1783–7.

46   Leung, K. H., Ip, M. M., and Koren, H. S. (1986). Regulation of human natural killing. IV. Role of lipoxygenase in regulation of natural killing activity. *Scand. J. Immunol.*, **24**, 371–82.

47   Sibbitt, W. L., Imir, T., and Bankhurst, A. D. (1986). Reversible inhibition of lymphokine-activated killer cell activity by lipoxygenase-pathway inhibitors. *Int. J. Cancer*, **38**, 517–22.

48   Gagnon, L., Girard, M., Sullivan, A. K., and Rola-Pleszczynski, M. (1987). Augmentation of human natural cytotoxic cell activity by leukotriene B_4 mediated by enhanced effector-target cell binding and increased lytic efficiency. *Cell. Immunol.*, **110**, 243–52.

49   Badr, K. F., DeBoer, D. K., Schwartzberg, M., and Serhan, C. N. (1989). Lipoxin A_4 antagonizes cellular and *in vivo* actions of leukotriene D_4 in rat glomerular mesangial cells: evidence for competition at a common receptor. *Proc. Natl. Acad. Sci. U.S.A.*, **86**, 3438–42.

50   Ramstedt, U., Serhan, C. N., Nicolaou, K. C., Webber, S. E., Wigzell, H., and Samuelsson, B. (1987). Lipoxin A-induced inhibition of human natural killer cell cytotoxicity: studies on stereospecificity of inhibition and mode of action. *J. Immunol.*, **138**, 266–70.

51   Goodwin, J. S. and Webb, D. (1980). Regulation of the immune response by prostaglandins. *Clin. Immunol. Immunopathol.*, **15**, 106–12.

52   Gordon, D., Bray, M. A., and Morley, J. (1976). Control of lymphokine secretion by prostaglandins. *Nature*, **262**, 401–3.

53   Knudsen, P. J., Dinarello, C., and Strom, T. B. (1986). Prostaglandins post-transcriptionally inhibit monocyte expression of interleukin-1 activity by increasing cyclic adenosine monophosphate. *J. Immunol.*, **137**, 3187–94.

54   Renz, H., Gong, J.-H., Schmidt, A., Nain, M., and Gemsa, D. (1988). Release of tumour necrosis factor-α from macrophages. Enhancement and suppression are dose-dependently regulated by prostaglandin E_2 and cyclic nucleotides. *J. Immunol.*, **141**, 2388–94.

55   Herman, J. and Rabson, A. R. (1984). Prostaglandin E_2 depresses natural cytotoxicity by inhibiting interleukin-1 production by large granular lymphocytes. *Clin. Exp. Immunol.*, **57**, 380–4.

56   Brunda, M. J., Herberman, R. B., and Holden, H. (1980). Inhibition of murine natural killer cell activity by prostaglandins. *J. Immunol.* **124**, 2682–6.

57   Koren, H. S., Anderson, S. J., Fischer, D. G., Copeland, G. S., and Jensen, P. (1981). Regulation of human natural killing. The role of monocytes, interferon, and prostaglandins. *J. Immunol.*, **127**, 2007–14.

58   Rola-Pleszczynski, M., Gagnon, L., Bolduc, D., and LeBreton, G. (1985). Evidence for the involvement of the thromboxane synthase pathway in human natural cytotoxic cell activity. *J. Immunol.* **135**, 4114–9.

59   Defreyn, G. H., Deckmyn, H., and Vermylen, J. (1982). A thromboxane synthetase inhibitor reorients endoperoxide metabolism in whole blood towards prostacyclin and prostaglandin E_2. *Thromb. Res.*, **26**, 389–95.

60   Farkas, G., Mandi, Y., Koltai, M., and Braquet, P. (1987). Role of PAF in splenic lymphocyte-induced impairment of Langerhans cells. *Prostaglandin*, **34**, 158–62.

61   Dobozy, A., Hunyadi, J., Kenderessy, A., Csato, M., and Braquet, P. (1988). Effects of lipid mediator inhibitors on the UV-B irradiation-induced elevated

Candida albicans killing activity of human keratinocytes and polymorphonuclear leucocytes. In *New trends in lipid mediator research* (ed. P. Braquet), Vol. 1 pp. 168–76. Karger, Basel.

62 McDonald, A. J., Mogbel, R., Wardlaw, A. J., and Kay, A. B. (1986). Platelet activating factor (PAF-acether) enhances eosinophils cytotoxicity *in vitro*. *J. All. Clin. Immunol.*, **77**, 227–33.

63 Rola-Pleszczynski, M. and Turcotte, S. (1987). Enhancement of human natural killer cell activity by platelet activating factor. *Immunobiology*, (Suppl.) **3**, 135.

64 Rola-Pleszczynski, M., Turcotte, S., Gagnon, L., Pignol, B., Braquet, P., Bolduc, D., and Bouvrette, L. (1988). Enhancement of natural killer (NK) cell activity by platelet activating factor. In *New trends in lipid mediator research* (ed. P. Braquet), Vol. 1, pp. 89–98. Karger, Basel.

65 Mandi, Y., Farkas, G., Koltai, M., Braquet, P., and Beladi, I. (1988). The effect of BN 52021, a PAF-acether antagonist, on natural killer activity. In *New trends lipid mediator research* (ed. P. Braquet), Vol. 1, 76–84. Karger, Basel.

66 Honda, Z.-I., Nakamura, M., Miki, I., Minami, M., Watanabe, T., Seyama, Y., Okado, H., Toh, H., Ito, K., Miyamoto, T., and Shimizu, T. (1991). Cloning by functional expression of platelet activating factor receptor from guinea pig lung. *Nature*, **349**, 342–6.

67 Thivierge, M. and Rola-Pleszczynski, M. (1991). Enhancement of pulmonary natural killer cell activity by platelet activating factor: mechanisms of activation involving Ca^{2+}, protein kinase C, and lipoxygenase products. *Am. Rev. Resp. Dis.*, **144**, 272–7.

68 Foegh, M. and Ramwell, P. (1987). PAF and transplant immunology. *Prostaglandins*, **34**, 186–95.

69 Foegh, M. L., Khirabadi, B. S., Rowles, J. R., Braquet, P., and Ramwell, P. W. (1986). Prolongation of cardiac allograft survival with BN 52021, a specific antagonist of platelet activating factor. *Transplantation*, **42**, 86–8.

70 Adams, D. O. and Hamilton, T. A. (1984). The cell biology of macrophage activation. *Annu. Rev. Immunol.*, **2**, 283–314.

71 Schade, U. F. (1986). Involvement of lipoxygenases in the activation of mouse macrophages by endotoxin. *Biochem. Biophys. Res. Commun.*, **138**, 842–7.

72 Feuerstein, N., Foegh, M., and Ramwell, P. W. (1981). Leukotrienes C_4 and D_4 induce prostaglandin and thromboxane release from rat peritoneal macrophages. *Br. J. Pharmacol.*, **72**, 389–96.

73 Schenkelaars, E. J. and Bonta, I. L. (1983). Effect of leukotriene C_4 on the release of secretory products by elicited populations of rat peritoneal macrophages. *Eur. J. Pharmacol.*, **86**, 477–86.

74 Schenkelaars, E. J. and Bonta, I. L. (1986). Cyclo-oxygenase inhibitors promote leukotriene C_4-induced release of beta-glucuronidase from rat peritoneal macrophages prostaglandin E_2 suppresses. *Int. J. Immunopharmacol.*, **8**, 305–12.

75 Ophir, R., Ben-Efraim, S., and Bonta, I. L. (1987). Leukotriene D_4 and indomethacin enhance additively the macrophage cytostatic activity *in vitro* towards MOPC-315 tumour cells. *Int. J. Tiss. Reac.*, **9**, 189–97.

76 Bonta, I. L. and Ben-Efraim, S. (1990). Interactions between inflammatory mediators in expression of anti-tumour cytostatic activity of macrophages. *Immunol. Lett.*, **25**, 295–302.

77 Gagnon, L., Fillion, L., Dubois, C., and Rola-Pleszczynski, M. (1989). Leukotrienes and macrophage activation: augmented cytotoxic activity and enhanced

interleukin-1, tumour necrosis factor, and hydrogen peroxide production. *Agents Actions*, **26**, 141–7.

78 Schultz, R. M., Pavlidis, N. A., Stylos, W. A., and Chirigos, M. A. (1978). Regulation of macrophage tumouricidal function: a role for prostaglandins of the E series. *Science*, **202**, 320–3.

79 Taffet, S. and Russel, S. W. (1981). Macrophage-mediated tumour cell killing: regulation of expression of cytolytic activity by prostaglandin E. *J. Immunol.*, **126**, 424–9.

80 Valone, F. H., Philip, R., and Debs, R. J. (1988). Enhanced human monocyte cytotoxicity by platelet activating factor. *Immunology*, **64**, 715–18.

81 Bonavida, B., Mencia-Huerta, J.-M., and Braquet, P. (1989). Effect of platelet activating factor on monocyte activation and production of tumour necrosis factor. *Int. Arch. Allergy Appl. Immunol.*, **88**, 157–60.

82 Gagnon, L., Filion, L. G., and Rola-Pleszczynski, M. (1989). Enhanced production of tumour necrosis factor (TNF)-alpha by human monocytes exposed to leukotriene B$_4$. *Int. J. Immunopathol. Pharmacol.*, **2**, 155–63.

83 Dubois, C., Bissonnette, E., and Rola-Pleszczynski, M. (1989). Platelet activating factor (PAF) stimulates tumour necrosis factor production by alveolar macrophages: prevention by PAF receptor antagonists and lipoxygenase inhibitors. *J Immunol.*, **143**, 964–71.

84 Schade, U. F., Ernst, M., Reinke, M., and Wolter, D. T. (1989). Lipoxygenase inhibitors suppress formation of tumour necrosis factor *in vitro* and *in vivo*. *Biochem. Biophys. Res. Commun.*, **159**, 748–54.

85 Horiguchi, J., Spriggs, D., Imamura, K., Stone, R., Luebbers, R., and Kufe, D. (1989). Role of arachidonic acid metabolism in transcriptional induction of tumour necrosis factor gene expression by phorbol ester. *Mol. Cell. Biol.*, **9**, 252–8.

86 Mohri, M., Spriggs, D. R., and Kufe, D. (1990). Effects of lipopolysaccharide on phospholipase A$_2$ activity and tumour necrosis factor expression in HL-60 cells. *J. Immunol.*, **144**, 2678–82.

87 Spriggs, D. R., Sherman, M. L., Imamura, K., Mohri, M., Rodriguez, C., Robbins, G., and Kufe, D. W. (1990). Phospholipase A$_2$ activation and auto-induction of tumour necrosis factor gene expression by tumour necrosis factor. *Cancer Res.*, **50**, 7101–7.

88 Hoffman, T., Lee, Y. L., Lizzio, E. F., Tripathi, A. K., Jessop, J. J., Taplits, M., Abrahamsen, T. G., Carter, C. S., and Puri, J. (1991). Absence of modulation of monokine production via endogenous cyclo-oxygenase or 5-lipoxygenase metabolites: MK-886 (3-[1-(4-chlorobenzyl)-3-*t*-butyl-thio-5-isopropylondol-2-yl]-2,2-dimethyl-propanoic acid), indomethacin, or arachidonate fail to alter immunoreactive interleukin-1β, or TNFα production by human monocytes *in vitro*. *Clin. Immunol. Immunopathol.*, **58**, 399–408.

89 Sirko, S. P., Schindler, R., Doyle, M. J., Weisman, S. M., and Dinarello, C. A. (1991). Transcription, translation, and secretion of interleukin-1 and tumour necrosis factor: effects of tebufelone, a dual cyclo-oxygenase/5-lipoxygenase inhibitor. *Eur. J. Immunol.*, **21**, 243–50.

90 Kunkel, S. L., Spengler, M., May, M. A., Spengler, R., Larrick, J., and Remick, D. (1988). Prostaglandin E$_2$ regulates macrophage-derived tumour necrosis factor gene expression. *J. Biol. Chem.*, **263**, 5380–5.

91 Gong, J.-H., Renz, H., Sprenger, H., Nain, M., and Gemsa, D. (1990). Enhancement of tumour necrosis factor-α gene expression by low doses of prostaglandin E$_2$ and cyclic GMP. *Immunobiology*, **182**, 44–55.

92   Kovacs, E. J., Radzioch, D., Young, H. A., and Varesio, L. (1988). Differential inhibition of IL-1 and TNFα mRNA expression by agents which block second messenger pathways in murine macrophages. *J. Immunol.*, **141**, 3101–4.

93   Scales, W. E., Chensue, S. W., Otterness, I., and Kunkel, S. L. (1989). Regulation of monokine gene expression: prostaglandin E$_2$ suppresses tumour necrosis factor but not interleukin-1α or β-mRNA and cell-associated bio-activity. *J. Leuk. Biol.*, **45**, 416–21.

94   Rola-Pleszczynski, M., Bossé, J., Bissonnette, E., and Dubois, C. (1988). PAF-acether enhances the production of tumour necrosis factor by human and rodent lymphocytes and macrophages. *Prostaglandins*, **35**, 802.

95   Poubelle, P., Gingras, D., Demers, C., Dubois, C., Harbour, D., and Rola-Pleszczynski, M. (1991). Platelet activating factor (PAF-acether) enhances the concomitant production of tumour necrosis factor alpha and interleukin-1 by subsets of human monocytes. *Immunology*, **72**, 181–7.

96   Rola-Pleszczynski, M. and Stankova, J. (1992). Differentiation-dependent modulation of TNF production by PAF in human HL-60 myeloid leukaemia cells. *J. Leuk. Biol.*, **51**, 609–16.

97   Barthelson, R. and Valone, F. (1990). Interaction of platelet activating factor with interferon-γ in the stimulation of interleukin-1 production by human monocytes. *J. Allergy Clin. Immunol.*, **86**, 193–201.

98   Kroegel, C., Yukawa, T., Westwick, J., and Barnes, P. J. (1989). Evidence for two platelet activating factor receptors on eosinophils: dissociation between PAF-induced intracellular calcium mobilization, degranulation, and superoxide anion generation in eosinophils. *Biochem. Biophys. Res. Commun.*, **162**, 511–21.

99   Rola-Pleszczynski, M. (1990). Priming of human monocytes with PAF augments their production of tumour necrosis factor. *J. Lipid Mediators*, **2**, S77–82.

100 Rola-Pleszczynski, M., Turcotte, S., and Gingras, D. (1990). Enhanced TNF production and cytotoxic activity of human monocytes primed with PAF: post-receptor events. In *Molecular and cellular biology of cytokines* (ed. J. J. Oppenheim, M. C. Powanda, M. J. Kluger, and C. A. Dinnarello), pp. 105–10. Alan R. Liss Inc.

101 Vercellotti, G. M., Yin, H. Q., Gustabson, K. S., Nelson, R. D., and Jacob, H. S. (1988). Platelet activating factor primes neutrophil responses to agonists: role in promoting neutrophil-mediated endothelial damage. *Blood*, **71**, 1100–7.

102 Paubert-Braquet, M., Lonchampt, M-O, Klotz, P., and Guilbaud, J. (1988). Tumour necrosis factor (TNF) primes platelet activating factor (PAF)-induced superoxide generation by human neutrophils (PMN): consequences in promoting PMN-mediated endothelial cell (EC) damages. *Prostaglandins*, **35**, 803.

103 Worthen, G. S., Seccombe, J. F., Clay, K. L., Guthrie, L. A., and Johnston Jr, R. B. (1988). The priming of neutrophils by lipopolysaccharide for production of intracellular platelet activating factor. *J. Immunol.*, **140**, 3553–9.

104 Rola-Pleszczynski, M. (1989). Leukotrienes and the immune system. *J. Lipid Mediators*, **1**, 149–59.

13 Lipid mediators in defence mechanisms

Z. HONDA AND T. SHIMIZU

1 Introduction

This chapter focuses on three classes of lipid mediators; platelet activating factor (PAF), leukotrienes (LTs), and prostaglandins (PGs). Since a comprehensive review of this actively expanding field of research is impossible, we will focus on recent outstanding advances. Attention will be directed to regulation of the phospholipase/5-lipoxygenase pathway, cloning of PAF receptor cDNA, and related signal transduction systems followed by activation of the PAF receptor. Biosyntheses and cellular activation mechanisms of other lipid mediators will be briefly reviewed and recently published reviews provide additional material (1–6). Chapter 12 covers the eicosanoids in particular.

In contrast to mediators such as amines or peptides, lipid mediators are synthesized from precursors when cells are stimulated with agonists. Key enzymes involved in the biosyntheses of lipid mediators, including phospholipase A_2, phospholipase C, and 5-lipoxygenase are switched on by subtle and transient changes in the intracellular environment and then turned off when cells return to the steady state. Fine regulation of these enzyme activities are typical characteristics of biosyntheses of lipid mediators. Recent progress in biochemical and molecular biological techniques has led to an insight into the regulations of these 'signal-transduction enzymes'. The fate of the synthesized mediators are also complicated. It seems that LTs are released from cells by an energy-dependent transport mechanism (7), while the major part of PAF is retained on cell membranes and organelles (8).

The role of intracellular PAF requires much more attention before it is understood fully but may, together with arachidonic acid, represent as yet uncharacterized intracellular (second) messenger systems.

Lipid mediators readily bind to plasma membranes of target cells and exert actions through specific receptor proteins. A series of studies have demonstrated the existence of specific receptors for PGs, LTs, and PAF, and the involvement of G proteins in the related signalling pathways. The primary structures of the PAF receptor (9) and thromboxane A_2 receptor (10) have been determined by molecular cloning. These studies revealed that both receptors belong to a G protein coupled receptor superfamily with seven transmembrane alpha-helices, exposed on the surface of cells, suggesting that these lipid-derived components are important extracellular, humoral, media-tors. The specificities of receptor–G protein interactions and the coupling of G proteins to intracellular effector systems are being intensively studied. The biosynthesis of eicosanoids and PAF, as well as their mode of action as inflammatory mediators, are related through this common mechanism although the particular specificities of the receptors, G proteins, and target enzymes are not fully defined in all cases.

2   Biosynthesis of eicosanoids and PAF

Activation of cells, for example as a result of occupation of the C5a receptor on a mast cells, causes dissociation of the alpha subunit of a G protein from the beta and gamma subunits. The alpha subunit releases GDP, and then binds GTP. This GTP-alpha subunit will either activate or inhibit target enzymes until the associated GTP is hydrolysed to GDP. The inter-mediary G proteins, which have been likened to messenger-boys (11), can be permanently activated experimentally by supplying a non-hydrolysable form of GTP (GTP-γ-S). ADP ribosylation of the alpha subunit will also permanently activate Gs, or dissociate receptor–Gi coupling. This covalent modification is catalysed by bacterial toxins (see also Chapter 1.3).

2.1   Phospholipid breakdown

2.1.1   *Phospholipase A$_2$*

Arachidonic acid is liberated from the *sn*-2 position of membrane glycero-phospholipids by the action of phospholipase A$_2$ (PLA$_2$). Inflammatory leuco-cytes contain a relatively large amount of 1-*O*-alkyl-glycerophosphocholine (GPC) (12, 13), and the 1-*O*-alkyl species is enriched in arachidonic acid (12). Thus, the agonist-stimulated inflammatory leucocytes simultaneously produce arachidonic acid and lyso-PAF (1-*O*-alkyl-lyso-GPC, a direct pre-cursor of PAF) by the action of PLA$_2$ (Figure 13.1).

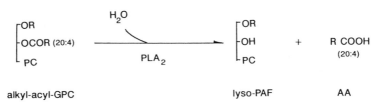

Fig. 13.1 Co-ordinate production of lyso-PAF and arachidonic acid (AA) from 1-*O*-alkyl-2-acyl (arachidonoyl)-GPC by PLA$_2$.

Several lines of evidence suggested the existence of an arachidonic acid-specific, cytosolic PLA$_2$ (cPLA$_2$) in inflammatory leucocytes (14, 15) which is entirely different from well characterized, secreted types of PLA$_2$s (sPLA$_2$s). sPLA$_2$s consist of a large isozyme family (16). These 14 kDa isozymes are mainly present extracellularly, are devoid of specificity on *sn*-2 fatty acid, and require millimolar concentrations of Ca^{2+} for activation (17). Therefore, agonist-induced arachidonic acid liberation has not been attributed to this type of PLA$_2$. The cytoplasmic form of PLA$_2$ requires for catalytic activity only submicromolar concentrations of Ca^{2+} (14, 15), and has been shown to translocate to membrane phospholipids at the physiologically relevant concentration of Ca^{2+} (18). Two reports also suggest the involvement of arachidonic acid-specific PLA$_2$ in the co-ordinate productions of PAF and eicosanoids from 1-*O*-alkyl-GPC; both PAF and eicosanoid syntheses were abolished in polymorphonuclear leucocytes (19) and HL-60 cells (20) depleted of arachidonic acid. These findings indicate that the cPLA$_2$ is probably responsible for arachidonic acid liberation in agonist-stimulated inflammatory cells.

cPLA$_2$ was purified from monocytic cell lines, U937 (21), and RAW264.7 (14), and the cDNA coding for the enzyme was cloned from a U937 cell cDNA library (22). Sequence analysis revealed that cPLA contains a putative calcium-dependent lipid binding domain that is shared among protein kinase C (PKC), phospholipase C (PLC) γ chain, GTPase activating protein (see Chapter 1-3), and several synaptic vesicle proteins (22). cPLA expressed in mammalian cells acts specifically on arachidonic acid, and also is activated and translocated to the membrane at submicromolar concentrations of Ca^{2+} (22). The translocation to the membrane might be a regulatory process augmenting accessibility of the enzyme to the substrate.

The calcium requirement of PLA$_2$ has led to the concept that PLC activation and subsequent inositol triphosphate and intracellular Ca^{2+} elevation are pre-requisites for PLA$_2$ activation. However, a series of experiments have shown that PLA$_2$ activation is regulated by G proteins and that PLC and PLA$_2$ activation are separate processes. The role of G proteins in PLA$_2$ activation has been suggested in studies showing that GTP or a non-hydrolysable GTP analogue, GTPγS, induced activation of PLA$_2$ in permeabilized cells (23–26). Agonist-induced arachidonic acid release has been shown to be sensitive to pertussis toxin (IAP) treatment in mouse 3T3 fibroblasts (27), rabbit platelets (24, 26), and a rat thyroid cell line, FRTL-5 (25), whereas PIP$_2$ hydrolysis was insensitive to the toxin treatment, in the same cells (25, 27). Studies with neomycin (a PLC inhibitor) or 12-*O*-tetradecanoyl-phorbol-13-acetate (TPA) which directly stimulates protein kinase C have revealed that the inhibition of PLC activity by these compounds did not affect PLA$_2$ activation in bradykinin-stimulated FRTL-5 cells (25) and in GTPγs-stimulated permeabilized MDCK-D1 canine kidney cells (28). Thus, PLA$_2$ and PLC activations seem to be regulated independently by different

G proteins. Gupta, *et al.* (29) showed the possible involvement of Gi in PLA₂ activation; they constructed a chimera of the α subunits of Gi and Gs in which the COOH-terminal 38 residues of α-S was substituted by the COOH-terminal 36 residues of a particular α-i, and expressed the chimeric protein in CHO cells. In the transformed cells, thrombin and ATP-induced arachidonic acid release was significantly decreased as compared to that in original CHO cells, thus, the chimeric subunit displayed a dominant inhibitory function which shuts off the coupling of receptors and PLA₂. It also showed that the COOH-terminal region of this α-i molecule was critically involved in receptor–PLA₂ coupling.

2.1.2 Phospholipase C

It is now well accepted that breakdown of phosphatidylinositol-4,5-biphosphate (PIP₂) by phosphoinositide-specific phospholipase C (PLC) is a primary event in intracellular signalling (30, 31). Hydrolysis of PIP₂ generates diacylglycerol (DAG) and inositol-1,4,5-triphosphate (IP₃) which serve as second messengers stimulating protein kinase C and Ca²⁺ mobilization from intracellular stores, respectively (Figure 13.2) (32, 33). At least two different mechanisms, phosphorylation of PLC and G protein-mediated PLC activation, appear to function in the regulation of PLC depending on the structures of receptors which lead to PLC activation (tyrosine kinase family or G protein-coupled receptor family, see below).

PLC activity is present in most mammalian cells (31), and cDNAs coding for five PLC isozymes (α, β, γ_1, γ_2 and δ) have been cloned and sequenced (31). Of particular interest is that PLCγ possesses a non-catalytic domain homologous to an oncogenic tyrosine kinase, *src* (SH2 domain) (34–36). A series of experiments revealed the involvement of PLCγ in PIP₂ hydrolysis induced by the activation of receptors for platelet-derived growth factor and epidermal growth factor (37). Ligand binding to these growth factor receptors augments tyrosine kinase activity of the receptors and induces receptor autophosphorylation on the tyrosine moiety (37). It was also shown that the SH2 domain of PLCγ and the phosphorylated receptors form high affinity complexes. PLCγ is phosphorylated by the receptor-tyrosine kinase (37, 38). The regulatory effects of the tyrosine phosphorylation on the activity of PLCγ remains controversial and at least two possible regulatory mechanism are

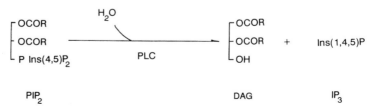

Fig. 13.2 PIP₂ hydrolysis by PLC. Both DAG and IP₃ are produced by the reaction.

reported. Nishibe *et al.* (39) reported that the catalytic activity of PLCγ was augmented by tyrosine phosphorylation, and Goldschmidt-Clermont *et al.* (40) considered that phosphorylation increased accessibility of the enzyme to substrate.

PLC regulation by heterotrimeric G proteins is well established (30), although the identity of the PLC-linked G protein, tentatively termed Gp (30), has not been fully established. A role for G proteins in PLC regulation has been suggested in experiments showing the stimulatory effects of GTP or GTPγS on agonist-induced PIP_2 hydrolysis in cell membranes or in permeabilized cells (41–43). IAP-sensitive, partially sensitive, and insensitive G proteins have been noted in a variety of cells stimulated with various agonists.

An IAP-sensitive G protein has been reported to regulate PIP_2 hydrolysis in various systems, including PAF-stimulated rabbit neutrophils (44), fMLP-stimulated HL-60 cell membrane (45), thrombin and PAF-stimulated human platelet membrane (46), thrombin-stimulated permeabilized rat vascular smooth muscle cells (47), and kyotorphin (tyrosine-arginine)-stimulated rat brain membrane (48). Since Gi and Go are both substrates for IAP and IAP-induced ADP ribosylation of Gi abolishes the Gi-mediated functions (49), both Gi and Go have been considered to be candidates for the G protein controlling PLC. Reconstitution of Gi (48), and Gi and Go (45) into IAP treated rat brain and HL-60 cell membranes, respectively, have been shown to restore the agonist-stimulated PIP_2 hydrolysis. These studies have been supported by other indirect measurements (50) but successful reconstitution of purified PLC and purified Go/Gi has not yet been reported.

IAP-insensitive G proteins controlling PLC have also been noted in a number of systems. PIP_2 hydrolysis was shown to be insensitive to IAP treatment in thrombin-stimulated mouse 3T3 fibroblasts (27), noradrenalin-stimulated FRTL thyroid cells (25), ATP-stimulated rat hepatocytes (51), U46619 (a thromboxane A_2 analogue)-stimulated human platelets (46), and the PAF-stimulated U937 monocytic cell line (52). In FRL5 thyroid cells and ATP-stimulated hepatocytes, IAP treatment partially inhibited PIP_2 hydrolysis (25, 51). These studies also indicate the existence of more than one Gp as identified by differences in IAP-sensitivity in the same cells (Figure 13.3a). In the human platelet membrane, PIP_2 breakdown induced by thrombin and PAF was sensitive to IAP treatment, but that induced by U46619 was not affected by the toxin treatment (46). In differentiated U937 cells, IP_3 synthesis by PAF was resistant to IAP treatment, whereas the toxin treatment inhibited LTB_4-induced IP_3 production, in the same cells (52).

The degeneracy in receptor–G protein coupling was also illustrated by Ashkenazi and colleagues (Figure 13.3b) who showed that muscarinic, acetylcholine (M1) receptors coupled to both IAP-sensitive and insensitive G proteins controlling PLC activation (53).

The IAP-insensitive Gp was merely a hypothesis until discovery of the Gq series of G proteins (54–58). Two laboratories purified the α subunit of

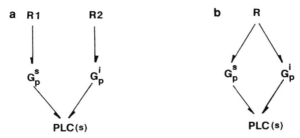

Fig. 13.3 (a) Different receptors, R1 and R2, in the same cell stimulate PLC via IAP-sensitive (Gp^s) and insensitive (Gp^i) G proteins, respectively. (b) Single receptor stimulates PLC via both IAP-sensitive (Gp^s) and insensitive (Gp^i) G proteins (53).

Gp which stimulates PI breakdown in reconstitution systems composed of GTPγs coupled Gα and partially purified PLC (54, 55). Pong and Sternweis purified Gp using immobilized βγ subunits, and determined several internal amino acid sequences (54) of the purified Gα which were not conserved among Gs, Gi, or Go. These sequences proved to be identical with two members of new family of Gα cloned by Strathmann and Simon using the homology-proving approach (56). Members of the new Gα family, termed Gq and G_{11}, are devoid of the COOH-terminal cysteine that is ordinarily the site of ADP ribosylation by IAP. Gq was shown to stimulate PI breakdown in a reconstitution system composed of Gq and PLCβ (58). Evidence supporting Gq activation by calcium-mobilizing agonists is now rapidly accumulating. GTPase activation of human platelet membrane by thromboxane A_2 was inhibited by an antiserum against the COOH-terminal region of Gq (59).

2.2   Cyclo-oxygenase pathway

Prostaglandin biosynthesis is initiated by the bis oxygenation of arachidonic acid by PGG/H synthase. PGG/H synthase catalyses PGG_2 formation (cyclo-oxygenase) and the reduction of the hydroperoxide in PGG_2 to hydroxide (peroxidase). Subsequently, PGH_2 is converted to various types of PGs, PGD_2, PGE_2, $PGF_{2\alpha}$, PGI_2, and thromboxane (TX) A_2 (Figure 13.4), (see references 3 and 6, for review).

Cyclo-oxygenase was purified from sheep and bovine seminal glands (60–62), and the primary structure of the enzyme was elucidated by cDNA cloning (63–65). Cyclo-oxygenase is a glycoprotein with one membrane spanning domain (63) and the site acetylated by the cyclo-oxygenase inhibitor, aspirin was identified to be at Ser 515. PGD synthase was purified (66–68) and cloned from rat brain (69). The primary structure showed that

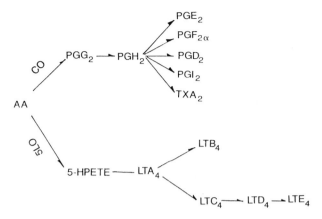

Fig. 13.4 Arachidonic acid metabolism through cyclo-oxygenase (CO) and 5-lip-oxygenase (5-LO) pathways.

it is an N-glycosylated membrane-bound enzyme with two carbohydrate chains (70). Immunohistochemical studies revealed that the enzyme is found in the endoplasmic reticulum and nuclear membranes (70). PGF synthase, which also catalyses the conversion of PGD_2 to 11-epi-$PGF_{2\alpha}$, was purified (71) and the cDNA was cloned from bovine lung (72). The primary structure of the enzyme showed an unexpected homology with aldehyde reductase and lens crystalline (72). PGI_2 synthase and TXA_2 synthase were purified to homogeneity and proved to be members of cytochrome P-450s (73, 74).

Several early studies demonstrated that peripheral and splenic lymphocytes produce cyclo-oxygenase metabolites, including PGE_2 and TXA_2 (75–77). However, lymphocytes are not considered to be a major source of PGs. Goldyne *et al.* and others critically re-evaluated those previous results using rigorously purified lymphocytes and a number of lymphocyte cell lines, and showed that PG production by lymphocytes was hardly detectable (78). The apparent PG synthesis by lymphocytes was presumably caused by macrophage/monocyte and platelet contamination in the 'purified' lymphocyte preparations (78). However, monocyte/macrophage is a well characterized source of PGE_2 and TXA_2 (3, 78).

Immunoregulatory effects of PGE_2 have been extensively studied. PGE_2 has been shown to inhibit lymphocyte proliferation (79), IL-2 production (80), natural killer cell activity (81), and immunoglobulin production (82). The immunosuppressive effects of PGE_2 are considered to function through the Gs-adenylate cyclase system, however precise molecular mechanisms of those actions have not been fully elucidated. The opposite actions of PGI_2 and TXA_2 on platelet aggregation and vascular tonus are also well recognized (3).

2.3   5-lipoxygenase pathway

The first step of LT biosynthesis is catalysed by the dual enzyme activities of 5-lipoxygenase; arachidonic acid is oxygenated to yield 5-hydroperoxy-eicosatetraenoic acid, and is further converted to LTA_4 by a single enzyme (83–86). LTA_4 is metabolized either to LTB_4 by LTA_4 hydrolase, or to LTC_4 by LTC_4 synthase. LTC_4 is further metabolized to LTD_4 by γ-glutamyl transferase, and then, to LTE_4 by dipeptidase (Figure 13.4) (see references 1–3, and 6, for review).

5-lipoxygenase was purified to homogeneity from human leucocytes, rat basophil leukaemic cells and murine mast cells (85–89), and cDNA coding for the enzyme was cloned (90, 91) and expressed in several systems (90, 92–94). During the purification steps, Rouzer and Samuelsson noted that intrinsic factors other than Ca^{2+} and ATP are required for the full enzyme activity (88). They also obtained evidence for the Ca^{2+}-dependent membrane trans-location of the enzyme (95) (see also Figure 12.2).

Recently, Miller *et al.* (96) and Dixon *et al.* (97) characterized a novel membrane protein required for cellular LT biosynthesis using as a probe the 5-lipoxygenase inhibitor, MK-886. Among the inhibitors of LT synthesis, an indole compound, MK-886 has unique characteristics; it inhibits cellular LT synthesis and 5-lipoxygenase translocation to the plasma membrane, but has no direct effects on the purified 5-lipoxygenase activity (96). They purified the target protein of MK-886, termed FLAP (five lipoxygenase activating protein), from rat neutrophil membranes (96), and cloned the cDNA from rat basophil leukaemia cell and human HL-60 cDNA libraries (97). They showed that co-expression of both FLAP and 5-lipoxygenase was required for LTA_4 production by calcium ionophore-stimulated mammalian cells, and that the cellular LT synthesis was inhibited by MK-886. They proposed that FLAP functions as a membrane anchor essential to the membrane association of activated 5-lipoxygenase.

LTA_4 hydrolase was purified from human leucocytes (98), human lung (99), and guinea pig lung (100), and the cDNA was cloned from human spleen and placental libraries (101, 102). The cDNA was expressed in *E. coli* with full enzyme activity (103). A large amount of the enzyme was purified from the bacterial source, and specific polyclonal antibody was prepared (104). Immunohistochemical studies using the antibody, detected localization of the enzyme in epithelial cells in the small intestine and trachea, macrophage, and smooth muscle of the aorta (104). Analysis of LTA_4 hydrolase cDNA revealed the existence of a sequence homologous to the zinc-binding domain of aminopeptidases (105, 106). Minami *et al.* demonstrated that purified LTA_4 hydrolase contained equimolar zinc ion and that the enzyme has a significant amount of aminopeptidase activity (107). The biological role of the dual enzyme activity remains to be clarified.

LTC_4 synthase, a microsomal enzyme catalyses the conjugation of LTA_4 with glutathione and has not yet been purified to homogeneity. Two groups, including ours, solubilized and partially purified the enzyme from guinea pig lung and rat basophilic leukaemia cells (108, 109). Both groups separated LTC_4 synthase activity and glutathione-S-transferase (GST) activity (1-chloro-2,4-dinitrobenzene as a substrate) by column chromatography. LTC_4 synthase activity was found mainly in the microsome fraction of spleen and lung; this tissue distribution is different from that of microsomal GST(109).

2.4   Cell-cell interactions in LT biosynthesis and the export system of LTC_4

LTA_4 hydrolase is a widely distributed enzyme, while 5-lipoxygenase which supplies the substrate, LTA_4, is present almost solely in leucocytes. This finding raised the possibility that LTB_4 is synthesized through the transfer of LTA_4 from leucocytes to cells devoid of 5-lipoxygenase. Human erythrocytes (110) and human endothelial cells (111) have been shown to convert LTA_4 supplied by calcium ionophore-stimulated leucocytes to LTB_4. Transcellular biosynthesis of LTC_4 by the same mechanisms were also reported. Bovine endothelial cells (112), murine mast cells (113), and human platelets (114) effectively converted exogenous LTA_4 to LTC_4. Net LT production may increase through such metabolic interactions, however, further studies are needed to evaluate the contribution of these mechanisms *in vivo*.

In a series of experiments, Lam *et al.*, William *et al.*, and Owen *et al.* showed that LT synthesis and the export of LTs to the extracellular space were separate biochemical steps (7, 115, 116). Eosinophils stimulated with calcium-ionophore or with fMLP accumulated LTC_4 intracellularly, then released LTC_4 in a time-dependent manner (116). As the next step, they incubated eosinophils with LTA_4 and separately measured extracellular and intracellular LTC_4 (7). They found that the LTC_4 *release* became saturated at a concentration of LTA_4, which did not saturate LTC_4 accumulation. It was also shown that the export of LTC_4 was time and temperature dependent and that the export was inhibited by LTC_5 but was only minimally inhibited by S-dinitrophenyl glutathione. Based on these findings, they proposed the existence of an LTC_4-specific transporter across the membrane.

2.5   Biosynthesis of platelet activating factor

PAF (1-*O*-alkyl-2-acetyl-*sn*-glycero-3-phosphocholine) was first recognized in two parallel studies as a lipophilic substance derived from the renal medulla that causes hypotension (117), and as a platelet-aggregating substance derived from rabbit basophilic leucocytes (118). These compounds proved to have identical structure, 1-*O*-alkyl-2-acetyl-GPC (119, 200).

PAF is synthesized via the phospholipase A_2/acetyltransferase pathway (remodelling pathway) or choline-phosphotransferase pathway (*de novo* synthesis) (Figure 13.5) (see reference 121, for review). Agonist-stimulated

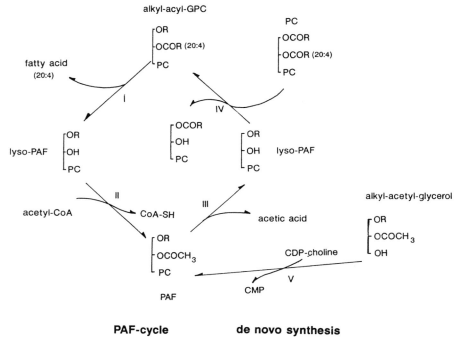

PAF-cycle   **de novo synthesis**

Fig. 13.5 Biosynthesis of PAF via re-modelling (PAF cycle) and *de novo* pathways. The enzymes catalysing the reactions are; I PLA$_2$, II acetyltransferase, III acetyl-hydrolase, IV acyltransferase, and V choline-phosphotransferase. Note that the trans-acylation by the acyltransferase (IV) and *sn*-2-fatty acid liberation by PLA$_2$ (I) are specific to arachidonic acid.

inflammatory leucocytes and platelets produce PAF through the remodelling pathway (8, 121). These cells contain considerable amounts of 1-*O*-alkyl-2-acyl-GPC (11–13), and arachidonic acid is a major constituent of *sn*-2 fatty acid of the alkyl-acyl-GPC (11, 12), thus PLA$_2$ simultaneously liberates lyso-PAF(1-*O*-alkyl-lyso-GPC) and arachidonic acid. Presumably, a recently cloned arachidonic acid-specific PLA$_2$ (22, see also Section 2.1.1) might be responsible for the reaction. The *sn*-2 position is acetylated by acetyltransferase to yield 1-*O*-alkyl-2-acetyl-GPC (PAF). PAF is inactivated when acetic acid at the *sn*-2 position is hydrolysd by acetyl hydrolase or PLA$_2$ and lyso-PAF is re-acylated to yield 1-*O*-alkyl-2-acyl-GPC (PAF cycle) (121).

In the *de novo* pathway, PAF is synthesized from 1-*O*-alkyl-2-acetyl-glycerol and CDP-choline by the action of a specific, dithiothreitol-insensitive choline-phosphotransferase (122). This is an analogous reaction to phosphatidylcholine (PC) synthesis, however choline-phosphotransferase catalysing PC synthesis is sensitive to dithiothreitol (122). The choline-phosphotransferase is distributed among spleen, kidney, liver, and lung (119). Since the *de novo* route can continuously produce PAF, this pathway may contribute to the regulation of blood pressure by PAF (123, 124).

3   Receptors for PAF and eicosanoids, and related signal transduction systems

3.1   Cellular biology of PAF and PAF receptor

PAF has been shown to induce a variety of actions on leucocytes and platelets (125). It causes shape change, serotonin release and aggregation of platelets (125–127), mediator release from inflammatory leucocytes, including neutrophils (128), eosinophils (129), and basophils (130), neutrophil and eosinophil chemotaxis (131), and oncogene expression and enhanced immunoglobulin production in B lymphocytes (132, 133). These actions are exerted through PAF receptors. Specific [^{3}H]PAF binding sites were detected in a number of cell types, including human and rabbit platelets (134, 135), human polymorphonuclear leucocytes (134), rat Kupffer cells (136), and a human Raji lymphoblast cell line (137). In most cases, PAF binding fits a single site model, however, high and low affinity sites were also found in rabbit platelets (135). Hwang found differential effects of a PAF antagonist, ONO-6209 and ions on [^{3}H]PAF bindings to human platelets and to human polymorphonuclear leucocytes (134). Na$^+$ and Li$^+$ augmented the ligand binding to polymorphonuclear leucocytes but inhibited binding to platelets, and ONO-6290 was six to ten times less potent in inhibiting [^{3}H]PAF binding and PAF-induced GTPase activation in human leucocytes than in human platelets. Based on the differences, the existence of receptor heterogeneity among tissues was proposed.

3.2   Signal transduction mechanisms following PAF receptor activation

Several studies indicated PAF receptor–G protein coupling by showing GTP-induced inhibition of specific [^{3}H]PAF binding to rabbit platelet membrane (135), and PAF-induced GTPase activation in human (134, 138) and rabbit (135) platelet membranes, and in human neutrophil membranes (134). The specificity of G proteins involved in PAF receptor–effector coupling was also studied using IAP as a probe. As shown in Section 2.1.2, a single receptor could govern two or more effectors via two or more G proteins. This seems to hold true for the PAF receptor and makes it difficult to obtain a straightforward understanding of the signalling system. Indeed, the PAF receptor appears to couple to at least three effectors, phospholipase C, phospholipase A$_2$, and adenylate cyclase.

In a variety of cells, PAF has been shown to elicit PIP$_2$ breakdown. PAF-induced PIP$_2$ hydrolysis was sensitive to IAP treatment in rabbit neutrophils (44), permeabilized human platelets (46), human macrophages

(139), and neurohybrid-NCB20 cells (140) but insensitive to the toxin treatment in rabbit platelets (141) and in a human monocytic cell line, U937 (62). Thus, both IAP-sensitive and insensitive G proteins are involved in the signalling pathway. PAF-induced inhibition of adenylate cyclase has been observed in human (138) and rabbit (142) platelets, and in mouse 3T3 fibroblasts (27), although the stimulation of cAMP phosphodiesterase by PAF (127, 142) was also claimed. The adenylate cyclase inhibition was sensitive to IAP in permeabilized human platelets (138) and mouse 3T3 fibroblasts (27). Phospholipase A_2 activation by PAF has also been noted in several systems including mouse 3T3 fibroblasts (27), a rat liver cell line, C-9 (143), and human polymorphonuclear leucocytes (144). The PAF-induced PLA_2 activation was sensitive to IAP in these systems (27, 144). Therefore, the PAF receptor appears to couple to PLA_2 and adenylate cyclase through IAP-sensitive G protein(s).

PAF causes an increase in intracellular Ca^{2+} through IP_3-induced Ca^{2+} release from intracellular stores (first phase) and through Ca^{2+} influx (second phase) (132, 145). Mechanisms involved in the Ca^{2+} influx are unknown, but several investigators proposed the involvement of a receptor operated Ca^{2+} channel (44, 146). However, the Ca^{2+} influx may be triggered by IP_3 itself, since (a) Ca^{2+} influx induced by PAF was abolished when PLC was inhibited by the PLC inhibitor, manoalide (52), and (b) micro-injection of IP_3 both in *Xenopus* oocytes (147) and mouse lacrimal acinar cells (148) elicited Ca^{2+} influx.

Recently, two groups reported PAF-induced tyrosine phosphorylation on several proteins in rabbit platelets (141) and in human neutrophils (149). The molecular weights of the phosphorylated proteins were found to be very similar to those phosphorylated in the presence of fMLP (149), suggesting that common tyrosine kinase(s) may be activated in both systems (149). Dhar *et al.* showed that PAF-induced IP_3 production was inhibited by the tyrosine kinase inhibitor, genistein (141) and suggested the involvement of tyrosine kinase in PAF receptor–PLC system. Since both PAF receptor (9) and fMLP receptor (150) have been shown by molecular cloning to belong to the G protein-coupled receptor superfamily, these findings may indicate 'cross-talk' between a G protein–PLC system and a tyrosine kinase pathway.

3.3 Roles of cell-associated PAF

In many cell types, PAF is retained intracellularly (8). The role of intracellular PAF is obscure, but two hypothetical roles have been proposed; a second messenger role of PAF (151), and a role of PAF/PAF receptor in cell adhesion (152). Stewart *et al.* (151) observed that production of eicosanoids and superoxide anion by agonist-stimulated bovine endothelial cells, guinea pig macrophages, and rabbit polymorphonuclear leucocytes were all preceded by PAF synthesis and that the release of mediators was inhibited by PAF receptor antagonists, WEB 2068 or CV6209. These results indicate that PAF synthesis is a pre-requisite for mediator release, and support the possible intracellular messenger role of PAF.

In bovine endothelial cells, PAF is synthesized and appears on the cell surface (8, 152). Zimmerman *et al.* (152) showed that polymorphonuclear leucocytes adhered to vascular endothelial cells through interaction of the PAF receptor or polymorphs and the PAF synthesized in the endothelial cell. The leucocyte adhesion to endothelial cells was shown to be abolished when these cells were treated with PAF antagonists or with acetyl hydrolase (152). This novel role of PAF may contribute to the pathogenesis of inflammation.

3.4   Molecular cloning of PAF receptor cDNA

3.4.1   Experimental design

As shown in the previous section, the signalling mechanisms following PAF receptor activation are complicated, and controversial observations have emerged. We intended to isolate cDNA coding for the PAF receptor in order to have a molecular basis for understanding of the PAF receptor and its signal transduction systems. Since the purification of the receptor had not been achieved, we employed an 'expression cloning' strategy using *Xenopus laevis* oocytes (153). Guinea pig lung PAF receptor cDNA was successfully cloned, as described (9) and was the first example of a lipid autacoid receptor to be cloned. A human homologue was also obtained from a leucocyte cDNA library (154). In the following sections, the cloning strategy, structures of the cloned cDNA, and pharmacological properties of the encoded receptors in various expression systems are described in detail.

3.4.2   Cloning strategy

Xenopus laevis oocyte has most efficient *in vivo* translation machinery (153). The oocytes effectively translate micro-injected mRNA, carry out the post-translational modifications, and transport foreign proteins to appropriate cellular compartments (153). Thus, functional receptor molecules are expressed on the oocytes' surface when the oocytes are injected with mRNA obtained from appropriate organs. The oocyte system has another advantage in the detection of G protein coupled receptor expression; the oocytes contain the Ca^{2+}-sensitive Cl^- channel that is operated by the intrinsic G protein–PLC pathway (147), thus, ligand-induced activation of 'foreign' receptors could elicit the Cl^- current via this pathway, given that the receptors effectively couple to the oocytes' G protein. The Cl^- current can be sensitively detected by electrophysiological methods. Several G protein coupled receptor cDNAs have been successfully cloned using the oocyte system (155–157).

Figure 13.6 illustrates the electrophysiological detection of PAF receptor expressed in the oocytes by the two electrode voltage clamp method. The oocytes injected with guinea pig lung mRNA was placed in a circulating bath, and voltage-clamped below the reversal potential of Cl^- (-25 to -30 mV)

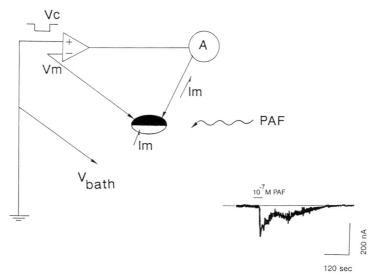

Fig. 13.6 Electrophysiological detection of PAF receptor expression. Membrane potential (Vm) is held below the equilibrium potential of Cl$^-$ in *Xenopus* oocytes (Vc) in modified Ringer's solution (115 mM NaCl/2 mM KCl/1.8 mM CaCl$_2$/5 mM Hepes, pH 7.4), and PAF-induced inward current (Im) is recorded (*inset*). The downward deflection indicates the inward current.

in a frog Ringer's solution (routinely −50 to −100 mV). Bath-applied PAF elicited a two phase inward current (Figure 13.6, inset), which is characteristic of G protein coupled receptors (147). We fractionated guinea pig mRNA by density gradient ultracentrifugation, and constructed a λ Zap II (Stratagene) phage library from the active fractions.

Phage DNA was then prepared from each 6 × 10^4 phage aliquot, digested at the *Not*I site located downstream of the T7 promoter, and the template was transcribed *in vitro* using T7 RNA polymerase. The transcript was injected into the oocytes and PAF receptor expression was detected electrophysiologically. The oocytes injected with the transcript derived from a group of 6 × 10^4 phages showed a positive response (Figure 13.7a). Then, we subdivided the phages by monitoring the PAF-induced response and isolated a functional phage clone (Figure 13.7b). We also isolated human leucocyte PAF receptor cDNA using guinea pig PAF receptor cDNA as a probe.

3.4.3   Primary structures of guinea pig and human PAF receptors

Both guinea pig and human PAF receptor are composed of 342 amino acids (calculated molecular weight around 39 kDa), and both the receptors have seven hydrophobic, putative membrane spanning domains, a characteristic

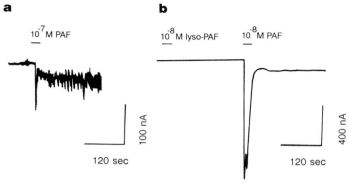

Fig. 13.7 PAF-induced inward current in oocytes. Response in an oocyte injected with about 50 ng of the transcript made from a mixture of 6×10^4 phage clones some of which contain PAF receptor cDNA (a) and that in an oocyte injected with about 5 ng of the transcript of the cloned PAF receptor cDNA (b).

feature of G protein coupled receptors (Figure 13.8). Amino acid identity between the two receptors is 83 per cent overall, and 90 per cent in the membrane spanning domains (shown in Figure 13.8 as single lettered circles). Several commonly observed amino acids among G protein coupled receptors are conserved in the PAF receptors, which include Asp in the 2nd membrane spanning domain, two Cys in the 2nd and 3rd extracellular loop which possibly form a disulfide-bond, and three Pro in the 6th and 7th membrane spanning domains which may contribute to bending of helices to form a ligand binding pocket (158). Interestingly, one Thr in the 3rd intracellular loop and five Ser and four Thr in the cytoplasmic tail are completely conserved between the guinea pig and the human PAF receptors. Since phosphorylation of these amino acids has been shown to result in a rapid receptor desensitization of the β_2 adrenergic receptor (158), these amino acid residues may contribute to the desensitization, commonly observed with PAF action. A possible glycosylation site in the NH_2-terminus of the guinea pig PAF receptor was not found in the human PAF receptor, hence, glycosylation of the N-terminus may not be required for function of the receptors.

3.4.4 Functions of guinea pig and human PAF receptors expressed in various systems

The PAF receptors encoded by the cloned cDNAs were expressed in *Xenopus* oocytes and COS-7 cells to determine pharmacological properties of the receptors. The oocytes injected with the transcript of the cloned guinea pig cDNA showed a dose-dependent increase in the amplitude of the PAF-induced response (Figure 13.9) with ED_{50} at around 10 nM, a value consistent with findings in human neutrophils (128), human eosinophils (129), and guinea pig and human platelets (134, 135). The responses elicited by 1-*O*-octadecyl-2-acetamido-2-deoxyglycero-3-phosphocholine (a partial agonist of

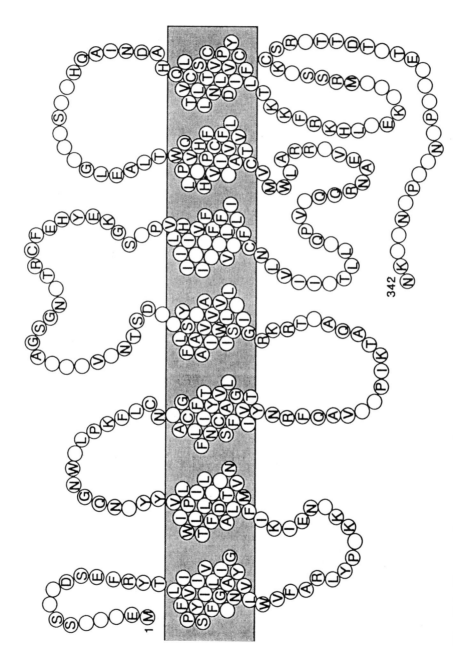

Fig. 13.8 Transmembrane structure of the PAF receptor. The conserved amino acids between guinea pig and human PAF receptors are shown by a single letter.

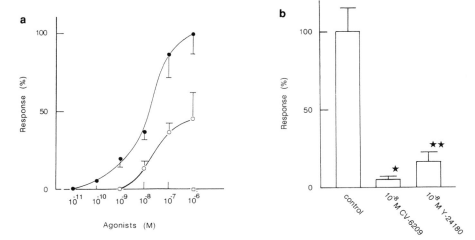

Fig. 13.9 (a) Dose–response curve of PAF (●) 1-*O*-octadecyl-2-acetamido-2-deoxy-glycero-3-phosphocholine (○), and lyso-PAF (□). The mean amplitude of the inward current induced by 10^{-6} M PAF was defined as 100%. (b) Inhibition of PAF-induced response by specific antagonists, CV-6209 and Y-24180. Oocytes were pre-treated with 10^{-8} M antagonists for 2 minutes, or not treated with antagonists (control), and stimulated with 10^{-8} M PAF. The mean amplitude in the control oocytes was defined as 100%.

PAF) were smaller than those elicited by PAF, and lyso-PAF induced no detectable response even at one μM (Figure 13.9). Two structurally different PAF antagonists, CV-6209 (159) and Y-24180 (160) almost completely inhibited the PAF-induced responses at equimolar concentration with PAF (0.1 μM) (Figure 13.9). A prior injection of the guanine nucleotide analogue, GDPβS into the oocyte reduced the response by about 70 per cent, thereby indicating that a G protein is involved in the PAF receptor-mediated Cl$^-$ channel opening. As shown in Figure 13.10, the PAF-induced response was desensitized by repeated bath-applications of PAF. We also found that several PKC inhibitors abolished the desensitization (unpublished observation), thus protein phosphorylation seems to be involved in the desensitization process.

Membrane fractions of COS-7 cells expressing the human PAF receptors displayed a dose-dependent and saturable binding of [^{3}H]PAF and [^{3}H]WEB 2086 (Figure 13.11). Dissociation constants for PAF and WEB 2086 of the expressed human PAF receptor were 1.3 nM and 9.1 nM, respectively, this being in good agreement with reported data (134–137, 161). Displacements of [^{3}H]WEB 2086 binding by several antagonists and by PAF revealed that the rank order of binding affinity was PAF > Y-24180 > CV-6209 > WEB 2086 (Figure 13.12). PAF induced a rapid, and transient IP$_3$ production in COS-7 cells expressing the human PAF receptor.

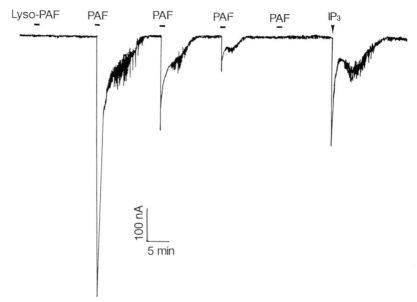

Fig. 13.10   Desensitization of the inward current by repeated application of 10^{-8} M PAF. Micro-injection of IP_3 evoked Cl^- current in the desensitized oocytes, showing that the refractoriness was not due to Ca^{2+} depletion.

3.5   Recent progress in eicosanoid receptor research

Thromboxane A_2 receptor has been purified from human platelets (162) and the cDNA from MEG-01 cell line was cloned (10). Structural analysis revealed that the TXA_2 receptor also belongs to a G protein coupled receptor super-family. The TXA_2 receptor expressed in *Xenopus* oocyte elicited Cl^- channel opening, thereby suggesting coupling of the TXA_2 receptor with PLC.

The LTD_4 receptor was solubilized in an active form from guinea pig lung and the receptor was shown to be coupled to IAP-sensitive G protein (163). The LTB_4 receptor was also shown to be linked to PLC via IAP-sensitive G protein (52, 164, 165). Gifford *et al.* (166) characterized the human LTB_4 receptor using anti-idiotypic antibody to a monoclonal anti-LTB_4 antibody. The PGE_2 receptor was partially purified from bovine renal medulla as a receptor–G protein complex (167). The molecular properties of the LT and PG receptors remain to be determined.

4   Summary

Lipid mediators possess variable and highly potent biological activities which are important in conditions of tissue damage and increased phagocytosis.

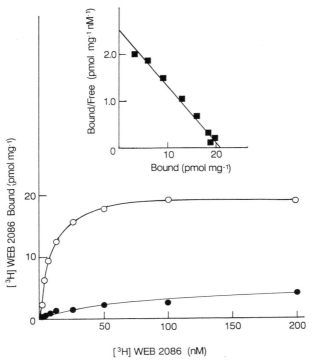

Fig. 13.11 Saturation isotherms and the derived Scatchard plots of [³H]WEB 2086 binding to COS-7 cell membranes expressing the human PAF receptor. ○ and ● indicate specific and non-specific binding, respectively.

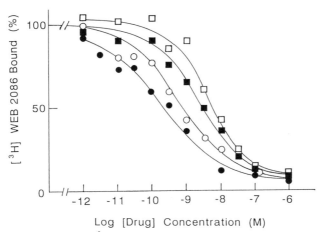

Fig. 13.12 Displacement of [³H]WEB binding to the human PAF receptor expressed in COS-7 cells by PAF and specific PAF antagonists (●:PAF, □:WEB 2086, ○:Y-24180, and ■:CV-6209). Data are expressed as a percentage of the [³H]WEB 2086 binding without the antagonists.

Extensive studies have been done in this area to elucidate the molecular mechanisms of biosyntheses and functions of these lipid autacoids. These lipid mediators may act both intracellularly and extracellularly. PAF which is released by endothelial cells may promote the interaction of polymorphonuclear leucocytes to the vascular endothelium via the newly identified PAF receptor. The growing knowledge in this field will lead to new insights in the understanding of physiological cellular functions and pathophysiology of clinical disorders.

Acknowledgement

We are grateful to Drs K. Tkahashi, K. Inoue, I. Kudo (University of Tokyo), and S. Nakanishi (Kyoto University) for suggestions and M. Ohara for comments.

References

1   Samuelsson, B. (1983). Leukotrienes: mediators of immediate hypersensitivity reactions and inflammation. *Science*, **220**, 568–75.
2   Samuelsson, B., Dahlén, S-E., Lindgren J-Å., Rouzer, C. A., and Serhan, C. N. (1987). Leukotrienes and lipoxins: structures, biosynthesis, and biological effects. *Science*, **237**, 1171–6.
3   Needleman, P., Turk, J., Jakschik, B. A., Morrison, A. R., and Lefkowith, J. B. (1986). Arachidonic acid metabolism. *Annu. Rev. Biochem.*, **55**, 69–102.
4   Hanahan, D. J. (1986). Platelet activating factor: a biologically active phosphoglyceride. *Annu. Rev. Biochem.*, **55**, 483–509.
5   Smith, W. L. (1989). The eicosanoids and their biochemical mechanisms of action. *Biochem. J.*, **259**, 315–24.
6   Shimizu, T. and Wolfe, L. S. (1990). Arachidonic acid cascade and signal transduction. *J. Neurochem.*, **55**, 1–15.
7   Lam, B. K., Owen Jr, W. F., Austen, K. F., and Soberman, R. J. (1989). The identification of a distinct export step following the biosynthesis of leukotriene C_4 by human eosinophils. *J. Biol. Chem.*, **264**, 12885–9.
8   Prescott, S. M., Zimmerman, G. A., and McIntyre, T. M. (1990). Platelet activating factor. *J. Biol. Chem.*, **265**, 17381–4.
9   Honda, Z., Nakamura, M., Miki, I., Minami, M., Watanabe, T., Seyama, Y., Okado, H., Toh, H., Ito, K., Miyamoto, T., and Shimizu, T. (1991). Cloning by functional expression of platelet activating factor receptor from guinea pig lung. *Nature*, **349**, 342–6.
10   Hirata, M., Hayashi, Y., Ushikubi, F., Yokota, Y., Kageyama, R., Nakanishi, S., and Narumiya, S. (1991). Cloning and expression of cDNA for a human thromboxane A_2 receptor. *Nature*, **349**, 617–20.
11   Rang, H. P. and Dale, M. M. (1991). 2nd Edition. In *Pharmacology* pp. 38–??. Churchill Livingstone.
12   Nakagaya, Y., Sugiura, T., and Waku, K. (1985). The molecular species composition of diacyl-, alkylacyl-, and alkenyl-acylglycerophospholipids in rabbit

alveolar macrophages. High amounts of 1-*O*-hexadecyl-2-arachidonyl molecular species in alkylacylglycerophosphocholine. *Biochim. Biophys. Acta*, **833**, 323–9.

13 Albert, D. H. and Snyder, F. (1983). Biosynthesis of 1-*O*-alkyl-2-acetyl-*sn*-glycero-3-phosphocholine (platelet activating factor) from 1-alkyl-2-acyl-*sn*-glycero-3-phosphocholine by rat alveolar macrophages. Phospholipase A$_2$ and acetyl-transferase activities during phagocytosis and ionophore stimulation. *J. Biol. Chem.*, **258**, 97–102.

14 Leslie, C. C., Voelker, D. R., Channon, J. Y., Wall, M. W., and Zelarney, P. T. (1988). Properties and purification of an arachidonoyl-hydrolysing phospholipase A$_2$ from a macrophage cell line RAW 264.7. *Biochim. Biopys. Acta*, **963**, 476–92.

15 Kim, D. K., Kudo, I., and Inoue, K. (1988). Detection in human platelets of phospholipase A$_2$ activity which preferentially hydrolyses an arachidonoyl residue. *J. Biochem.* (Tokyo), **104**, 492–4.

16 Davidson, F. F. and Dennis, E. A. (1990). Evolutionary relationships and implications for the regulation of phospholipase A$_2$ from snake venom to human secreted forms. *J. Mol. Evol.*, **31**, 228–38.

17 Hara, S., Kudo, I., Chang, H. W., Matsuta, K., Miyamoto, T., and Inoue, K. (1989). Purification and characterization of extracellular phospholipase A$_2$ from human synovial fluid in rheumatoid arthritis. *J. Biochem.* (Tokyo), **105**, 395–9.

18 Channon, J. Y. and Leslie, C. C. (1990). A calcium-dependent mechanism for associating a soluble arachidonoyl-hydrolysing phospholipase A$_2$ with membrane in the macrophage cell line RAW 264.7. *J. Biol. Chem.*, **265**, 5409–13.

19 Ramesha, C. S. and Pickett, W. C. (1986). Platelet activating factor and leukotriene biosynthesis is inhibited in polymorphonuclear leucocytes depleted of arachidonic acid. *J. Biol. Chem.*, **261**, 7592–5.

20 Suga, K., Kawasaki, T., Blamk, M. L., and Snyder, F. (1990). An arachidonoyl (polyenoic)-specific phospholipase A$_2$ activity regulates the synthesis of platelet activating factor in granulocytic HL-60 cells. *J. Biol. Chem.*, **265**, 12363–71.

21 Clark, J. D., Milona, N., and Knopf, J. L. (1990). Purification of a 110-kilodalton cytosolic phospholipase A$_2$ from the human monocytic cell line U937. *Proc. Natl. Acad. Sci. U.S.A.*, **87**, 7708–12.

22 Clark, J. D., Lin, L-L., Kriz, W. R., Ramesha, C. S., Sultzman, L. A., Lin, A. Y., Milona, N., and Knopf, J. L. (1991). A novel arachidonic acid-selective cytosolic PLA$_2$ contains a Ca^{2+}-dependent translocation domain with homology to PKC and GAP. *Cell*, **65**, 1043–51.

23 Nakashima, S., Tohmatsu, T., Hattori, H., Suganuma, A., and Nozawa, Y. (1987). Guanine nucleotides stimulate arachidonic acid release by phospholipase A$_2$ in saponin-permeabilized human platelets. *J. Biochem.* (Tokyo), **101**, 1055–8.

24 Kajiyama, Y., Murayama, T., and Nomura, Y. (1989). Pertussis toxin sensitive GTP-binding protein may regulate phospholipase A$_2$ in response to thrombin in rabbit platelets. *Arch. Biochem. Biophys.*, **274**, 200–8.

25 Burch, R. M., Luini, A., and Axelrod, J. (1986). Phospholipase A$_2$ and phospholipase C are activated by distinct GTP-binding proteins in response to β-adrenergic stimulation in FRTL5 thyroid cells. *Proc. Natl. Acad. Sci. U.S.A.*, **83**, 7201–5.

26 Murayama, T., Kajiyama, Y., and Nomura, Y. (1990). Histamine-stimulated and GTP-binding proteins-mediated phospholipase A_2 activation in rabbit platelets. *J. Biol. Chem.*, **265**, 4290–5.

27 Murayama, T. and Ui, M. (1985). Receptor-mediated inhibition of adenylate cyclase and stimulation of arachidonic acid release in 3T3 fibroblasts. Selective susceptibility to islet-activating protein, pertussis toxin. *J. Biol. Chem.*, **260**, 7226–33.

28 Slivka, S. R. and Insel, P. A. (1988). Phorbol ester and neomycin dissociate bradykinin receptor-mediated arachidonic acid release and polyphosphoinositide hydrolysis in Madin–Darby canine kidney cells. Evidence that bradykinin mediates non-interdependent activation of phospholipase A_2 and C. *J. Biol. Chem.*, **263**, 14640–7.

29 Gupta, S. K., Diez, E., Heasley, L. E., Osawa, S., and Johnson, G. L. (1990). A G protein mutant that inhibits thrombin and purinergic receptor activation of phospholipase A_2. *Science*, **249**, 662–6.

30 Cockroft, S. (1987). Phosphoinositide phosphodiesterase: regulation by a novel guanine nucleotide binding protein Gp. *Trends Pharmacol. Sci.*, **12**, 75–8.

31 Rhee, S. G., Suh, P-G., Ryu, S-H., and Lee, S. Y. (1989). Studies of inositol phospholipid-specific phospholipase C. *Science*, **244**, 546–50.

32 Berridge, M. J. (1987). Inositol triphosphate and diacyl glycerol: two interacting second messengers. *Annu. Rev. Biochem.*, **56**, 159–93.

33 Nishizuka, Y. (1988). The molecular heterogeneity of protein kinase C and its implications for cellular regulation. *Nature*, **334**, 661–5.

34 Sadowski, I., Stone, J. C., and Pawson, T. (1986). A non-catalytic domain conserved among cytoplasmic protein tyrosine kinases modifies the kinase function and transforming activity of Fujinami sarcoma virus p130 *gag-fps*. *Mol. Cell. Biol.*, **6**, 4396–408.

35 Stahl, M. L., Ferenz, C. R., Kelleher, K. L., Kriz, R. W., and Knopf, J. L. (1988). Sequence similarity of phospholipase C with the non-catalytic region of *src*. *Nature*, **332**, 269–72.

36 Suh, P. G., Ryo, S. H., Moon, K. H., Suh, H. W., and Rhee, S. G. (1988). Inositol phospholipid-specific phospholipase C: complete cDNA and protein sequences and sequence homology to tyrosine kinase-related oncogene products. *Proc. Natl. Acad. Sci. U.S.A.*, **85**, 5419–23.

37 Cantley, L. L., Auger, K. R., Carpenter, C., Duckworth, B., Graziani, A., Kapeller, R., and Soltoff, S. (1991). Oncogenes and signal transduction. *Cell*, **64**, 281–302.

38 Anderson, D., Koch, C. A., Gray, L., Ellis, C., Moran, M. F., and Pawson, T. (1990). Binding of SH2 domains of phospholipase C-γ1, GAP, and *src* to activated growth factor receptors. *Science*, **250**, 979–82.

39 Nishibe, S., Wahl, M. I., Hernandes-Sotomayor, S. M. T., Tonks, N. K., Rhee, S. G., and Carpenter, G. (1990). Increase of the catalytic activity of phospholipase C-γ1 by tyrosine phosphorylation. *Science*, **250**, 1253–6.

40 Goldschmidt-Clermont, P. J., Kim, J. W., Machesky, L. M., Rhee, S. G., and Pollard, T. D. (1991). Regulation of phospholipase C-γ1 by profilin and tyrosine phosphorylation. *Science*, **251**, 1231–3.

41 Barrowman, M. M., Cockroft, S., and Gomperts, B. D. (1985). Two roles for guanine nucleotides in the stimulus–secretion sequence of neutrophils. *Nature*, **319**, 504–7.

42 Straub, R. E. and Gershengorn, M. C. (1986). Thyrotropin-releasing hormone and GTP activate inositol triphosphate formation in membranes isolated from rat pituitary cells. *J. Biol. Chem.*, **261**, 2712–17.

43 Smith, C. D., Lane, B. C., Kusaka, I., Verghese, M. W., and Snyderman, R. (1985). Chemoattractant receptor-induced hydrolysis of phosphatidylinositol-4, 5-biphosphate in human polymorphonuclear leucocyte membranes. *J. Biol. Chem.*, **260**, 5875–8.

44 Naccache, P. H., Molski, M. M., Volpi, M., Becker, E. L., and Sha'afi, R. I. (1985). Unique inhibitory profile of platelet activating factor induced calcium mobilization, polyphosphoinositide turnover, and granule enzyme secretion in rabbit neutrophils towards pertussis toxin and phorbol ester. *Biochem. Biophys. Res. Commun.*, **130**, 677–84.

45 Kikuchi, A., Kozawa, O., Kaibuchi, K., Katada, T., Ui, M., and Takai, Y. (1986). Direct evidence for involvement of a guanine nucleotide-binding protein in chemotactic peptide-stimulated formation of inositol biphosphate and triphosphate in differentiated human leukaemic (HL-60) cells. Reconstitution with Gi or Go of the plasma membranes ADP ribosylated by pertussis toxin. *J. Biol. Chem.*, **261**, 11558–62.

46 Brass, L. F,. Woolkalis, M. J., and Manning, D. R. (1988). Interactions in platelets between G proteins and the agonists that stimulate phospholipase C and inhibit adenylate cyclase. *J. Biol. Chem.*, **263**, 5348–55.

47 Huang, C-L. and Ives, H. E. (1989). Guanosine 5'-O-(3-thiotriphosphate) potentiates both thrombin and platelet-derived growth factor-induced inositol phosphate release in permeabilized vascular smooth muscle cells. *J. Biol. Chem.*, **264**, 4391–7.

48 Ueda, H., Yoshihara, Y., Misawa, H., Fukushima, N., Katada, T., Ui, M., Takagi, H., and Satoh, M. (1989). The kyotorphin (tyrosine-arginine) receptor and a selective reconstitution with purified Gi, measured with GTPase and phospholipase C assays. *J. Biol. Chem.*, **264**, 3732–41.

49 Ui, M. (1984). Islet-activating protein, pertussis toxin: a probe for the function of the inhibitory guanine nucleotide regulatory component of adenylate cyclase. *Trends Pharmacol. Sci.*, **5**, 277–9.

50 Moriarty, T. M., Padrell, E., Carty, D. J., Omri, G., Landau, E. M., and Iyengar, R. (1990). Go protein as signal transducer in the pertussis toxin-sensitive phosphatidylinositol pathway. *Nature*, **343**, 79–82.

51 Okajima, F., Tokumitsu, Y., Kondo, Y., and Ui, M. (1987). P2-purinergic receptors are coupled to two signal transduction systems leading to inhibition of cAMP generation and to production of inositol triphosphate in rat hepatocytes. *J. Biol. Chem.*, **262**, 13483–90.

52 Barzaghi, G., Sarau, H. M., and Mong, S. (1989). Platelet activating factor-induced phosphoinositide metabolism in differentiated U937 cells in culture. *J. Pharmac. Exp. Ther.*, **248**, 559–65.

53 Ashkenazi, A., Peralta, E. G., Winslow, J. W., Ramachandran, J., and Capon, D. J. (1990). Functionally distinct G proteins selectively couple different receptors to PI hydrolysis in the same cell. *Cell*, **56**, 487–93.

54 Pong, I-H. and Sternweis, P. C. (1990). Purification of unique α subunits of GTP-binding regulatory proteins (G protein) by affinity chromatography with immobilized βγ subunits. *J. Biol. Chem.*, **265**, 18707–12.

55 Taylor, S. J., Smith, J. A., and Exton, J. H. (1990). Purification from bovine liver membranes of a nucleotide-dependent activator of phosphoinositide-specific phospholipase C. *J. Biol. Chem.*, **265**, 17150–6.

56 Strathmann, M. and Simon, M. I. (1990). G protein diversity: a distinct class of subunits is present in vertebrates and invertebrates. *Proc. Natl. Acad. Sci. U.S.A.*, **87**, 9113–7.

57 Smrcka, A. V., Hepler, J. R., Brown, K. O., and Sternweis, P. C. (1991). Regulation of polyphosphoinositide-specific phospholipase C activity by purified Gq. *Science*, **251**, 804–7.

58 Taylor, S. J., Chae, H. Z., Rhee, S. G., and Exton, J. H. (1991). Activation of the βI isozyme of phospholipase C by α subunits of the Gq class of G proteins. *Nature*, **350**, 516–18.

59 Shenker, A., Goldsmith, P., Unson, C. G., and Spiegel, A. M. (1991). The G protein coupled to the thromboxane A_2 receptor in human platelets is a member of the novel Gq family. *J. Biol. Chem.*, **266**, 9309–13.

60 Roth, G. J., Siok, C. J., and Ozols, J. (1980). Structural characteristics of prostaglandin synthetase from sheep vesicular gland. *J. Biol. Chem.*, **255**, 1301–4.

61 DeWitt, D. L., Rollins, T. E., Day, J. S., Gauger, J. A., and Smith, W. L. (1981). Orientation of the active site and the antigenic determinants of prostaglandin endoperoxide synthase 1n the endoplasmic reticulum. *J. Biol. Chem.*, **256**, 10375–82.

62 Miyamoto, T., Ogino, N., Yamamoto, S., and Hayaishi, O. (1976). Purification of prostaglandin endoperoxide synthetase from bovine vesicular gland microsomes. *J. Biol Chem.*, **251**, 2629–36.

63 DeWitt, D. L. and Smith, W. L. (1988). Primary structure of prostaglandin G/H synthase from sheep vesicular gland determined from the complementary DNA sequence. *Proc. Natl. Acad. Sci. U.S.A.*, **85**, 1412–6.

64 Merlie, J. P., Fagan, D., Mudd, J., and Needleman, P. (1988). Isolation and characterization of the complementary DNA for sheep seminal vesicle prostaglandin endoperoxide synthase (cyclo-oxygenase). *J. Biol. Chem.*, **263**, 3550–3.

65 Yokoyama, C., Takai, T., and Tanabe, T. (1988). Primary structure of sheep prostaglandin endoperoxide synthase deduced from cDNA sequence. *FEBS Lett.*, **231**, 347–50.

66 Christ-Hazelhof, E. and Nugteren, D. H. (1979). Purification and characterization of prostaglandin endoperoxide D-isomerase, a cytoplasmic, glutathione requiring enzyme. *Biochim. Biophys. Acta*, **572**, 43–51.

67 Shimizu, T., Yamamoto, S., and Hayaishi, O. (1979). Purification and properties of prostaglandin D synthetase from rat brain. *J. Biol. Chem.*, **254**, 5222–8.

68 Urade, Y. Fujimoto, N., and Hayaishi, O. (1985). Purification and characterization of rat brain prostaglandin D synthetase. *J. Biol. Chem.*, **260**, 12410–5.

69 Urade, Y., Nagata, A., Suzuki, Y., Fujii, Y., and Hayaishi, O. (1989). Primary structure of rat brain prostaglandin D synthetase deduced from cDNA sequence. *J. Biol. Chem.*, **264**, 1041–5.

70 Urade, Y., Fujimoto, N., Kaneko, T., Konishi, A., Mizuno, O., and Hayaishi, O. (1987). Post-natal changes in the localization of prostaglandin D synthetase from neurons to oligodendrocytes in the rat brain. *J. Biol. Chem.*, **262**, 15132–6.

71 Watanabe, K., Yoshida, R., Shimizu, T., and Hayaishi, O. (1985). Enzymic formation of prostaglandin $F_{2\alpha}$ from prostaglandin H_2 and D_2. Purification and properties of prostaglandin F synthase from bovine lung. *J. Biol. Chem.*, **260**, 7035–51.

72 Watanabe, K., Fujii, Y., Nakayama, K., Ohkubo, H., Kuramitsu, S., Kagami-yama, H., Nakanishi, S., and Hayaishi, O. (1988). Structural similarity of bovine prostaglandin F synthase to lens crystalline of the Europian common frog. *Proc. Natl. Acad. Sci. U.S.A.*, **85**, 11–5.

73 DeWitt, D. J. and Smith, W. T. (1983). Purification of prostacyclin synthase from bovine aorta by immunoaffinity chromatography. Evidence that the enzyme is a haemoprotein. *J. Biol. Chem.*, **258**, 3285–93.

74 Haurand, M. and Ullrich, B. (1985). Isolation and characterization of throm-boxane synthase from human platelets as a cytochrome P-450 enzyme. *J. Biol. Chem.*, **260**, 15059–67.

75 Webb, D. R. and Nowowiejski, I. (1978). Mitogen-induced changes in lympho-cyte prostaglandin levels: a signal for the induction of suppressor cell activity. *Cell Immunol.*, **41**, 72–85.

76 Phillips, C. A., Girit, E. Z., and Kay, J. E. (1978). Changes in intracellular prostaglandin content during activation of lymphocytes by phytohaemagglutinin. *FEBS Lett.*, **94**, 115–9.

77 Rapoport, B., Pillarisetty, R. J., Herman, E. A., and Congco, E. G. (1977). Evidence for prostaglandin production by human lymphocytes during culture with human thyroid cells in monolayer: a possible role for prostaglandins in the pathogenesis of Graves disease. *Biochem. Biophys. Res. Commun.*, **77**, 1245–50.

78 Goldyne, M. E. (1988). Lymphocytes and arachidonic acid metabolism. *Prog. Allergy*, **44**, 140–52.

79 Goodwin, J. S., Bankhurst, A. D., and Messner, R. P. (1977). Suppression of human T cell mitogenesis by prostaglandin. Existence of a prostaglandin producing suppressor cells. *J. Exp. Med.*, **146**, 1719–34.

80 Gordon, D., Bray, A. M, and Morley, J. (1976). Control of lymphokine secre-tion by prostaglandins. *Nature*, **262**, 401–2.

81 Droller, M. J., Perlmann, P., and Schneider, M. U. (1978). Enhancement of natural and antibody-dependent lymphocyte cytotoxicity by drugs which inhibit prostaglandin production by tumour target cells. *Cell. Immunol.*, **39**, 154–64.

82 Thompson, P. A., Jelinek, D. F., and Lipsky, P. E. (1984). Regulation of human B cell proliferation by prostaglandin E_2. *J. Immunol.*, **133**, 2446–53.

83 Shimizu, T., Rådmark, O., and Samuelsson, B. (1984). Enzyme with dual lipoxygenase activities catalyzes leukotriene A_4 synthesis from arachidonic acid. *Proc. Natl. Acad. Sci. U.S.A.*, **81**, 689–93.

84 Rouzer, C. A., Matsumoto, T., and Samuelsson, B. (1986). Single protein from human leucocytes possesses 5-lipoxygenase and leukotriene A_4 synthase activities. *Proc. Natl. Acad. Sci. U.S.A.*, **83**, 857–61.

85 Ueda, N., Kaneko, S., Yoshimoto, T., and Yamamoto, S. (1986). Purification of arachidonate 5-lipoxygenase from porcine leucocytes and its reactivity with hydopeoxy-eicosatetraenoic acid. *J. Biol. Chem.*, **261**, 7982–8.

86 Shimizu, T., Izumi, T., Seyama, Y., Tadokoro, K., Rådmark, O., and Samuels-son, B. (1986). Characterization of leukotriene A_4 synthase from murine mast cells: evidence for its identity to arachidonate 5-lipoxygenase. *Proc. Natl. Acad. Sci. U.S.A.*, **83**, 4175–9.

87 Hogaboon, G. K., Cook, M., Newton, J. F., Varrichio, A., Shorr, R. G., Sarau, H. M., and Crooke, S. T. (1986). Purification, characterization, and structural properties of a single protein from rat basophilic leukaemia cells

(RBL-1) possessing 5-lipoxygenase and leukotriene A$_4$ synthase activities. *Mol. Pharmacol.*, **30**, 510–19.

88   Rouzer, C. A. and Samuelsson, B. (1985). On the nature of 5-lipoxygenase in human leucocytes: enzyme purification and requirements for multiple stimulatory factors. *Proc. Natl. Acad. Sci. U.S.A.*, **82**, 6040–4.

89   Goetze, A. W., Fayer, L., Bouska, J., Bornemeier, D., and Carter, G. W. (1985). Purification of a mammalian 5-lipoxygenase from rat basophilic leukaemia cells. *Prostaglandins*, **29**, 689–701.

90   Dixon, R. A. F., Jones, R. E., Diehl, R. E., Bennett, C. D., Kargman, S., and Rouzer, C. A. (1988). Cloning of the cDNA for human 5-lipoxygenase. *Proc. Natl. Acad. Sci. U.S.A.*, **85**, 416–20.

91   Matsumoto, T., Func, C. D., Rådmark, O., Höög, J-O., Jörnvall, H., and Samuelsson, B. (1988). Molecular cloning and amino acid sequence of human 5-lipoxygenase. *Proc. Natl. Acad. Sci. U.S.A.*, **85**, 26–30.

92   Funk, C. D., Gunne, H., Steiner, H., Izumi, T., and Samuelsson, B. (1989). Native and mutant 5-lipoxygenase expression in a baculovirus/insect cell system. *Proc. Natl. Acad. Sci. U.S.A.*, **86**, 2592–6.

93   Noguchi, M., Matsumoto, T., Nakamura, M., and Noma, M. (1989). Expression of human 5-lipoxygenase cDNA in *Escherichia coli*. *FEBS Lett.*, **249**, 1365–70.

94   Nakamura, M., Matsumoto, T., Noguchi, M., Yamashita, I., and Noma, M. (1990). Expression of a cDNA encoding human 5-lipoxygenase under control of the *STA1* promoter in *Saccharomyces cerevisiae*. *Gene*, **89**, 231–7.

95   Kargeman, S. K. and Rouzer, C. A. (1989). Studies on the regulation, and activation of 5-lipoxygenase in differentiated HL-60 cells. *J. Biol. Chem.*, **264**, 13313–20.

96   Miller, D. K., Gilard, J. W., Vickers, P. J, Sadowski, S., Leveille, C., Mancini, J. A., Charleson, P., Dixon, R. A. F., Ford-Hutchinson, A. W., Fortin, R., Gauthier, J. Y., Rodkey, J., Rosen, R., Rouzer, C., Sigal, I. S., Strader, C. D., and Evans, J. F. (1991). Identification and isolation of a membrane protein necessary for leukotriene production. *Nature*, **343**, 278–81.

97   Dixon, R. A. F., Diehl, R. E., Opas, E., Rands, E., Vickers, P. J., Evans, J. F., Gillard, J. W., and Miller, D. K. (1991). Requirement of a 5-lipoxygenase-activating protein for leukotriene synthesis. *Nature*, **343**, 282–4.

98   Rådmark, O., Shimizu, T., Jörnvall, H., and Samuelsson, B. (1984). Leukotriene A$_4$ hydrolase in human leucocytes. Purification and properties. *J. Biol. Chem.*, **259**, 12339–45.

99   Ohishi, N., Izumi, T., Minami, M., Kitamura, S., Seyama, Y., Ohkawa, S., Terao, S., Yotsumoto, H., Takaku, F., and Shimizu, T. (1987). Leukotriene A$_4$ hydrolase in human lung: inactivation of the enzyme with leukotriene A$_4$ isomers. *J. Biol. Chem.*, **262**, 10200–5.

100   Bito, H., Ohishi, N., Miki, I., Minami, M., Tanabe, T., Shimizu, T. J., and Seyama, Y. (1989). Leukotriene A$_4$ hydrolase from guinea pig lung: the presence of two catalytically active forms. *J. Biochem.* (Tokyo), **105**, 261–4.

101   Minami, M., Ohno, S., Kawasaki, H., Rådmark, O., Samuelsson, B., Jornvall, H., Shimizu, T., Seyma, Y., and Suzuki, K. (1987). Molecular cloning of a cDNA coding for human leukotriene A$_4$ hydrolase. *J. Biol. Chem.*, **262**, 13873–6.

102 Funk, C. D., Rådmark, O., Fu, J. Y., Matsumoto, T., Jornvall, H., Shimizu, T., and Samuelsson, B. (1987). Molecular cloning and amino acid sequence of leukotriene A$_4$ hydrolase. *Proc. Natl. Acad. Sci. U.S.A.*, **84**, 6677–81.

103 Minami, M., Minami, Y., Emori, Y., Kawasaki, H., Ohno, S., Suzuki, K., Ohishi, N., Shimizu, T., and Seyama, Y. (1988). Expression of human leukotriene A$_4$ hydrolase in *Escherichia coli*. *FEBS Lett.*, **229**, 279–82.

104 Ohishi, N., Minami, M., Kobayashi, J., Seyama, Y., Hata, J., Yotsumoto, H., Takaku, F., and Shimizu, T. (1990). Immunological quantitation and immunohistochemical localization of leukotriene A$_4$ hydrolase in guinea pig tissues. *J. Biol. Chem.*, **265**, 7520–5.

105 Toh, H., Minami, M., and Shimizu, T. (1990). Molecular evolution and zinc ion binding motif of leukotriene A$_4$ hydrolase. *Biochem. Biophys. Res. Commun.*, **171**, 216–21.

106 Valle, B. and Auld, D. S. (1990). Zinc co-ordination, function, and structure of zinc enzymes and other proteins. *Biochemistry*, **29**, 5647–59.

107 Minami, M., Ohishi, N., Mutoh, H., Izumi, T., Bito, H., Wada, H., Seyama, Y., Toh, H., and Shimizu, T. (1990). Leukotriene A$_4$ hydrolase is a zinc-containing aminopeptidase. *Biochem. Biophys. Res. Commun.*, **173**, 620–6.

108 Yoshimoto, T., Soberman, R. J., Spur, B., and Austen, K. F. (1988). Properties of highly purified leukotriene C$_4$ synthase of guinea pig lung. *J. Clin. Invest.*, **81**, 866–71.

109 Izumi, T., Honda, Z., Ohishi, N., Kitamura, S., Tsuchida, S., Sato, K., Shimizu, T., and Seyama, Y. (1988). Solubilization and partial purification of leukotriene C$_4$ synthase from guinea pig lung: a microsomal enzyme with high specificity towards 5,6-epoxide leukotriene A$_4$. *Biochim. Biophys. Acta*, **959**, 305–15.

110 Fitzpatrick, F., Liggett, W., McGee, J., Bunting, S., Morton, D., and Samuelsson, B. (1984). Metabolism of leukotriene A$_4$ by human erythrocytes. A novel cellular source of leukotriene B$_4$. *J. Biol. Chem.*, **259**, 11403–7.

111 Claesson, H. E. and Haeggstrom, J. (1988). Human endothelial cells stimulate leukotriene synthesis and convert granulocyte released leukotriene A$_4$ into leukotriene B$_4$, C$_4$, D$_4$, and E$_4$. *Eur. J. Biochem.*, **173**, 93–100.

112 Feinmark, S. J. and Cannon, P. J. (1986). Endothelial cell leukotriene C$_4$ synthesis results from intercellular transfer of leukotriene A$_4$ synthesized by polymorphonuclear leucocytes. *J. Biol. Chem.*, **261**, 16466–72.

113 Dahinden, C. A., Clancy, R. M., Gross, M., Chiller, J. M., and Hugli, T. E. (1985). Leukotriene C$_4$ production by murine mast cells: evidence of a role for extracellular leukotriene A$_4$. *Proc. Natl. Acad. Sci. U.S.A.*, **82**, 6632–6.

114 Maclof, J. A. and Murphy, R. C. (1988). Transcellular metabolism of neutrophil-derived leukotriene A$_4$ by human platelets. A potential cellular source of leukotriene C$_4$. *J. Biol. Chem.*, **263**, 174–81.

115 Williams, J. D., Lee, T. H., Lewis, R. A., and Austen, F. (1985). Intracellular retention of the 5-lipoxygenase pathway product, leukotriene B$_4$ by human neutrophils activated with opsonized zymosan. *J. Immunol.*, **134**, 2624–30.

116 Owen Jr, W. F., Soberman, R. J., Yoshimoto, T., Sheffer, A. L., Lewis, R. A., and Austen, K. F. (1987). Synthesis and release of leukotriene C$_4$ by human eosinophils. *J. Immunol.*, **138**, 532–8.

117 Prewitt, R. L., Leach, B. E., Byers, L. W., Brooks, B., Lands, W. E., and Muirhead, E. E. (1979). Anti-hypertensive polar renomedullary lipid, a semi-synthetic vasodilator. *Hypertension*, **1**, 299–308.

118 Benveniste, J., Henson, P. M., and Cochrane, C. G. (1972). Leucocyte-dependent histamine release from rabbit platelets. The role of IgE, basophils, and a platelet activating factor. *J. Exp. Med.*, **136**, 1356–77.

119 Blank, M. L., Snyder, F., Byers, L. W., Brooks, B., and Muirhead, E. E. (1979). Anti-hypertensive activity of an alkyl ether analogue of phosphatidylcholine. *Biochem. Biophys. Res. Commun.*, **90**, 1194–200.

120 Demopoulos, C. A., Pinckard, R. N., and Hanahan, D. J. (1979). Platelet activating factor. Evidence for 1-*O*-alkyl-2-acetyl-*sn*-glycero-3-phosphocholine as the active component, (a new class of lipid chemical mediator). *J. Biol Chem.*, **254**, 9355–8.

121 Snyder, F. (1987). Enzymatic pathways for platelet activating factor, related alkyl glycerolipids, and their precursors. In *Platelet activating factor and related lipid mediators* (ed. F. Snyder), pp. 89–113. Plenum Press, New York.

122 Renooij, W. and Snyder, F. (1981). Biosynthesis of 1-alkyl-2-acetyl-*sn*-glycero-3-phosphocholine (platelet activating factor and a hypotensive lipid) by choline-transferase in various rat tissues. *Biochim. Biophys. Acta*, **663**, 545–56.

123 Masugi, F., Ogihara, T., Saeki, S., Otsuka, A., and Kumahara, Y. (1985). Role of acetyl glyceryl ether phosphorylcholine in blood pressure regulation in rats. *Hypertension*, **7**, 742–6.

124 Woodard, D. S., Lee, T-C., and Snyder, F. (1987). The final step in the *de novo* biosynthesis of platelet activating factor. Properties of a unique CDP-choline:1-alkyl-2-acetyl-*sn*-glycerol choline-phosphotransferase in microsomes from the renal inner medulla of rats. *J. Biol Chem.*, **262**, 2520–7.

125 Braquet, P., Touqui, L., Shen, T. Y., and Vargaftig, B. B. (1987). Perspectives in platelet activating factor research. *Pharmacol. Rev.*, **39**, 97–145.

126 Shukla, S. D. and Hanahan, D. J. (1982). AGEPC (platelet activating factor) induced stimulation of rabbit platelets: effects on phosphatidylinositol, di- and triphosphoinositides, and phosphatidic acid metabolism. *Biochem. Biophys. Res. Commun.*, **106**, 697–703.

127 Haslam, R. J. and Vanderwel, M. (1982). Inhibition of platelet adenylate cyclase by 1-*O*-alkyl-2-*O*-acetyl-*sn*-glyceryl-3-phosphorylcholine (platelet activating factor). *J. Biol. Chem.*, **257**, 6879–85.

128 Lad, P. M., Olson, C. V., and Greval, I. S. (1985). Platelet activating factor mediated effects on human neutrophil function are inhibited by pertussis toxin. *Biochem. Biophys. Res. Commun.*, **129**, 632–8.

129 Kroegel, C., Yukawa, T., Dent, G., Venge, P., Chung, K. F., and Barnes, P. J. (1989). Stimulation of degranulation from human eosinophils by platelet activating factor. *J. Immunol.*, **142**, 3518–26.

130 Brunner, T., De Weck, A. L., and Dahinden, C. A. (1991). Platelet activating factor induces mediator release by human basophils primed with IL-3, granulocyte macrophage colony-stimulating factor, or IL-5. *J. Immunol.*, **147**, 237–42.

131 Wardlaw, A. J., Moqbel, R., Cromwell, O., and Kay, A. B. (1986). Platelet activating factor. A potent chemotactic and chemokinetic factor for human eosinophils. *J. Clin. Invest.*, **78**, 1701–6.

132 Mazer, B., Domenico, J., Sawami, H., and Gelfand, E. W. (1991). Platelet activating factor induces an increase in intracellular calcium and expression of regulatory genes in human B lymphoblastoid cells. *J. Immunol.*, **146**, 1914–20.

133 Mazer, B., Clay, K. L., Renz, H., and Gelfand, E. W. (1990). Platelet activating factor enhances Ig production in B lymphoblastoid cell lines. *J. Immunol.*, **145**, 2602–7.

134 Hwang, S-B. (1988). Identification of a second putative receptor of platelet activating factor from human polymorphonuclear leucocytes. *J. Biol. Chem.*, **263**, 3225–33.

135 Hwang, S-B., Lam, M-H., and Pong, S-S. (1986). Ionic and GTP regulation of binding of platelet activating factor to receptors and platelet activating factor-induced activation of GTPase in rabbit platelet membranes. *J. Biol. Chem.*, **261**, 532–7.

136 Chao, W., Liu, H., DeBuysere, M., Hanahan, D. J., and Olson, M. S. (1989). Identification of receptors for platelet activating factor in rat Kupffer cells. *J. Biol. Chem.*, **264**, 13591–8.

137 Travers, J. B., Li, Q., Kniss, D. A., and Fertel, R. H. (1989). Identification of functional platelet activating factor receptors in Raji lymphoblasts. *J. Immunol.*, **143**, 3708–13.

138 Houslay, M. D., Bojanic, D., Gawler, D., O' Hagan, S., and Wilson, A. (1986). Thrombin, unlike vasopressin, appears to stimulate two distinct guanine nucleotide regulatory proteins in human platelets. *Biochem.*, **238**, 109–13.

139 Huang, S. J., Monk, P. N., Downes, C. P., and Whetton, A. D. (1988). Platelet activating factor-induced hydrolysis of phosphatidyl-inositol-4,5-bi-phosphate stimulates the production of reactive oxygen intermediates in macrophages. *Biochem.*, **249**, 839–45.

140 Yue, T. L., Stadel, J. M., Sarau, H. M., Friedman, E., Gu, J. L., Powers, D. A., Gleason, M. M., Feuerstein, G., and Wang, H. Y. (1992). Platelet-activating factor stimulates phosphoinositide turnover in neurohybrid NCB-20 cells: Involvement of pertussis toxin-sensitive guanine nucleotide binding proteins and inhibition by protein kinase C. *Mol. Pharmacol.* **41**, 281–9.

141 Dhar, A., Paul, A. K., and Shkla, S. D. (1990). Platelet activating factor stimulation of tyrosine kinase and its relationship to phospholipase C in rabbit platelets: studies with genistein and monoclonal antibody to phosphotyrosine. *Mol. Pharmacol.*, **37**, 519–25.

142 Sugatani, J., Miwa, M., and Hanahan, D. J. (1987). Platelet activating factor stimulation of rabbit platelets is blocked by serine protease inhibitor (chymotryptic protease inhibitor) *J. Biol. Chem.*, **262**, 5740–7.

143 Levine, L. (1988). Platelet activating factor stimulates arachidonic acid metabolism in rat liver cells (C-9 cell line) by a receptor-mediated mechanism. *Mol. Pharmacol.*, **34**, 791–9.

144 Nakashima, S., Suganuma, A., Sato, M., Tohmatsu, T., and Nozawa, Y. (1989). Mechanism of arachidonic acid liberation in platelet activating factor-stimulated human polymorphonuclear neutrophils. *J. Immunol.*, **143**, 1295–302.

145 Randriamampita, C. and Trautmann, A. (1989). Biphasic increase in intracellular calcium induced by platelet activating factor in macrophages. *FEBS Lett.*, **249**, 199–206.

146 Avdonin, P. V., Cheglakov, I. B., Boogry, E. M., Svitina-Ulitina, I. V., Mazaev, A. V., and Tkachuk, V. A. (1987). Evidence for the receptor-operated calcium channels in human platelet plasma membrene. *Thrombosis Res.*, **46**, 29–37.

147 Sugiyama, H., Ito, I., and Hirono, C. (1987). A new type of glutamate receptor linked to inositol phospholipid metabolism. *Nature*, **325**, 531–3.

148   Bird, G. St. J., Rossier, M. F., Hughes, A. R., Shears, S. B., Armstrong, D. J., and Putney Jr, J. W. (1991). Activation of Ca^{2+} entry into acinar cells by a non-phosphorylatable inositol triphosphate. *Nature*, **352**, 162–5.

149   Gomez-Cambronero, J., Wang, E., Johnson, G., Huang, C. K., and Sha'afi, R. I. (1991). Platelet activating factor induces tyrosine phosphorylation in human neutrophils. *J. Biol. Chem.*, **266**, 6240–5.

150   Thomas, K. M., Pyun, H. Y., and Navarro, J. (1990). Molecular clonong of the fMet-Leu-Phe receptor from neutrophils. *J. Biol. Chem.*, **265**, 20061–4.

151   Stewart, A. G., Dubbin, P. N., Harris, T., and Dusting, G. J. (1990). Platelet activating factor may act as a second messenger in the release of eicosanoids and superoxide anions from leucocytes and endothelial cells. *Proc. Natl. Acad. Sci. U.S.A.*, **87**, 3215–9.

152   Zimmerman, G. A., McIntyre, T. M., Mehra, M., and Prescott, S. M. (1990). Endothelial cell-associated platelet activating factor: a novel mechanism for signalling intercellular adhesion. *J. Cell. Biol.*, **110**, 529–40.

153   Colman, A. (1984). Translation of eukaryotic messenger RNA in *Xenopus* oocytes. In *Transcription and translation* (ed. B. D. Hames and S. J. Higgins), pp. 271–300. IRL Press, Oxford.

154   Nakamura, M., Honda, Z., Izumi, T., Sakanaka, C., Mutoh, H., Minami, M., Bito, H., Seyama, Y., Matsumoto, T., Noma, M., and Shimizu, T. (1991). Molecular cloning of platelet activating factor receptor from human leucocytes. *J. Biol. Chem.*, **266**, 20400–5.

155   Masu, Y., Nakayama, K., Tamaki, H., Harada, Y., Kuno, M., and Nakanishi, S. (1987). cDNA cloning of bovine substance-K receptor through oocyte expression system. *Nature,* **329**, 836–8.

156   Julius, D., MacDermott, A. B., Axel, R., and Jessell, T. M. (1988). Molecular characterization of a functional cDNA encoding the serotonin 1c receptor. *Science*, **241**, 558–64.

157   Vu, T-K. H., Hung, D. T., Wheaton, V. I., and Coughlin, S. R. (1991). Molecular cloning of a functional thrombin receptor reveals a novel proteolytic mechanism of receptor activation. *Cell*, **64**, 1057–68.

158   Dohlman, H. G., Caron, M. G., and Lefkowitz, R. J. (1987). A family of receptors coupled to guanine nucleotide regulatory proteins. *Biochemistry*, **26**, 2657–64.

159   Terashita, Z., Imura, Y., Takatani, M., Tsushima, S., and Nishikawa, K. (1987). CV-6209, a highly potent antagonist of platelet activating factor *in vivo* and *in vitro*. *J. Pharmacol. Exp. Ther.* **242**, 263–8.

160   Terasawa, M., Mikashima, H., Takehara, S., Moriwaki, M., Setoguchi, M., and Tahara, T. (1989). Potent and selective PAF antagonistic activity of a new thienotriazolodiazepine. In *Third international conference on platelet activating factor and structurally related alkyl ether lipids*, (Tokyo), pp. 10 (abstract).

161   Dent, G., Ukena, D., Sybrecht, G. W., and Barnes, J. B. (1989). [^{3}H]WEB 2086 labels platelet activating factor receptors in guinea pig and human lung. *Eur. J. Pharmacol.*, **169**, 313–6.

162   Ushikubi, F., Nakajima, M., Hirata, M., Okuma, M., Fujiwara, M., and Narumiya, S. (1989). Purification of the thromboxane A_2/prostaglandin H_2 receptor from human blood platelets. *J. Biol. Chem.*, **264**, 16496–501.

163   Watanabe, T., Shimizu, T., Miki, I., Sakanaka, C., Honda, Z., Seyama, Y., Teramato, T., Matsushima, T., Ui, M., and Kurokawa, K. (1990). Characterization of guinea pig lung membrane leukotriene D_4 receptor solubilized in an

active form. Association and dissociation with an islet-activating protein-sensitive guanine nucleotide-binding protein. *J. Biol. Chem.*, **265**, 21237–41.

164 Holian, A. (1986). Leukotriene B_4 stimulation of phosphatidyl-inositol turnover in macrophages and inhibition by pertussis toxin. *FEBS Lett.*, **201**, 15–19.

165 Miki, I., Watanabe, T., Nakamura, M., Seyama, Y., Ui, M., Sato, F., and Shimizu, T. (1990). Solubilization and characterization of leukotriene B_4 receptor–GTP binding protein complex from porcine spleen. *Biochem. Biophys. Res. Commun.*, **166**, 342–8.

166 Gifford, L. A., Chernov-Rogan, T., Harvey, J. P., Koo, C. H., Goldman, D. W., and Goetzl, E. J. (1987). Recognition of human polymorphonuclear leucocyte receptors for leukotriene B_4 by rabbit anti-idiotypic antibodies to a mouse monoclonal anti-leukotriene B_4. *J. Immunol.*, **138**, 1184–9.

167 Negishi, M., Ito, S., Yokohama, H., Hayashi, H., Katada, T., Ui, M., and Hayaishi, O. (1988). Functional reconstitution of prostaglandin E receptor from bovine adrenal medulla with guanine nucleotide binding proteins. *J. Biol. Chem.*, **263**, 6893–900.

Index